Infection in the cancer patient

Infection in the cancer patient
A practical guide

Edited by

Roy AJ Spence, OBE, JP, MA, MD, FRCS
Consultant Surgeon,
Belfast City Hospital,
Honorary Professor,
Queen's University Belfast, and
Honorary Professor, University of Ulster

Roderick J Hay MA (Oxon), BM, BCh, DM, FRCP, FRCPath, F.Med.Sci
Head, School of Medicine and Dentistry,
Queen's University Belfast,
Professor of Dermatology,
Queen's University Belfast

Patrick G Johnston MD, PhD, FRCP, FRCPI
Professor of Oncology,
Belfast City Hospital, and
Queen's University Belfast, and
Director of the Centre for Cancer Research and Cell Biology,
Queen's University Belfast

OXFORD
UNIVERSITY PRESS

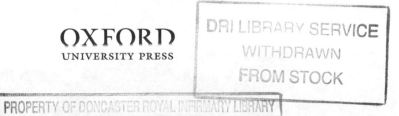

OXFORD

UNIVERSITY PRESS

Great Clarendon Street, Oxford OX2 6DP

Oxford University Press is a department of the University of Oxford.
It furthers the University's objective of excellence in research, scholarship,
and education by publishing worldwide in

Oxford New York

Auckland Cape Town Dar es Salaam Hong Kong Karachi
Kuala Lumpur Madrid Melbourne Mexico City Nairobi
New Delhi Shanghai Taipei Toronto

With offices in

Argentina Austria Brazil Chile Czech Republic France Greece
Guatemala Hungary Italy Japan Poland Portugal Singapore
South Korea Switzerland Thailand Turkey Ukraine Vietnam

Oxford is a registered trade mark of Oxford University Press
in the UK and in certain other countries

Published in the United States
by Oxford University Press Inc., New York

British Library Cataloguing in Publication Data

Data available

Library of Congress Cataloging in Publication Data

Data available

Typeset by Newgen Imaging Systems (P) Ltd., Chennai, India
Printed in Great Britain
on acid-free paper by
Biddles Ltd., King's Lynn

ISBN 0–19–856632–8 (pbk.: alk.paper)   978–0–19–856632–8 (Pbk.)

10 9 8 7 6 5 4 3 2 1

Contents

List of Contributors

Professor Elie Azoulay MD, PhD
Service de réanimation médicale
Hôspital Saint-Louis, Université
Paris 7
1 Avenue Claude Vellefaux, 75010
PARIS, France
Elie.azoulay@sls.ap-hop-paris.fr

**Dr. Julia C Chisholm
BA, PhD, FRCPCH**
Department of Oncology,
Great Ormond Street Hospital,
London, UK

**Dr. Vicky Coyle
MB, BCh, MRCP(UK)**
Department of Oncology
Belfast City Hospital
Lisburn Road
Belfast
BT9 7AB
vmcoyle@hotmail.com

Dr. Rachel Dommett
Clinical Research Fellow Infectious
Diseases and Microbiology Unit
Institute of Child Health
30 Guildford Street
London WC1N 1EH
Tel: 0207 9052392
Fax: 0207 813 8494

**Dr. Elizabeth Graham FRCP,
FRCOphth**
Consultant Medical
Ophthalmologist

The Medical Eye Unit, St Thomas'
Hospital SE1 7EH and
The National Hospital for Neurology
and Neurosurgery WC1N 3BG
Elizabeth.Graham@gstt.sthames.
nhs.uk

Professor Roderick J. Hay DM, FRCP
School of Medicine and Dentistry,
Queens University Belfast
Whitla Medical Building, 97 Lisburn
Road, Belfast BT9 7BL
r.hay@qub.ac.uk
r.hay@Queens-Belfast.AC.UK

**Mr. David J Howard BSc, FRCS,
FRCSEd**
Senior Head & Neck Surgeon
University College Hospital and
Honorary Consultant Head and
Neck Surgeon
Royal National Throat, Nose and
Ear Hospital
National Hospital for Nervous
Diseases
Great Ormond Street Hospital for
Children and Senior Lecturer
Institute of Laryngology & Otology
University College Hospital

**Mr. Hari Jayaram MA, MRCSEd,
MRCOphth**
Medical Eye Unit, St Thomas'
Hospital, London
SE1 7EH
hari@doctors.org.uk

Dr. Dakshika Jeyaratnam MSc, MRCPCH, MRCPath
Department of Infection,
Guy's and St.Thomas' NHS
Foundation Trust, St. Thomas'
Hospital, Lambeth Palace Road,
London SE1 7EH.
Dakshika.jeyaratnam@gstt.sthames.nhs.uk

Professor Jim Johnston, PhD
Head, Infection and Immunity,
Centre for Cancer Research & Cell
Biology, Rm 226 Whitla Medical
building, Queens University Belfast,
97 Lisburn Rd. Belfast
Northern Ireland, BT8 6YH
Jim.johnston@qub.ac.uk

**Professor Patrick G Johnston
FRCP, FRCPI, PhD, MD,
MB, BCh, BAO (Hons)**
Professor of Oncology
Centre for Cancer Research & Cell
Biology
Queen's University Belfast
p.johnston@qub.ac.uk

Dr Lionel Karlin
Resident
Service de réanimation médicale
Hôspital Saint-Louis, Université
Paris 7
1 Avenue Claude Vellefaux, 75010
PARIS, France

**Mr. Michael D. Laverick FRCS(Ed)
FRCS(Orth)**
Consultant Orthopaedic Surgeon
Ulster Hospital
Dundonald
Belfast and Musgrave Park Hospital
Stockmans Lane
Belfast
md.laverick@btinternet.com

Dr Aurelie Lefebvre
Fellow
Service de réanimation médicale
Hôspital Saint-Louis, Université
Paris 7
1 Avenue Claude Vellefaux, 75010
PARIS, France

**Professor Valerie J Lund MS,
FRCS, FRCSEd**
Professor of Rhinology
Institute of Laryngology & Otology
University College Hospital
Honorary Consultant ENT Surgeon
Royal National Throat Nose and
Ear Hospital
330 Grays Inn Road
London WC1X 8DA and
Honorary Consultant ENT Surgeon
Moorfields Eye Hospital
v.lund@ucl.ac.uk

**Dr. Eithne MacMahon MD,
FRCPath, FRCPI, DCH**
Consultant Virologist, Department
of Infection, Guy's & St Thomas'
NHS Foundation Trust,
St Thomas' Hospital,
Lambeth Palace Road,
London SE1 7EH, United Kingdom
Honorary Senior Lecturer,
Department of Infectious Diseases,
King's College London School of
Medicine at Guy's, King's College

and St Thomas' Hospitals,
Lambeth Palace Road,
London SE1 7EH,
United Kingdom
Eithne.macmahon@gstt.nhs.uk

Dr. Caroline McLoughlin
MB. BaO. BCH, MRCP
Specialist Registrar
West Midlands Palliative Medicine
Training Scheme
St.Giles Hospice
Lichfield
UK

Dr Ronan McMullan MB, BCh,
MRCP(UK), MRCPath
Department of Microbiology
Kelvin Laboratories
The Royal Hospitals
Grosvenor Road
Belfast
Ronan.mcmullan@bll.n-i.nhs.uk

Mr Thiagarajan NambiRajan MS,
DNB, MCh, FRCS(Urol), FEBU
Consultant Urologist Belfast City
Hospital Belfast
BT9 7AB
tnambirajan@hotmail.com

Dr. Joe O'Sullivan MD, MRCPI,
FFR(RCSI)
Consultant/Senior Lecturer in
Clinical Oncology
Queen's University Belfast/Northern
Ireland Cancer Centre
Belfast
BT9 7AB
Joe.osullivan@qub.ac.uk

Mr. James Powles FRCS
SpR in Otolaryngology
Royal National Throat Nose and
Ear Hospital
330 Grays Inn Road
London WC1X 8DA

Dr Geoffrey Scott
University College London Hospitals
Acute Foundation Trust;
University College London and
London School of Hygiene and
Tropical Medicine, UK
geoff.scott@uclh.nhs.uk

Dr. Mike Sharland
Consultant Paediatrician
Paediatric Infectious Diseases Unit
5th Floor, Lanesborough Wing
St George's Hospital
Blackshaw Road
London
SW17 0QT
mike.sharland@stgeorges.nhs.uk

Dr. Nigel J Stevenson, PhD
Research Fellow
Dept Immunology, Queen's
University Belfast
Centre for Cancer Research and
Cell Biology
Whitla Medical Building
97 Lisburn Road
Belfast BT9 7BL
n.stevenson@qub.ac.uk

Dr. Henk J van Leeuwen MD, PhD
internist-intensivist
Ziekenhuis Gelderse Vallei
(Gelderse Vallei Hospital)

Intensive Care Willy
Brandtlaan 10
6716 RP EDE
PO box 9025
6710 HN EDE
The Netherlands
LeeuwenH@zgv.nl

Jan Verhoef, MD, PhD
Professor of Clinical Microbiology
and Infectious Diseases
Head, EijKman - Winkler Centre

University Medical Centre Utrecht
The Netherlands
j.verhoef@umcutrecht.nl

**Dr. Max Watson, BD, MB.ChB,
MRCGP, MSc. DRCOG, DCH, DMH**
Honorary Consultant Palliative
Medicine
The Princess Alice Hospice Esher
Orthobiotech Research Fellow
Belfast City Hospital
email alimaxuk@yahoo.com

Chapter 1

Pathogenesis of sepsis

H.J. van Leeuwen and J. Verhoef

Introduction

Infection and refractory malignancy are the most common causes of death in patients with cancer (Safdar and Armstrong 2001). Once an infection evolves into the systemic inflammatory response syndrome (SIRS) this is called sepsis. For patients admitted to the intensive care unit (ICU) sepsis remains a major contributor to mortality. Despite remarkable progress in unravelling the mechanisms behind this enigmatic condition, mortality has hardly changed over the past decades (Friedman *et al.* 1998; Martin *et al.* 2003). The treatment of sepsis today remains supportive: antibiotics or surgical treatment of the focus of infection, replacing or supporting the function of failing organs, nutritional support, and prophylactic measures to reduce the occurrence of complications (Cross and Opal 2003). Recently, a number of large random-ized clinical trials have shown a reduction in mortality in patients with sepsis and allied conditions. The administration of activated protein C (aPC) (Bernard *et al.* 2001), early goal-directed cardiovascular therapy (Rivers *et al.* 2001), tight glycaemic control (Van den Berghe *et al.* 2001), steroid supple-mentation in adrenal failure (Annane *et al.* 2002) and mechanical ventilation with low tidal volumes (Brower *et al.* 2000) have all been shown to reduce mortality in critically ill patients. These results revive hope in the quest for the optimal treatment of patients with sepsis, based on the insights gained from thorough basic research in sepsis and systemic inflammation.

Sepsis definition

The word sepsis is derived from the Greek verb σηπειν (se pein) meaning to putrefy. According to Hippocrates, πέψις (pepsis) and σηψις (sepsis) stood on opposite sides of biological breakdown: pepsis meant fermentation and was helpful, whereas sepsis meant putrefaction and was dangerous (Majno 1991).

Today, sepsis is used to describe a clinical condition caused by an infection. Although an experienced clinician can recognize when a patient is 'septic', sepsis is a clinical diagnosis that is hard to define. As opposed to a local inflammatory reaction, sepsis involves an additional systemic response to an infection. Sepsis is therefore not a disease but a complex of acute humoral and cellular changes in an organism in response to the invasion of micro-organisms. This set of reactions is a phylogenetically ancient host defence mechanism and part of innate immunity, an immune system that vertebrates, invertebrates, and plants have in common (Magor and Magor 2001). It is designed to maintain the integrity of the organism. Without this response the organism is unable to survive. However, an exaggerated systemic response triggered by an overwhelming infection can lead to damage to organs that are not involved in the primary focus of infection. Peritonitis for example can cause damage to the lung, presenting as acute respiratory distress syndrome, damage to the kidney presenting as acute tubular necrosis, or damage to the brain presenting as septic encephalopathy. By definition this is called severe sepsis. Involvement of the cardiovascular system ultimately leads to a state of persistent hypotension defined as septic shock.

The inflammatory response can also be triggered by non-infectious stimuli such as trauma, burns or pancreatitis. This syndrome is SIRS. Both SIRS and sepsis can eventually lead to the so-called multiple organ dysfunction syndrome, which has a high associated mortality (Beal and Cerra 1994). Sepsis/SIRS and multiple organ dysfunction syndrome actually constitute both ends of the spectrum of systemic inflammation with increasing organ involvement and increasing mortality (Rangel Frausto et al. 1995).

In 1992 the American College of Chest Physicians and the Society of Critical Care Medicine published definitions of sepsis and SIRS, which were elaborated as a result of a consensus conference (Bone et al. 1992) and confirmed during the latest consensus conference in 2001 (Levy et al. 2003) (Table 1.1). The criteria were set up to help researchers and clinicians to identify patients with sepsis or SIRS and to create guidelines for the use of innovative therapies. Three years after the first consensus conference the late Roger Bone, one of the principal initiators of this meeting, developed metastases from an earlier diagnosed renal cell carcinoma. He was treated with immune-enhancing therapy containing the cytokine interleukin (IL)-2. He personally described the symptoms and signs of SIRS while he received immune therapy (Bone 1996a):

> My symptoms and signs of SIRS began immediately after the administration of IL-2. I experienced hypothermia that was followed by chills and then hyperthermia. My blood pressure decreased from the preadministration values; this hypotension was associated with a relative tachycardia and tachypnea. Over the next 1 to 2 days, I gained 8 pounds of edema fluid associated with hyponatremia. On listening to my

Table 1.1 The 1992 SCCM/ACCP consensus conference criteria for SIRS, sepsis, severe sepsis and septic shock

SIRS	• Tachycardia (>90/min)
	• Tachypnoea (>20/min, pCO_2 < 32 mmHg)
	• Temperature(>38°C, <36°C)
	• Leucocytosis(>12 × 10^6/ml) or
	leucocytopenia (<4 × 10^6/ml) or
	>10% immature neutrophils (bands)

Sepsis = SIRS + documented infection

Severe sepsis = sepsis + signs of altered organ perfusion

- Oliguria (<0.5 ml/kg/min)
- Lactic acidosis
- Altered mental status

Septic shock = severe sepsis + persistent hypotension despite adequate fluid resuscitation or the need for vasopressors

lungs, I found more distinct respiratory sounds with a prolonged expiratory phase and inspiratory crackles. The sensation of dyspnea was a troublesome feeling of breathing discomfort that was alleviated by the administration of narcotics.

My face was red due to the loss of vasoregulation and presumed high cardiac output. I noted the subsequent progressive development of multiple organ dysfunction syndrome (MODS) over the next 24 hrs, characterized by oliguria and azotemia (manifested by increased blood urea nitrogen and creatinine concentrations), liver dysfunction (manifested by increased ASAT, ALAT, and alkaline phosphatase), nausea and vomiting, and a relative neutropenia (with a total neutrophil count of 800 neutrophils/mm³). Neurologic symptoms consisted of increased irritability and difficulty concentrating.

Roger Bone died in 1997. His memory lives on in the 'Bone' criteria for sepsis.

The criteria for sepsis are all clinical and broad and therefore lack specificity. The criteria were designed to improve early detection of patients with sepsis and allow specific therapeutic intervention. However, the same criteria were used in the design of large randomized controlled clinical trials in sepsis that were carried out during the last decade. These criteria failed to identify the patients who were most likely to respond to specific intervention. New strategies have been proposed in treatment modalities and trial design to identify the appropriate patient category for a specific therapeutic agent (Cohen *et al.* 2001). Recent trials have introduced biochemical parameters of inflammation to define further the targeted patient population (Reinhart *et al.* 2001) and other promising markers merit further investigation. In a recent meta-analysis for instance, the diagnostic accuracy of serum procalcitonin was higher than other markers of inflammation in the diagnosis of serious bacterial infection (Simon *et al.* 2004). Furthermore in haemato-oncology patients and neutropenic fever, serum procalcitonin helped identify patients who had microbiologically proven (bloodstream) infection (Kallio *et al.* 2000; Schuttrumpf *et al.* 2003; Jimeno *et al.* 2004; Lilienfeld-Toal *et al.* 2004).

Sepsis incidence

Derek Angus has made a major contribution towards our insight into the incidence of sepsis (Angus *et al.* 2001). From a discharge registry of all hospitals in seven states in the USA he retrospectively identified 192 980 cases of sepsis in adults in 1995. From these data an incidence of three cases per 1000 population was deducted, with an average hospital mortality rate of 28.6%. Both incidence and mortality were higher in males. In more than half of cases an underlying illness was present. In these patients, neoplasms were the most frequent underlying illness with an associated hospital mortality of 36.9% for non-metastatic and 43.4% for metastatic disease. The major focus of infection and also the most frequent organ with dysfunction was the lung. However, only half of the patients with sepsis were admitted to the ICU. This indicates that the other half of patients must have lacked organ failure, which is the most frequent sign prompting ICU admission. This again highlights the broadness of the definition of sepsis.

From the same database 9675 cases of severe sepsis in children were identified, leading to an incidence of 0.56 cases per 1000 population per year with an associated hospital mortality of 10.3%. As in adults, males were more affected, half of the children had an underlying comorbidity, neoplasms were the most frequent comorbidity in adolescents (10–19 years), the respiratory tract was the most common site of infection, and staphylococcus the most commonly isolated pathogen (Watson *et al.* 2003). A prospective study of 11 828 admissions in 170 French ICUs during 2 months in 1993 documented an incidence of 9% of clinically suspected severe sepsis with an associated 28-day mortality of 56% for patients with a documented infection and 60% for patients with culture negative severe sepsis (Brun Buisson *et al.* 1995). The most recent retrospective study on the epidemiology of sepsis in the USA reported an increase in the incidence from 0.83 cases per 1000 population in 1979 to 2.4 cases per 1000 population in 2000. Cancer was the most frequent coexisting condition over the years, only surpassed by diabetes and hypertension in the last half decade (Martin *et al.* 2003).

During the past decades both the focus of infection and the involved microorganisms have changed from Gram-negative infections below the diaphragm to Gram-positive infections above the diaphragm (Friedman *et al.* 1998).

Pathophysiology of sepsis

Sepsis is initiated by the inflammatory response of the host to invading micro-organisms (Figure 1.1). If the infection is caused by Gram-negative micro-organisms, endotoxin or lipopolysaccharide (LPS) is supposed to be the triggering molecule recognized by the innate immune system (Bone 1991). The triggering molecules in Gram-positive infections are less clear but lipoteichoic acid and capsular proteoglycans have both been implicated (Bone 1994; Opal and Cohen 1999). Interestingly, the same level of endotoxaemia can be detected in patients with sepsis irrespective of the infecting micro-organism (Opal *et al.* 1999) or even in patients without a culture documented infection (Casey *et al.* 1993). This observation has given rise to the paradigm that, once a systemic inflammatory response has started and has given rise to gut barrier dysfunction, translocation of bacteria or bacterial products from the intestinal lumen are the 'motor of sepsis' (Fink and Aranow 1997).

The receptors involved in recognizing bacterial molecules are called pattern recognition receptors (Medzhitov and Janeway 2002). These receptors recognize molecules widely expressed by a number of different micro-organisms

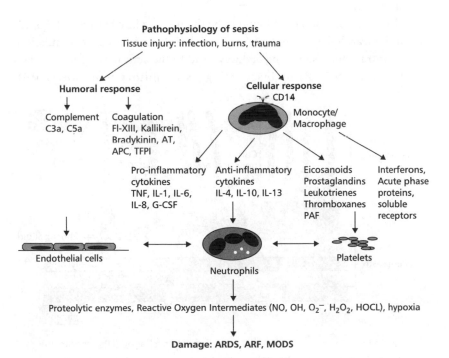

Fig 1.1 Schematic representation of the cascade of inflammatory cells and mediators eventually leading to organ dysfunction in sepsis.

and are designed to immediately differentiate infectious non-self from non-infectious self. Alternatively, the micro-organism can be recognized by the immune system after opsonization with antibodies or complement.

Most of the research in sepsis has focussed on LPS (Figure 1.2). The molecule can be easily isolated from bacteria and is remarkably stable. LPS is a structural component of the outer membrane of Gram-negative micro-organisms. It consists of a highly conserved lipid core, a core oligosaccharide and a variable polysaccharide containing side-chain. The lipid core is part of the bacterial phospholipid bilayer and is also the toxic moiety of the molecule. The polysaccharide side-chain determines the serotype of the bacterium and is the antibody binding moiety.

The innate immunity on the other hand recognizes LPS by CD14, a receptor found on the membrane of cells of the immune system (mCD14) or circulating in plasma in soluble form (sCD14) (Wright *et al.* 1990). The binding of LPS to CD14 is markedly enhanced by a soluble protein called LPS-binding protein (Schumann *et al.* 1990). CD14 is phosphatidylinositol linked to the outer membrane of the cell and has no transmembrane domain. Therefore, the transmembrane signalling pathway after binding to LPS remained an enigma until recently.

Toll-like receptor has been found to be the missing link between LPS binding and intracellular signalling (Yang *et al.* 1998). After receptor stimulation, several intracellular signalling pathways lead to the activation of nuclear factor-kappa B (NF-κB) by inactivating its inhibitory molecule (I-κB).

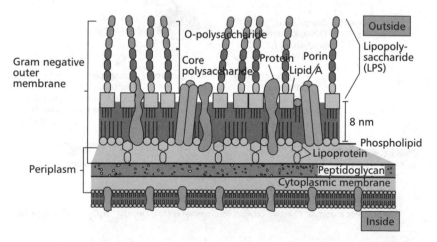

Fig. 1.2 Cell wall of gram-negative bacteria: lipopolysaccharide (LPS, endotoxin) is part of the outer membrane. Note: O-polysaccharide, core polysaccharide and lipid A.

Consequently, NF-κB is translocated from the cytosol to the nucleus where it binds to DNA and acts as a promoter of a multitude of inflammatory genes (Barnes and Karin 1997; Hatada, Krappmann, and Scheidereit 2000). In this way, NF-κB plays a pivotal role in the production of cytokines, adhesion receptors, and acute phase proteins, mediators essential in the inflammatory response (Christman *et al.* 1998) (Figure 1.3). Recently, alternative LPS signalling pathways have been described. Triggering receptor expressed on

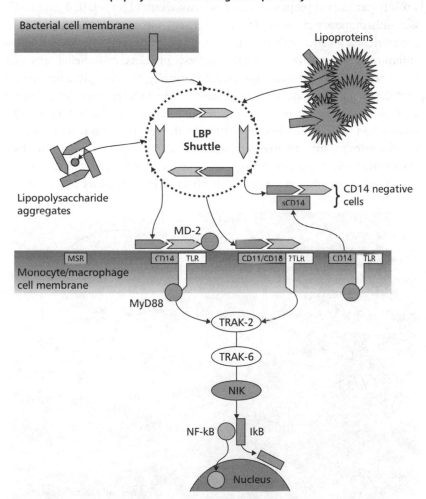

Fig. 1.3 Pathophysiology of sepsis: receptor recognition. LPS is bound in plasma to LBP, lipoproteins, CD14, etc. Binding to lipoproteins leads to neutralization, binding to LBP to activation via receptors.

myeloid cells (TREM-1) is upregulated in the presence of various micro-organisms (Cohen 2001; Nathan and Ding 2001). Its ligand remains to be identified. The monocytic intracellular NOD (nucleotide-binding oligomer-ization domain) receptor proteins have been found to bind to and confer cellular responsiveness to LPS (Inohara *et al.* 2002) (Figure 1.4).

In neutrophilic granulocytes, LPS enhances the production of reactive oxygen species (oxidative burst) caused by other inflammatory mediators, a process called priming (Condliffe *et al.* 1998). Stimulation of monocytes and macrophages by LPS leads to the production of inflammatory mediators like proinflammatory cytokines (tumour necrosis factor (TNF)-α, IL-1, and IL-6), anti-inflammatory cytokines (IL-4 and IL-10), eicosanoids (prostaglandins, leukotrienes, platelet-activating factor), nitric oxide, and interferons. These inflammatory mediators will further activate platelets, endothelial cells, and the already activated neutrophils. Additionally, the complement system and the coagulation cascade become activated by LPS (Haeney 1998; Vincent *et al.* 2001). The interplay between these humoral and cellular factors can ulti-mately lead to organ dysfunction, either by the enzymes and reactive oxygen species released by activated immune cells, or by hypoxia as a result of an insufficient microcirculation (hypoxic hypoxia) (De Backer *et al.* 2002; Ince 2002) or hypoxia due to a direct toxic effect of inflammatory mediators on

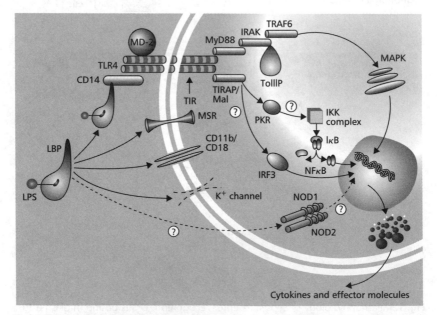

Fig. 1.4 Summary of receptor recognition pathways of the LPS-macrophage interaction (For details see Cohen J, *Nature* **420**, December 2002).

mitochondrial function (cytopathic hypoxia) (Sair *et al.* 2001; Brealey *et al.* 2002; Fink 2002).

The development of sepsis from a local infection is dependent on the balance between the amount of bacteria and their virulence on the one hand and the quality of the immune system (immune competence) of the host on the other hand. The inflammatory response is designed to confine the infection to the organ that is involved in the infection. At the site of the infection, tissue macrophages produce cytokines and chemokines to attract leucocytes to that particular site (Schluger and Rom 1997; Luster 1998). This is accomplished by the upregulation of receptors (selectins) on endothelial cells of the local post-capillary venules, which slow down passing leucocytes and receptors for firm adhesion of leucocytes to the luminal side of the endothelial cells (intercellular adhesion molecules) (Springer 1990; Hogg 1992). Subsequently the leucocytes pass the endothelial layer by a process called leucodiapedesis (Parkos 1997) (Figure 1.5). At tissue level, the leucocytes are further attracted by the concentration gradient of chemokines produced by tissue macrophages. The inflammatory cells phagocytize and kill live bacteria, remove dead bacteria and cellular debris, and play an important part in tissue repair. The inability of the immune system to keep the infection localized or a massive inflammatory response to a severe localized infection will lead to sepsis. Cytokines and

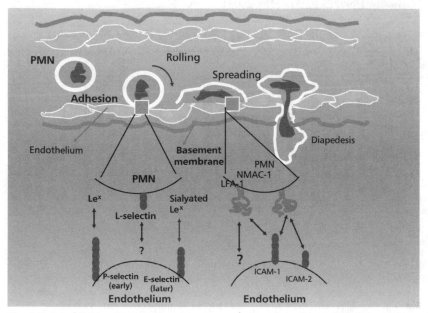

Fig. 1.5 Schematic representation of leukocyte interaction with endothelial cells in post-capillary venules and the receptors involved in this process.

chemokines, normally produced locally to have an autocrine or paracrine effect on adjacent cells, enter the circulation (cytokinaemia) and produce 'endocrine' effects in distant organs.

Circulating cytokines and chemokines will induce upregulation of receptors on all endothelial cells leading to influx of neutrophils in non-involved organ systems. The combination of neutrophil-, cytokine-, and hypoxia-induced endothelial and organ damage will eventually lead to multiple organ dysfunction with a high associated mortality.

Sepsis and inflammation

The clinical signs of sepsis and the associated biochemical changes can be induced by LPS and a number of pro-inflammatory cytokines. The development of recombinant antibodies against these mediators eventually led to a number of large randomized clinical trials in patients with (severe) sepsis (Figure 1.6). Several antibodies against LPS, TNF, and Enterobacteriaceae Common Antigen, soluble TNF receptors, IL-1 receptor antagonist, a platelet-activating factor receptor antagonist, a non-steroidal anti-inflammatory drug, and a bradykinin antagonist, however, all failed to show reduced mortality in human studies, despite proven efficacy in animal models. A number of explanations have been proposed why these sepsis trials failed (Zeni *et al.* 1997; Nasraway, 1999; Eichacker *et al.* 2002).

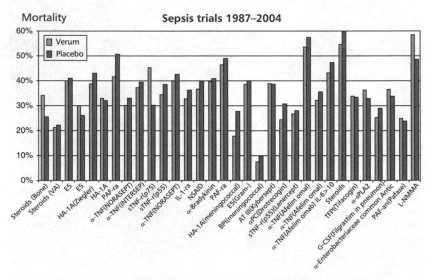

Fig. 1.6 Mortality data from all the large phase III multicenter randomized controlled trials in patients with severe sepsis. Data are expressed as percentage mortality in the intervention group and in the placebo group.

The broad study entry criteria can lead to a heterogeneous group of patients with a wide range of bacterial infections, different underlying diseases, and different mortality risks. The higher the mortality risk the more likely the intervention will show benefit. In this light it is remarkable that actuated protein C (aPC) was able to show benefit in a group of severe sepsis patients with a substantially lower mortality rate (30.8% control mortality) compared with patients in trials with other anti-inflammatory agents (average 39% control mortality) (Figure 1.6). Additionally, selecting patients at an anti-inflammatory stage of sepsis will lead to a counterproductive effect of anti-inflammatory therapy. It is therefore essential to select patients in the inflammatory stage of sepsis for trials with anti-inflammatory therapy. For this purpose immunological monitoring has been proposed (Volk *et al.* 1999). IL-10 and HLA-DR expression on monocytes have been proposed as the most promising parameters to monitor.

Sepsis and anti-inflammation

The inflammatory response induced by pro-inflammatory cytokines, is accompanied by a compensatory anti-inflammatory response induced by anti-inflammatory cytokines (Bone 1996b; Bone *et al.* 1997). At a cellular level this stage is characterized by a shift from a T-helper lymphocyte (Th)-1 response to a Th-2 response. Th-1 lymphocytes characteristically mediate enhanced cellular immune response by releasing pro-inflammatory cytokines (IL-2, TNF α, and interferon-γ), while Th-2 lymphocytes mediate the humoral immune response and secrete a number of anti-inflammatory cytokines (IL-4, IL-10, IL-13) (Hotchkiss and Karl 2003). In this phase of sepsis, leucocytes from patients are less responsive to LPS challenge *in vitro* (endotoxin tolerance), monocytes have a reduced HLA-DR expression, and patients are more susceptible to secondary infections (West and Heagy 2002). Patients in this stage of immunoparalysis in sepsis might be amenable for treatment with immune-enhancing therapy such as interferon-γ (Volk *et al.* 1996; Docke *et al.* 1997; Kox *et al.* 1997; Haveman *et al.* 1999). The failure of certain anti-inflammatory interventions in sepsis might be explained by a selection of patients in this stage of immune paralysis (Bone 1996c; Dellinger *et al.* 1997; Abraham 1999; Nasraway 1999; Abraham *et al.* 2000; Martin *et al.* 2003).

Sepsis and coagulation

The relation between sepsis and coagulation has been extensively studied (Levi and ten Cate 1999). During sepsis the extrinsic coagulation pathway is activated. LPS-induced expression of tissue factor on endothelial cells and monocytes leads to the activation of coagulation factor VII. Together with activated factor X it forms a complex that activates prothrombin that eventually leads to the production of fibrin. During this process both coagulation factors and anticoagulation factors are consumed, leading to low serum levels, which are correlated with mortality (Brandtzaeg *et al.* 1989). Clinically, patients present with signs of diffuse intravascular coagulation: low platelet count, prolonged prothrombin time and elevated fibrin degradation products (D-dimer). Recently, three large randomized clinical trials have investigated the effectiveness of the anticoagulation factors antithrombin (Warren *et al.* 2001), aPC (Bernard *et al.* 2001), and tissue factor pathway inhibitor (TFPI) (Abraham *et al.* 2003) in reducing mortality in patients with severe sepsis. While antithrombin and TFPI did not show mortality reduction, the aPC study was terminated prematurely after the second interim analysis because of a significantly reduced 28-day mortality in patients who received aPC (30.8% in the placebo group versus 24.7% in the intervention group). Although a number of questions remain (Eichacker and Natanson 2003), aPC (Xigris®) is presently the first and only drug registered for the treatment of patients with severe sepsis.

Sepsis and lipoproteins

The relation between sepsis and lipoproteins has received more attention recently (Alvarez and Ramos 1986; Bentz and Magnette 1998; Fraunberger *et al.* 1999; Carpentier and Scruel 2002). This is not surprising, considering the fact that a multitude of molecules that play an important part in mediating the inflammatory response in sepsis are associated with lipoproteins. Two of these molecules (TFPI and platelet-activating factor acetylhydrolase) have recently been tested in large phase 3 multicentre sepsis trials. High-density lipoprotein plays an important part in the neutralization of endotoxin in vitro (Van Leeuwen *et al.* 2001). In patients with severe sepsis, plasma levels of both high- and low-density lipoprotein are markedly decreased (Van Leeuwen *et al.* 2003). Patients with severe sepsis may therefore be at increased risk for the deleterious effects of endotoxaemia. The administration of lipoproteins may be able to restore innate immunity in patients with sepsis and may also be useful in the prevention of sepsis in patients at risk of developing sepsis (i.e. hypocholesterolaemia in patients with malignancies). Figure 1.7 shows the relation between inflammatory mediators, coagulation factors, and molecules associated with lipoprotein metabolism.

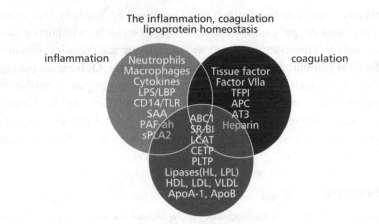

Fig. 1.7 Relation between inflammatory mediators, coagulation factors and molecules associated with lipoprotein metabolism. LPS: lipopolysaccharide; LBP: LPS binding protein; TLR: Toll-like receptor; SAA: serum amyloid A; PAF-ah: platelet activating factor acetyl hydrolase; sPLA2: secretory phospholipase A2; TFPI: tissue factor pathway inhibitor; aPC: activated protein C; AT3: antithrombin 3; ABC1: ATP binding cassette transporter 1; SR-B1: scavenger receptor B1; LCAT: lecithin-cholesterol acyltransferase; CETP: cholesteryl ester transfer protein; PLTP: phospholipid transfer protein; HL: hepatic lipase; LPL: Lipoprotein lipase; HDL: high density lipoprotein; LDL: low density lipoprotein; VLDL: very low density lipoprotein.

Sepsis and oncology

Patients with haematological malignancies or solid neoplasms are at increased risk for developing sepsis. This susceptibility is associated with both the underlying disease as well as the complications associated with therapy. Host defence mechanisms in cancer patients are hampered by anatomical barrier dysfunction (e.g. intravascular catheters, gut mucosal barrier disruption), disturbances of cellular immunity (e.g. neutropenia, lymphoma, bone marrow transplant) as well as humoral immunity (hypogammaglobulinaemia, hypocomplementaemia, hypocholesterolaemia, splenic dysfunction). This renders the patient susceptible to invading micro-organisms. Both Gram-negative micro-organisms, Gram-positive micro-organisms, yeast, and fungi are involved. Similar to the causative micro-organisms in a general sepsis population, the epidemiology of nosocomial bloodstream infections in cancer patients also shows a shift from Gram negative towards a predominance of Gram-positive micro-organisms over the past decades (Wisplinghoff *et al.* 2003). In both neutropenic and non-neutropenic patients coagulase negative staphylococci are most frequently isolated, followed by *Staphylococcus aureus*, *Enterocci, Candida* species, and *Escherichia coli*. As sepsis is an important cause of morbidity and mortality in patients with underlying malignancies, prevention of infectious complications is of the utmost importance. Options for management strategies include gut decontamination and prophylactic antibiotics, immunonutrition, probiotics, hyperoxia, and growth factors (Ellis 2004). In patients who develop sepsis, guidelines can prove helpful in the provision of optimal care and outcome improvement in these critically ill patients (Dellinger *et al.* 2004).

References

Abraham E (1999). Why immunomodulatory therapies have not worked in sepsis. *Intensive Care Medicine*, 25(6), 556–566.

Abraham E, Matthay MA, Dinarello CA, *et al.* (2000). Consensus conference definitions for sepsis, septic shock, acute lung injury, and acute respiratory distress syndrome: time for a reevaluation. *Critical Care Medicine*, 28, 232–235.

Abraham E, Reinhart K, Opal S, *et al.* (2003). Efficacy and safety of tifacogin (recombinant tissue factor pathway inhibitor) in severe sepsis—A randomized controlled trial. *JAMA*, 290(2), 238–247.

Alvarez C. and Ramos A. (1986). Lipids, lipoproteins, and apoproteins in serum during infection. *Clinical Chemistry*, 32, 142–145.

Angus DC, Linde-Zwirble WT, Lidicker J, Clermont G, Carcillo J, and Pinsky MR. (2001). Epidemiology of severe sepsis in the United States: Analysis of incidence, outcome, and associated costs of care. *Critical Care Medicine*, 29(7), 1303–1310.

Annane D, Sebille V, Charpentier C, *et al.* (2002). Effect of treatment with low doses of hydrocortisone and fludrocortisone on mortality in patients with septic shock. *JAMA*, 288(7), 862–871.

Barnes PJ and Karin M. (1997). Nuclear factor-kappaB: a pivotal transcription factor in chronic inflammatory diseases. *New England Journal of Medicine*, 336(15), 1066–1071.

Beal AL and Cerra FB. (1994). Multiple organ failure syndrome in the 1990s. Systemic inflammatory response and organ dysfunction [see comments]. *JAMA*, 271(3), 226–233.

Bentz MH and Magnette J. (1998). [Hypocholesterolemia during the acute phase of an inflammatory reaction of infectious origin. 120 cases] Hypocholesterolemie au cours de la phase aigue de la reaction inflammatoire d'origine infectieuse. A propos de 120 cas. *Revue de Medecine Interne*, 19(3), 168–172.

Bernard GR, Vincent JL, Laterre P, *et al.* (2001). Efficacy and safety of recombinant human activated protein C for severe sepsis. *New England Journal of Medicine*, 344(10), 699–709.

Bone RC. (1991). Gram-negative sepsis. Background, clinical features, and intervention. *Chest*, 100(3), 802–808.

Bone RC. (1994). Gram-positive organisms and sepsis. *Archives of Internal Medicine*, 154, 26–34.

Bone RC. (1996a). A personal experience with SIRS and MODS. *Critical Care Medicine*, 24(8), 1417–1418.

Bone RC. (1996b). Sir Isaac Newton, sepsis, SIRS, and CARS. *Critical Care Medicine*, 24(7), 1125–1128.

Bone RC. (1996c). Why sepsis trials fail [see comments]. *JAMA*, 276(7), 565–566.

Bone RC, Balk RA, Cerra FB, *et al.* (1992). American College of Chest Physicians/Society of Critical Care Medicine Consensus Conference: definitions for sepsis and organ failure and guidelines for the use of innovative therapies in sepsis [see comments]. *Critical Care Medicine*, 20(6), 864–874.

Bone RC, Grodzin CJ, and Balk RA. (1997). Sepsis: a new hypothesis for pathogenesis of the disease process. *Chest*, 112, 235–243.

Brandtzaeg P, Sandset PM, Joo GB, Ovstebo R, Abildgaard U, and Kierulf P. (1989). The quantitative association of plasma endotoxin, antithrombin, protein C, extrinsic pathway inhibitor and fibrinopeptide A in systemic meningococcal disease. *Thrombosis Research*, 55(4), 459–470.

Brealey D, Brand M, Hargreaves I, *et al.* (2002). Association between mitochondrial dysfunction and severity and outcome of septic shock. *Lancet*, 360(9328), 219–223.

Brower RG, Matthay MA, Morris A, *et al.* (2000). Ventilation with lower tidal volumes as compared with traditional tidal volumes for acute lung injury and the acute respiratory distress syndrome. *New England Journal of Medicine*, 342(18), 1301–1308.

Brun Buisson C, Doyon F, Carlet J, *et al.* (1995). Incidence, risk factors, and outcome of severe sepsis and septic shock in adults. A multicenter prospective study in intensive care units. French ICU Group for Severe Sepsis. *JAMA*, 274(12), 968–974.

Carpentier YA and Scruel O. (2002). Changes in the concentration and composition of plasma lipoproteins during the acute phase response. *Current Opinion in Clinical Nutrition and Metabolic Care*, 5(2), 153–158.

Casey LC, Balk RA, and Bone RC. (1993). Plasma cytokine and endotoxin levels correlate with survival in patients with the sepsis syndrome [see comments]. *Annals of Internal Medicine*, 119(8), 771–778.

Christman JW, Lancaster LH, and Blackwell TS. (1998). Nuclear factor kappa B: a pivotal role in the systemic inflammatory response syndrome and new target for therapy [see comments]. *Intensive Care Medicine*, 24(11), 1131–1138.

Cohen J. (2001). TREM-1 in sepsis. *Lancet*, 358(9284), 776–778.

Cohen J, Guyatt G, Bernard GR, *et al.* (2001). New strategies for clinical trials in patients with sepsis and septic shock. *Critical Care Medicine*, 29(4), 880–886.

Condliffe AM, Kitchen E, and Chilvers ER. (1998). Neutrophil priming: pathophysiological consequences and underlying mechanisms. *Clinical Science*, 94(5), 461–471.

Cross AS and Opal SM. (2003). A new paradigm for the treatment of sepsis: is it time to consider combination therapy? *Annals of Internal Medicine*, 138(6), 502–505.

De Backer D, Creteur J, Preiser JC, Dubois MJ, and Vincent JL. (2002). Microvascular blood flow is altered in patients with sepsis. *American Journal of Respiratory and Critical Care Medicine*, 166, 98–104.

Dellinger RP, Opal SM, Rotrosen D, Suffredini AF, and Zimmerman JL. (1997). From the bench to the bedside: the future of sepsis research. Executive summary of an American College of Chest Physicians, National Institute of Allergy and Infectious Disease, and National Heart, Lung, and Blood Institute Workshop. *Chest*, 111(3), 744–753.

Dellinger RP, Carlet JM, Masur H, *et al.* (2004). Surviving Sepsis Campaign guidelines for management of severe sepsis and septic shock. *Intensive Care Medicine*, 30(4), 536–555.

Docke WD, Randow F, Syrbe U, *et al.* (1997). Monocyte deactivation in septic patients: restoration by IFN-gamma treatment. *Nature Medicine*, 3(6), 678–681.

Eichacker PQ and Natanson C. (2003). Recombinant human activated protein C in sepsis: inconsistent trial results, an unclear mechanism of action, and safety concerns resulted in labeling restrictions and the need for phase IV trials. *Critical Care Medicine*, 31(1 Suppl.), S94–S96.

Eichacker PQ, Parent C, Kalil A, *et al.* (2002). Risk and the efficacy of antiinflammatory agents: retrospective and confirmatory studies of sepsis. *American Journal of Respiratory and Critical Care Medicine*, 166(9), 1197–1205.

Ellis M. (2004). Preventing microbial translocation in haematological malignancy. *British Journal of Haematology*, 125(3), 282–293.

Fink MP. (2002). Cytopathic hypoxia. Is oxygen use impaired in sepsis as a result of an acquired intrinsic derangement in cellular respiration? *Critical Care Clinics*, 18, 165–175.

Fink MP and Aranow JS. (1997). Gut barrier dysfunction and sepsis. In: *Sepsis and Multiorgan Failure* (eds AM Fein *et al.*), pp. 383–407. Williams and Wilkins.

Fraunberger P, Schaefer S, Werdan K, Walli AK, and Seidel D. (1999). Reduction of circulating cholesterol and apolipoprotein levels during sepsis. *Clinical Chemistry and Laboratory Medicine*, 37(3), 357–362.

Friedman G, Silva E, and Vincent JL. (1998). Has the mortality of septic shock changed with time [see comments]. *Critical Care Medicine*, 26(12), 2078–2086.

Haeney MR. (1998). The role of the complement cascade in sepsis. *Journal of Antimicrobial Chemotherapy*, 41(Suppl. A), 41–46.

Hatada EN, Krappmann D, and Scheidereit C. (2000). NF-kappa B and the innate immune response. *Current Opinions in Immunology*, 12, 52–58.

Haveman JW, Kobold AC, Tervaert JW, *et al.* (1999). The central role of monocytes in the pathogenesis of sepsis: consequences for immunomonitoring and treatment. *Netherlands Journal of Medicine*, 55(3), 132–141.

Hogg N. (1992). Roll, roll, roll your leucocyte gently down the vein. *Immunology Today*, 13(4), 113–115.

Hotchkiss RS and Karl IE. (2003). The pathophysiology and treatment of sepsis. *New England Journal of Medicine*, 348(2), 138–150.

Ince C. (2002). The microcirculation unveiled. *American Journal of Respiratory and Critical Care Medicine*, 166, 1–2.

Inohara N, Ogura Y, and Nunez G. (2002). Nods: a family of cytosolic proteins that regulate the host response to pathogens. *Current Opinion in Microbiology*, 5, 76–80.

Jimeno A, Garcia-Velasco A, del Val O, *et al.* (2004). Assessment of procalcitonin as a diagnostic and prognostic marker in patients with solid tumors and febrile neutropenia. *Cancer*, 100(11), 2462–2469.

Kallio R, Surcel HM, Bloigu A, and Syrjala H. (2000). C-reactive protein, procalcitonin and interleukin-8 in the primary diagnosis of infections in cancer patients. *European Journal of Cancer*, 36(7), 889–894.

Kox WJ, Bone RC, Krausch D, *et al.* (1997). Interferon gamma-1b in the treatment of compensatory anti-inflammatory response syndrome. A new approach: proof of principle. *Archives of Internal Medicine*, 157(4), 389–393.

Levi M and ten Cate H. (1999). Disseminated intravascular coagulation. *New England Journal of Medicine*, **341**(8), 586–592.

Levy MM, Fink MP, Marshall JC, *et al.* (2003). (2001 SCCM/ESICM/ACCP/ATS/SIS) International Sepsis Definitions Conference. *Critical Care Medicine*, **31**(4), 1250–1256.

Lilienfeld-Toal M, Dietrich MP, Glasmacher A, *et al.* (2004). Markers of bacteremia in febrile neutropenic patients with hematological malignancies: procalcitonin and IL-6 are more reliable than C-reactive protein. *European Journal of Clinical Microbiology and Infectious Diseases*, **23**(7), 539–544.

Luster AD. (1998). Chemokines–chemotactic cytokines that mediate inflammation. *New England Journal of Medicine*, **338**(7), 436–445.

Magor BG and Magor KE. (2001). Evolution of effectors and receptors of innate immunity. *Developmental and Comparative Immunology*, **25**(8–9), 651–682.

Majno G. (1991). The ancient riddle of sigma eta psi iota sigma (sepsis). *Journal of Infectious Diseases*, **163**(5), 937–945.

Martin GS, Mannino DM, Eaton S, and Moss M. (2003). The epidemiology of sepsis in the United States from 1979 through 2000. *New England Journal of Medicine*, **348**(16), 1546–1554.

Medzhitov R and Janeway CA, Jr. (2002). Decoding the patterns of self and nonself by the innate immune system. *Science*, **296**(5566), 298–300.

Nasraway SA, Jr. (1999). Sepsis research: we must change course [see comments]. *Critical Care Medicine*, **27**(2), 427–430.

Nathan C and Ding A. (2001). TREM-1: a new regulator of innate immunity in sepsis syndrome. *Nature Medicine*, **7**(5), 530–532.

Opal SM and Cohen J. (1999). Clinical gram-positive sepsis: does it fundamentally differ from gram-negative bacterial sepsis? *Critical Care Medicine*, **27**(8), 1608–1616.

Opal SM, Scannon PJ, Vincent JL, *et al.* (1999). Relationship between plasma levels of lipopolysaccharide (LPS) and LPS-binding protein in patients with severe sepsis and septic shock. *Journal of Infectious Diseases*, **180**(5), 1584–1589.

Parkos CA. (1997). Molecular events in neutrophil transepithelial migration. *Bioessays*, **19**(10), 865–873.

Rangel Frausto MS, Pittet D, Costigan M, Hwang T, Davis CS, and Wenzel RP. (1995). The natural history of the systemic inflammatory response syndrome (SIRS). A prospective study [see comments]. *JAMA*, **273**(2), 117–123.

Reinhart K, Menges T, Gardlund B, *et al.* (2001). Randomized, placebo-controlled trial of the anti-tumor necrosis factor antibody fragment afelimomab in hyperinflammatory response during severe sepsis: The RAMSES Study. *Critical Care Medicine*, **29**(4), 765–769.

Rivers E, Nguyen B, Havstad S, *et al.* (2001). Early goal-directed therapy in the treatment of severe sepsis and septic shock. *New England Journal of Medicine*, **345**(19), 1368–1377.

Safdar A and Armstrong D. (2001). Infectious morbidity in critically ill patients with cancer. *Critical Care Clinics*, **17**(3), 531–570, VII, VIII.

Sair M, Etherington PJ, Winlove CP, and Evans TW. (2001). Tissue oxygenation and perfusion in patients with systemic sepsis. *Critical Care Medicine*, **29**(7), 1343–1349.

Schluger NW and Rom WN. (1997). Early responses to infection: chemokines as mediators of inflammation. *Current Opinion in Immunology*, **9**(4), 504–508.

Schumann RR, Leong SR, Flaggs GW, *et al.* (1990). Structure and function of lipopolysaccharide binding protein. *Science*, **249**(4975), 1429–1431.

Schuttrumpf S, Binder L, Hagemann T, Berkovic D, Trumper L, and Binder C. (2003). Procalcitonin: a useful discriminator between febrile conditions of different origin in hemato-oncological patients? *Annals of Hematology*, **82**(2), 98–103.

Simon L, Gauvin F, Amre DK, Saint-Louis P, and Lacroix J. (2004). Serum procalcitonin and C-reactive protein levels as markers of bacterial infection: a systematic review and meta-analysis. *Clinical Infectious Diseases*, **39**(2), 206–217.

Springer TA. (1990). Adhesion receptors of the immune system. *Nature*, **346**(6283), 425–434.

Van den Berghe G, Wouters P, Weekers F, *et al.* (2001). Intensive insulin therapy in the critically ill patients. *New England Journal of Medicine*, **345**(19), 1359–1367.

Van Leeuwen HJ, van Beek AP, Dallinga-Thie GM, van Strijp JA, Verhoef J, and van Kessel KP. (2001). The role of high density lipoprotein in sepsis. *Netherlands Journal of Medicine*, **59**(3), 102–110.

Van Leeuwen HJ, Heezius EC, Dallinga GM, van Strijp JA, Verhoef J, and van Kessel KP. (2003). Lipoprotein metabolism in patients with severe sepsis. *Critical Care Medicine*, **31**(5), 1359–1366.

Vincent JL, Levi M, Fisher C, and Reinhart K. (2001). Rationale for restoration of physiological anticoagulant pathways in patients with sepsis and disseminated intravascular coagulation—Question and answer session after scientific review. *Critical Care Medicine*, **29**(7), S94.

Volk HD, Reinke P, Krausch D, *et al.* (1996). Monocyte deactivation—rationale for a new therapeutic strategy in sepsis. *Intensive Care Medicine*, **22** (Suppl. 4), S474–481.

Volk HD, Reinke P, and Docke WD. (1999). Immunological monitoring of the inflammatory process: Which variables? When to assess? *European Journal of Surgery*, **163** (Suppl. 584), 70–72.

Warren BL, Eid A, Singer P, *et al.* (2001). Caring for the critically ill patient. High-dose antithrombin III in severe sepsis: a randomized controlled trial. *JAMA*, **286**(15), 1869–1878.

Watson RS, Carcillo JA, Linde-Zwirble WT, Clermont G, Lidicker J, and Angus DC. (2003). The epidemiology of severe sepsis in children in the United States. *American Journal of Respiratory and Critical Care Medicine*, **167**(5), 695–701.

West MA and Heagy W. (2002). Endotoxin tolerance: a review. *Critical Care Medicine*, **30**(1 Suppl.), S64–S73.

Wisplinghoff H, Seifert H, Wenzel RP, and Edmond MB. (2003). Current trends in the epidemiology of nosocomial bloodstream infections in patients with hematological malignancies and solid neoplasms in hospitals in the United States. *Clinical Infectious Diseases*, **36**(9), 1103–1110.

Wright SD, Ramos RA, Tobias PS, Ulevitch RJ, and Mathison JC. (1990). CD14, a receptor for complexes of lipopolysaccharide (LPS) and LPS binding protein [see comments]. *Science*, **249**(4975), 1431–1433.

Yang RB, Mark MR, Gray A, *et al.* (1998). Toll-like receptor-2 mediates lipopolysaccharide-induced cellular signalling. *Nature*, **395**(6699), 284–288.

Zeni F, Freeman B, and Natanson C. (1997). Anti-inflammatory therapies to treat sepsis and septic shock: a reassessment [editorial; comment]. *Critical Care Medicine*, **25**(7), 1095–1100.

Chapter 2

The role of the immune system in cancer

Nigel J. Stevenson and Jim Johnston

Introduction

Infection and chronic inflammation predisposes us to many forms of cancer and the response to malignant disease shows many parallels with inflammation and wound healing. The cells involved in inflammation are detected in a range of common cancers, together with the inflammatory cytokines and members of the chemokine ligand/receptor systems.

Many cancers occur more frequently with certain infectious diseases; examples include *Helicobacter pylori* infection, human immunodeficiency virus, hepatitis, and human papillomavirus (HPV). The longer the infection and inflammation persist, the higher the risk of associated cancer. Chronic inflammatory conditions such as inflammatory bowel disease, have a five- to sevenfold higher incidence of colon cancer, as a result of the immune response causing colonic epithelium to become transformed. Therefore, understanding these disease processes may lead to better prevention and treatment for cancer.

The theory of immune surveillance suggests that the immune system continually recognizes and eliminates tumours; when a tumour escapes immune surveillance and grows too large for the immune system to kill, cancer can result. Immune surveillance is most likely to be successful against virus-induced cancers that express foreign peptides. However, tumours vary greatly in their immunogenicity, and even those with antigens, which can be recognized by the host immune system, can evade immune elimination.

Lack of tumour rejection by intact immune systems is not always due to the absence of antigens that can be recognized or to the absence of T cells that can recognize those antigens. Tumour-specific lymphocytes can be found in the blood, draining lymph nodes, and in the tumour itself of patients with actively growing tumours. These lymphocytes can kill tumour cells *in vitro* but fail to do so *in vivo*. The presence of these cells has allowed immunologists to identify antigens on some tumour cells.

The relationship between cancer and infection is not well defined. Malignancy can develop from chronic inflammation, when aberrant cell proliferation occurs in a milieu rich with proinflammatory cytokines and growth factors which are most frequently detected in chronic inflammatory states. During the acute inflammatory response anti-inflammatory homeostatic cytokines, such as interleukin (IL)-10 and intracellular inhibitors, such as the suppressors of cytokine signalling, are produced to help resolve the acute inflammation. In chronic inflammation, however, the inflammation persists, frequently due to the lack of anti-inflammatory mediators, and can result in increased production of reactive oxygen species, leading to oxidative DNA damage, reduced DNA repair, and the bypass of normal cell cycle checkpoints.

This chapter describes recent important developments in our understanding of how infection and inflammation lead to malignancy and the possible use of immune targets in the treatment of cancer.

Chronic inflammation and the progression of gastric cancer

With gastric cancer, low levels of stomach acid can be just as dangerous as too much. Both extremes create inflammatory changes in the stomach lining and a condition called chronic atrophic gastritis that can promote neoplasia. A recent publication (Zavros *et al.* 2005) demonstrated that chronic gastritis progresses to gastric cancer in mice with abnormally low levels of gastrin that stimulates stomach parietal cells to secrete hydrochloric acid. Other researchers have shown that overproduction of gastrin in mice stimulates uncontrolled growth of cells in the stomach lining and the development of gastric tumours. Moreover infection with *H. pylori*, if left untreated, is associated with stomach cancer. These findings suggest that inflammation, regardless of the cause is a fundamental trigger for the development of gastric cancer.

Prostate cancer and chronic inflammation

Latent prostate cancer may develop from lesions generally associated with chronic inflammation. In prostate cancer, the glutathione S-transferase p (GSTP1) gene is deactivated by hypermethylation. When various stages of normal and malignant prostate cells were screened for GSTP1 methylation status it was observed that 'hyper'methylation on the GSTP1 gene shuts off its cancer-preventing properties, as the prostate tissue fails to produce these critical protective enzymes. Examination of GSTP1 hypermethylation in normal and prostate cancers tissue samples as well as in inflammatory prostate lesions known as proliferative inflammatory atrophy (PIA) and prostate intraepithelial neoplasia found increasing levels of GSTP1 methylation during prostate cancer development. Early PIA lesions associated with inflammation have high GSTP1 expression. It may be that hypermethylation of the GSTP1 gene begins in PIA lesions leaving prostatic tissue unable to repair damage from carcinogens. Further carcinogenic insults over time cause PIA lesions to progress to the precancerous prostate intraepithelial neoplasia. These observations suggest that prostate cancer could be preventable/reversible with anti-inflammatory drugs.

Two direct links between chronic inflammation and colon cancer

Many studies have identified DNA damage caused by chronic infection and inflammation as a potential risk factor for colorectal cancer. Work reported in the *Proceedings of the National Academy of Sciences USA* shows how overproduction of the inflammation-causing enzyme cyclooxygenase-2 (COX-2) may contribute to cancer and conversely, how aspirin-like drugs that block COX-2 might help treat or prevent cancer. During oxidative stress, free radicals can mutate DNA. These mutations delete a small portion of DNA, effectively throwing off the 'reading frame' through which the genes' instructions are interpreted and resulting in an abnormal protein. Interestingly, these types of mutations are common in an inherited form of colon cancer, hereditary non-polyposis colon cancer. This work suggests that these mutations, caused by inflammation and other sources of oxidative stress, might also contribute to colorectal cancer.

Some reports suggest that bowel cancer may arise because of a lack of inhibitory control in the immune system. I-κB kinase (IKKb) is a proinflammatory kinase required for the activation of the transcription factor nuclear factor (NF)-κB, a master switch that turns on inflammation in response to bacterial or viral infections. In epithelial cells, IKKb can promote cancer by inhibiting apoptosis. Karin and colleagues found that in mice lacking IKKb intestinal epithelial cells, the incidence decreased by 80%, and chemical induction of inflammation occurred even without activation of NF-κB, and further analysis showed markedly enhanced apoptosis. These findings prove that blocking the inflammatory response can significantly reduce tumour incidence and indicate that this pathway is a key molecular mechanism linking chronic inflammation, particularly colitis, and colon cancer.

Skin cancer

Skin cancer from sun overexposure affects millions each year. One in 87 will develop malignant melanoma, the most serious type of skin cancer. The ultraviolet rays destroy epidermal cells, damaging capillaries and cellular DNA, and repeated DNA damage can lead to cancer. Natural killer (NK) cells and cyto-toxic T cells can identify the damaged cells as foreign. A weakened immune system leaves individuals at higher risk for skin cancer, particularly patients with AIDS, cancer, or those on immune-suppressant drugs.

Daniel and colleagues (Daniel D *et al.* 2003) have found that by crossing mice that ordinarily develop invasive skin carcinomas with another strain lacking a particular type of T immune cell, resulted in reduced tumour formation, rather than the expected increase. Similarly, Lin and colleagues (Lin *et al.* 2001) have evidence that macrophage infiltration can promote both the development of breast cancers and their eventual spread. Targeting the gene for colony-stimulating factor 1, a cytokine that attracts macrophages, resulted in progression to malignancy being slowed, and there was almost no metastases. Therefore, activating macrophages appears to be especially dangerous, as many of the weapons these immune system scavengers release can promote cancer. The noxious substances include highly reactive forms of oxygen that can cause carcinogenic mutations. Cells are especially vulnerable to these assaults when they are dividing rapidly, as may be the case when tissues try to repair the damage caused by viral or bacterial infections.

Cervical cancer and macrophages

Smouldering beneath many latent tumours is a chronic inflammation that drives malignancy. de Visser *et al.* (2005) demonstrate that specialized cells from the 'adaptive' immune system orchestrate the innate inflammation that promotes tumour progression.

Further studies found that cancer-associated inflammation actually promotes tumour growth and progression. For instance, tumour-associated macrophages work their way into precancerous tissue, and can promote tumour growth and metastases and infiltration of large numbers of macrophages can be associated with poor prognosis. Moreover, increased expression of genes associated with macrophage infiltration (such as CD68) form part of the molecular signatures that herald poor prognosis in certain cancers (Paik *et al.* 2004).

The best-studied examples of inflammation-associated cancer are colon cancer and cervical carcinoma. Cervical carcinoma is caused by infection with HPV. Innate immune cells, such as macrophages, infiltrate the premalignant epithelial tissues and drive a chronic inflammatory process that promotes overproliferation of epithelial cells, tissue remodelling, and angiogenesis, followed eventually by invasive carcinoma.

Work by adaptive immune cells called B cells produce the signal that kindles inflammation in the epidermal layer of the skin. By genetic elimination of these adaptive cells, de Visser *et al.* (2005) showed blocked recruitment of innate cells, and subsequent tissue remodelling and angiogenesis. Carcinogenesis was arrested at the stage of epithelial overproliferation. When B cells from HPV16 mice were transferred into the immune-deficient HPV16 cross-bred animals, the expected inflammatory response and cancer progression were restored, showing that these cells are the perpetrators. This is surprising as we expect T cells to be implicated, but B-cell antibodies were found in the underlying dermis layer suggesting they may trigger responses by recognizing molecules on the surface of the tumour cells.

Causal role of viruses and bacteria in cancer

H. pylori, found in the stomachs of a third of all adults causes inflammation of the mucous membrane of the stomach and can induce gastric ulcers (Marshall 1989). Peptic ulcer disease, a chronic inflammatory condition of the stomach and duodenum, affects as many as 10% of people in the United States at some time in their lives. Infection of humans with *H. pylori* is causally associated with the risk of developing adenocarcinoma of the stomach, one of the most common malignancies in the world (24 000 new cases and 14 000 deaths per year). The strongest evidence that *H. pylori* is associated with gastric cancer comes from prospective studies indicating that *H. pylori* infected persons have a significantly increased rate of gastric cancer (Marshall 1989).

H. pylori is also associated with less common forms of cancer, non-Hodgkin's lymphoma and mucosa-associated lymphoid tissue lymphomas of the stomach (Marshall 1989). These types of lymphomas in the stomach only arise in the setting of *H. pylori* inflammation. In 70% of *H. pylori*-infected patients with lymphoma, treatment with appropriate antibiotics leads to regression, suggesting that treatment of a bacterial infection can actually result in regression of cancer.

Another landmark study, published in June, 1997, showed that a 12-year nation-wide vaccination programme against hepatitis B virus in Taiwan resulted in a significant reduction in the number of cases of childhood liver cancer. (Chang MH *et al.* 1997).

Immunotherapy

Immunotherapy for cancer can stimulate the host's antitumour response by increasing the number of effector cells or by producing cytokines to decrease host-suppressor mechanisms, thus making the tumour cells more susceptible to damage by immunological processes. These mechanisms that represent manipulation of immunological processes are considered immunotherapy.

Cellular immunotherapy

Passive cellular immunotherapy is the term used when activated, specific effector cells are directly infused into a patient and are not induced or expanded within the patient. Early attempts involved reinfusion of the patient's lymphocytes after expansion *in vitro* by exposure to IL-2 (T-cell growth factor) (Figure 2.1). These cells are called *lymphokine-activated killer* (LAK) *cells* and can be expanded by a variety of lymphokines. The availability of purified recombinant IL-2 in large quantities has made the LAK cell/IL-2 therapy feasible, and some melanoma and renal carcinoma patients have shown good responses. However, as infusion of IL-2 after LAK cell infusions is associated with significant toxicity, variations of these methods are being explored. One approach is to isolate and expand populations of lymphocytes that have infiltrated tumours *in vivo* and have specificity (termed *tumour-infiltrating lymphocytes* (TILs)). Infusion of TILs reduces the IL-2 dose required. The use of *interferon (IFN)-γ*, can enhance the expression of major histocompatibility complex (MHC) antigens and tumour-associated antigens (TAAs) on tumour cells, thus enhancing killing of tumour cells by the infused effector cells.

Humoral immunotherapy

The use of antitumour antibodies as a form of passive immunotherapy (in contrast to active stimulation of the host's immune system) is at least a century old. Hybridoma technology has increased the potential of this approach to human immunotherapy, because it permits *in vitro* detection and production of monoclonal antitumour antibodies directed against a variety of animal and human neoplasms.

A number of monoclonal antibodies such as rituximab, a chimeric anti-CD20 monoclonal, activates complement-mediated cytotoxicity and antibody-dependent cellular cytotoxicity. Rituximab has direct antitumour effects, has synergistic activity with chemotherapy and appears to sensitize chemoresistant cell lines. It is being used in follicular non-Hodgkin's lymphoma and diffuse large B-cell lymphoma with some success. Table 2.1 describes antibodies currently approved for therapy.

Another variation is conjugation of monoclonal antitumour antibodies with toxins (e.g. ricin, diphtheria) or with radioisotopes, so that the antibodies will deliver these toxic agents specifically to the tumour cells. A new approach, using cellular and humoral mechanisms, is the development of bispecific antibodies, which links one antibody reacting with the tumour cell to a second

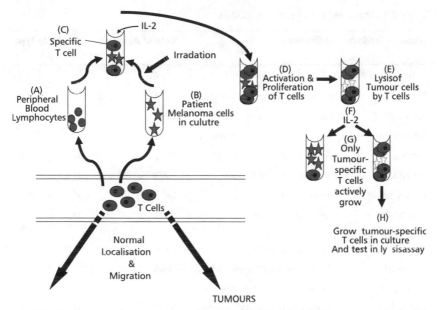

Fig. 2.1 Generation of Lymphokine-activated Killer cells. (A) T cells isolated from the blood are (B) stimulated in vitro with (C) irradiated autologous tumour cells. The T-cell growth factor Interleukin-2 (IL-2) is added, allowing (D) the proliferation of the T cells that are specifically activated because they recognize their target antigen on the tumour cells. The tumour-specific T cells then differentiate into cytotoxic T lymphocytes and (E) lyse the tumour cells. (F) These responder T cells can be cloned by limiting dilution: small numbers of cells are distributed into multiple new culture wells and stimulated by the addition of tumour cells and IL-2, so that (G) T-cell growth is observed in only a small proportion of the wells, ensuring that each growing culture derives from a single T cell. (H) These T cell clones are amplified in culture and their lytic activity can be tested before use in immunotherapy.

antibody reacting with a cytotoxic effector cell, thus targeting the latter more specifically to the tumour.

Specific immunotherapy

Approaches designed to induce therapeutic cellular immunity in the tumour-bearing host are more promising than passive immunotherapy techniques. Inducing immunity in a host that failed to develop an effective response in the first place requires special procedures to present the tumour antigens to the host effectors. Intact tumour cells, defined tumour antigens, or general immunostimulants are used.

Autologous tumour cells (cells taken from the host) have been used—after irradiation, neuraminidase treatment, hapten conjugation, or hybridization

Table 2.1 Approved therapeutic antibodies

Name of Product	Indications	Date of Approval	Antibody Type (2)
Orthoclone-OKT®	Organ Transplant Rejection	1986	M
ReoPro®	Acute Cardiac Conditions	1994	C
Rituxan®	Non-Hodgkin's Lymphoma	1997	C
Zevalin™	Non-Hodgkin's Lymphoma	2002	M
Zenapax®	Acute Transplant Rejection	1997	H
Synagis®	Viral Respiratory Disease	1998	H
Herceptin®	Breast Cancer	1998	H
Avastin ®	Colorectal Cancer	2004	H
Remicade®	Crohn's disease, Rheumatoid Arthritis	1998	C
Simulect®	Acute Transplant Rejection	1998	C
Mylotarg™	Acute Myeloid Leukemia	2000	H
Campath®	Chronic Lymphocytic Leukemia	2001	H
Humira™	Rheumatoid Arthritis	2002	PD
Xolair®	Asthma	2003	H
Raptiva™	Psoriasis	2003	H
Bexxar®	Non-Hodgkin's Lymphoma	2003	M
Erbitux™	Colorectal Cancer	2004	C

Mouse (M), Chimeric (C), Human (H)

with long-term cell lines *in vitro*—in kidney carcinoma and malignant melanoma patients, among others. More recently, approaches using tumour cells genetically modified to produce immunostimulatory molecules (including cytokines, such as granulocyte-macrophage colony-stimulating factor or IL-2, co-stimulatory molecules such as B7–1, and allogeneic class I MHC molecules) have been used successfully in animal studies and are being evaluated in human clinical trials.

Allogeneic tumour cells (cells taken from other patients) have been used in patients with acute lymphoblastic and acute myeloblastic leukaemia. Remission is induced by intensive chemotherapy and radiotherapy; irradiated allogeneic tumour cells are then injected with Bacille Calmette-Guérin (BCG) vaccine or other adjuvants (see 'Non-specific immunotherapy' section). Prolonged remissions and/or improved re-induction rates have been reported in some series.

Defined tumour antigen-based vaccines are among the most promising approaches in cancer immunotherapy. One advantage of using defined antigens is that the immunization technique can be readily evaluated for effectiveness because a defined endpoint is available (i.e. measurable responses to a specific peptide). An increasing number of tumour antigens have been unequivocally identified as the target of specific T cells grown from cancer patients. These include antigens that have a normal sequence but are inappropriately expressed in the tumour and antigens derived from genes that have mutated during tumour development (e.g. oncogenes). B-cell lymphomas have a unique antigen derived from the variable region of the clonally expressed immunoglobulin sequence (the idiotype). This is unique to the tumour cells but varies among patients.

Cellular immunity (involving cytotoxic T cells) to specific, very well defined antigens can be induced using short synthetic peptides in adjuvant or bound to autologous antigen-presenting cells *in vitro* (antigen pulsing). These antigen-pulsed, antigen-presenting cells are reintroduced intravenously and stimulate the patient's T cells to respond to the pulsed peptide antigen. Early results in clinical trials have shown significant responses and immunization with the custom-synthesized idiotype sequences expressed by the patient's B-cell lymphoma cells has shown significant response rates.

Antigen-specific immunity can also be induced with recombinant viruses (e.g. adenovirus, vaccinia virus) expressing such TAAs as carcinoembryonic antigen (CEA). These antigen-delivery viruses are being tested for antitumour effectiveness.

Non-specific immunotherapy

Cytokines are the messengers of the immune system and are sometimes called immune hormones. They can act either locally or at a distance. Cytokines can either enhance or suppress immunity and in cancer treatment they are generally used to enhance immunity.

Two cytokines, IL-2 and IFN-a 2b are approved by the Federal Drug Administration (FDA) for use against certain cancers. IL-2 is used to treat renal cell carcinoma, melanoma, lymphoma, and leukaemia. IFN has been useful against a number of diseases, including Kaposi's sarcoma, chronic myelogenous leukaemia, and hairy cell leukaemia.

Cytokines are produced by white blood cells (WBCs) in combinations and in nature they work together. However, the response rate of individual cytokines is generally low. Studies using combined cytokines in the ratios they are produced naturally have shown that the combinations have synergistic effects. For instance, IL-2 is used to stimulate certain WBCs to divide and when used alone, a very high dose of IL-2 is required to make the cells divide. However, high doses of IL-2 can cause serious negative side-effects. When a natural combination of cytokines produced by WBCs is used, the dose of IL-2 can be lowered by a factor of 5000 producing minimal side-effects.

IFNs derived from WBCs (IFN-α and IFN-γ) or from fibroblasts (IFN-β) or synthesized in bacteria by recombinant genetic techniques, are glycoproteins that have antitumour and antiviral activity, which may originate partially from immunologically mediated mechanisms. Depending on the dosage, IFNs may either enhance or decrease cellular and humoral immune functions and may affect macrophage and NK cell activity. IFNs also inhibit division and certain synthetic processes in a variety of cells. As mentioned above human clinical trials have indicated that IFNs have antitumour activity in hairy cell leukaemia, chronic myelocytic leukaemia, and AIDS-associated Kaposi's sarcoma, but some response has been seen to a lesser degree in non-Hodgkin's lymphoma, multiple myeloma, and ovarian carcinoma. However, IFNs are quite toxic and patients may develop fever, malaise, leucopenia, alopecia, and myalgia.

Bacterial adjuvants (e.g. attenuated tubercle bacilli (BCG)), extracts of BCG (e.g. methanol-extracted residue), or killed suspensions of *Corynebacterium parvum* have been used in randomized trials. They have been used with, or without, added tumour antigen to treat a wide variety of cancers, usually along with intensive chemotherapy or radiotherapy. Direct injection of BCG into melanoma nodules almost always leads to regression of the injected nodules and, occasionally, of distant, non-injected nodules. Intravesicular instillation of BCG in patients with superficial bladder carcinoma has prolonged disease-free intervals, possibly as a result of immunological mechanisms. Some studies suggest that methanol-extracted residue may help prolong drug-induced remission in acute myeloblastic leukaemia and that BCG added to combination chemotherapy may increase survival in patients with ovarian carcinoma and possibly with non-Hodgkin's lymphoma. However, many studies have shown no benefit.

Tumour antigens

The concept of immune surveillance is based on the assumption that the function of the immune system is to recognize and destroy clones of cells before they grow into tumours and to kill tumours after they form. Immunological surveillance is also based on the theory that the immune system is able to discriminate between self and foreign antigens and that tumour-specific antigens are identified as non-self.

Cancer cells express proteins that are either not expressed at all or are present in much lower quantities in normal cells, that is why these proteins appear foreign to a tumour host. These proteins are termed 'tumour antigens' or 'tumour markers'. Therefore, a tumour antigen can be viewed as a substance in the body that may indicate the presence of cancer. Interest in tumour immunology has increased with the identification of numerous tumour antigens and their possible use in vaccination.

Dr Bence-Jones pioneered the concept of a tumour marker into medical science more than 150 years ago, by using a specific protein to aid in the diagnosis of multiple myeloma. This is now called the Bence-Jones protein and is currently one of the serum markers used to detect monoclonal tumour cell products in cancer patients (Beetham 2000).

Tumour antigens are secreted from the tumour itself or are produced by the body in response to the cancer. A tumour marker can be detected in a solid tumour, in circulating tumour cells, in peripheral blood, in bone marrow, in lymph nodes or in other body fluids, such as urine. Tumour markers are used to confirm the diagnosis of cancer, to determine the response to therapy, to detect recurrent disease and have significance in cancer screening programmes.

Studies in the 1950s with murine tumours, induced by chemical carcinogens or radiation, provided the first cellular evidence that tumour cells express antigens that trigger a specific immune response. In these experiments sarcomas were induced in mice by painting the skin with the chemical carcinogen methylcholanthrene (MCA). Transplantation of these tumours into syngeneic mice was successful and resulted in tumour growth and eventual death. However, reintroduction of the same tumour into the original host resulted in immunological rejection of the tumour, indicating that immunity had developed and was memorized. Furthermore, T cells from the tumour-bearing mice could be transferred and generated protection to tumour-free mice, suggesting that the immunity was T-cell mediated. To confirm that immunity could be developed in response to a specific tumour, irradiated cells of a tumour were used to immunize the tumour-free mice and resulted in rejection of the cancerous implant. However, the mice that had become immune to their tumour were unable to reject MCA-induced tumours transplanted from other mice, or even other tumours from a different site in their own body, demonstrating that the immunity was tumour-specific. In summary, these studies provided significant evidence that responses to chemically or radioactively-induced carcinomas were tumour-specific, generated a memory response and were mediated by lymphocytes (Chiplunkar 2001).

Identification of tumour antigens

Another significant step in tumour immunology research was the development of techniques to identifying tumour antigens. The genetic approach to identify human tumour antigens was pioneered by Boon (Van der Bruggen *et al.* 1991). One method of identification is transfecting cDNA libraries from tumour cell lines into target cells and subsequently testing the transfected cells for their recognition by autologous tumour-specific cytotoxic lymphocytes (CTLs). Once the gene is identified the antigenic peptide region can be isolated by transfecting gene fragments. The exact amino acid sequence is used to produce synthetic oligopeptides, which are subsequently tested for recognition by the original tumour-specific CTL clone (Boon *et al.* 1997).

Another method uses biochemical procedures to elute antigenic peptides bound to MHC class I molecules of tumour cells, which are recognized by CTLs. The peptides are separated by reverse-phase high-performance liquid chromatography (RP-HPLC) and mass spectrometry. The peptide fragments are then tested for their ability to stimulate CTLs by being pulsed into MHC-matched antigen-presenting cells. After a number of further fractionations, the individual peptide sequences are obtained (Rotzschke *et al.* 1990).

The search for antibodies that target tumour antigens is extremely important in the field of tumour immunology. Immunization of animals with human tumour cells and the removal of antibodies reactive with normal tissue antigens by serial absorption is a technique used to recognize tumour antigens. This approach was used to identify two important markers, Alpha fetoprotein (AFP) from liver cancer (Abelev *et al.* 1963) and carcino-embryonic antigen from colon and epithelial cancers (Gold and Freedman 1965). Monoclonal antibodies have been used to identify a number of specific markers, including CA19-9 for human pancreatic cancer and CA-125 for ovarian cancer.

Tumour-specific antigens

Tumour antigens that are detected by a rejection of transplanted tumour cells are termed 'tumour transplantation antigens'. However, as mentioned, one MCA-induced sarcoma will not induce protective immunity against another MCA-induced sarcoma, even if the tumours are derived from the same mouse, resulting in these antigens being called 'tumour-specific transplantation antigens' (TSTAs) (Figure 2.2).

TSTAs are unique to tumour cells and do not occur on normal cells of the body. TSTAs may result from mutations in tumour cells and after cytosolic processing are presented with MHC I molecules. The presentation of these antigens results in a cell-mediated response by tumour-specific lymphocytes.

Tumour-specific antigens have been identified on tumours induced with chemical, physical, or viral carcinogens. In contrast to chemically-induced tumours, a specific virus will induce the same antigens in all tumours. For example, if a syngeneic mouse is injected with killed cells from a specific

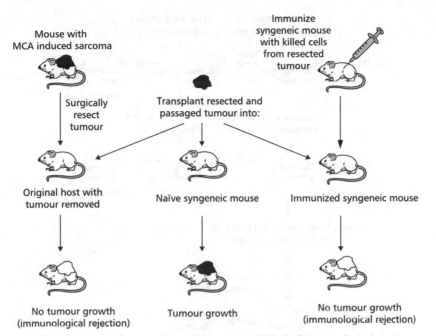

Fig. 2.2 Tumour specific transplantation antigens (TSTAs) of chemically-induced sarcoma. A mouse treated with the chemical carcinogen Methylcholanthrene (MCA) develops a sarcoma. If this tumour is resected and transplanted into a normal syngeneic mouse, the tumour will grow. In contrast, the original tumour-bearing animal that was cured by surgical resection will reject a subsequent transplant of the same tumour. Injection of killed cells from the same tumour into a syngeneic mouse induce the same type of protective immunity.

polyoma-induced tumour, the recipient mouse will develop immunity against live cells from any polyoma-induced tumours (Figure 2.3). Furthermore, when lymphocytes are transferred from mice with a virus-induced tumour into normal syngeneic mice, the recipient is given immunity and will reject subsequent transplants from any tumours generated by the same virus (Sjoegen 1964).

In both Simian virus 40 (SV40)-induced tumours and polyoma-induced tumours, the presence of the tumour antigens is related to the neoplastic state of the cell. Examples of virally-induced neoplasia resulting in antigen presentation include, Burkitt's lymphoma cells expressing nuclear antigen of the Epstein–Barr virus, hepatitis B and C viruses inducing hepatocellular carcinoma, HPV proteins, which are present on over 80% of invasive cervical cancers and in anal carcinomas and human T-lymphotropic virus inducing T-cell leukaemia.

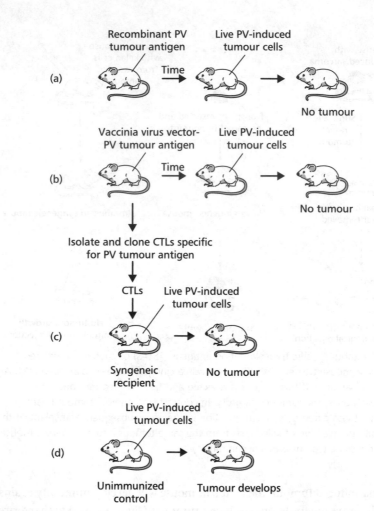

Fig. 2.3 Tumour specific transplantation antigens (TSTAs) of virally-induced sarcoma. Experimental induction of immunity against tumour cells induced by polyoma virus (PV) has been achieved by immunising mice with recombinant polyoma tumour antigen (A), with a vaccinia vector vaccine containing the gene encoding the PV tumour antigen (B), or with CTLs specific for the PV tumour antigen (C). Naive mice (D) develop tumours when injected with live polyoma-induced tumour cells, whereas the immunised mice do not.

The fact that one virus induces the same antigens in all its tumours makes these antigens valuable targets in the immunization against viral tumours. In fact mice immunized with genetically engineered polyoma virus tumour antigen, or a vaccinia virus vaccine engineered with the gene encoding the polyoma tumour antigen, have been seen to develop immunity to subsequent administrations of polyoma-induced tumour cells.

Tumour-associated antigens

The majority of tumour antigens are not unique to tumour cells and are also present on normal cells and are thus referred to as 'tumour-associated antigens' (TAAs). Many of these molecules do not stimulate immune responses, but are important in the diagnosis and possible treatment of cancer. TAAs may be proteins usually expressed on fetal cells, but not on normal adult cells, or they may be proteins expressed at low levels by normal cells, but at much higher levels in tumour cells.

Oncofetal tumour antigens

Oncofetal tumour antigens are found both on cancerous cells and normal fetal cells. These antigens appear early in embryonic development, before the mechanisms of self-tolerance are operative. When these genes are deregulated as a consequence of malignant transformation of a cell and are expressed inappropriately in the wrong tissues, at the wrong time of life, they behave as tumour antigens and induce an immunological response. Two well studied oncofetal antigens are the previously mentioned AFP and CEA.

Serum concentrations of AFP drop from milligram levels in fetal serum to nanogram levels in normal adult serum. An elevated serum AFP level is a useful indicator of advanced hepatocellular carcinoma or of recurrence of these tumours after treatment. Raised AFP levels can also be an indication of benign tumours or even pregnancy, making cancer diagnosis less straightforward. AFP is also expressed in testicular and ovarian cancer. Recent investigations have shown that murine vaccinations with AFP-DNA, inhibited growth of AFP-expressing hepatic tumours. These results indicate that AFP may be used in the future to not only identify tumours, but also to trigger an immune response against them (Hanke et al. 2002).

CEA is a membrane glycoprotein found on gastrointestinal and liver cells of 2–6-month-old fetuses. Approximately 90% of patients with advanced colo-rectal cancer and 50% of patients with early colorectal cancer have increased levels of CEA in their serum. However, other types of cancer can also poten-tially exhibit increased CEA levels. In 1981, a National Institute of Health Consensus Conference concluded that CEA was the best available, non-invasive technique for detection of recurrence in patients with previously diagnosed colorectal cancer. This led to CEA being widely used in the follow-up of colorectal cancer patients. Detection of CEA by polymerase chain reaction analysis of lymph node samples, taken during colorectal cancer sur-gery, is used as a prognostic factor in stage II of the disease, and may therefore help in the identification of patients who will benefit from adjuvant treat-ment. A recent study has shown CEA serum levels to be a strong indicator for postoperative breast cancer-free survival. Despite CEA determination being able to detect recurrent disease with a sensitivity of approximately 80% and a specificity of approximately 70% (Duffy 2001), its use remains controversial and its benefit in the clinic is still under discussion.

Tumour-related overexpression of normal self proteins

Many tumours cells abundantly express normal self proteins at higher levels than normal cells, including growth factor receptors and oncogene-encoded proteins. Immune reactions against these 'self-antigens' may result in damage of normal tissue. However, experiments with peptide immunization in patients with MART (melanoma-associated antigen recognized by T cells)-1, which is a melanocyte differentiation antigen present in melanoma and normal melanocytes, have not shown any drastic adverse reactions against normal tissue.

Human epidermal growth factor receptor (HER)-2/neu is a trans-membrane growth factor receptor, with tyrosine kinase activity, which is overexpressed in 30% of breast and ovarian cancers and a number of other adenocarcinomas. HER-2/neu has been documented to be essential for tumour growth and survival. In breast cancer overexpression of HER-2/neu was associated with aggressive disease and can be used an indicator of survival (Bewick *et al.* 2001). Spontaneous humoral and cellular immune response in patients with HER-2/neu expressing tumours have been observed. In fact, recognition and lysis of ovarian cancer cells by circulating tumour lymphocytes (CTL's) have been shown to correlate with the expression levels of HER-2/neu in tumour cells. Therefore, in the future these responses may be harnessed using immunization strategies leading to tumour regression.

A variety of tumours express the epidermal growth factor receptor at levels 100 times greater than that in normal cells, making it an ideal tumour marker for the detection of a number of tumour types. Recent findings have shown that epidermal growth factor receptor inhibitors could stabilize advanced non-small cell lung carcinomas, further indicating that tumour antigens can act as markers and potential treatments of cancer (Hirsch and Witta 2005).

Prostate-specific antigen is found in normal adult cells, but is highly expressed by prostate cancer cells. Both prostate-specific antigen and prostate-specific membrane antigen are routinely used in the diagnosis and relapse monitoring of prostate cancer. Screening for prostate carcinoma is carried out to detect early signs of the disease and therefore prevent or delay its progression (Bunting 2002).

Growth factors can also act as tumour markers. The transferrin growth factor, p97, aids the transport of iron into cells and is expressed at less than 8000 molecules per cell, but is found at 50 000–500 000 molecules per cell in melanoma cells. It has been documented as a reliable tumour antigen for the prognosis of a number of carcinomas, including gastric and hepatocellular tumours.(Yamamoto *et al.* 2003).

Tumour antigens encoded by oncogenes or tumour suppressor genes

Progress in understanding the mechanisms of cancer has arisen from the discovery of oncogenes, proto-oncogenes and tumour suppressor genes. Oncogenes are cellular genes whose expression can cause neoplasm and proto-oncogenes are normal cellular genes which can convert to oncogenes. Tumour suppressor gene expression may suppress tumour growth and their inactivation increases the likelihood of tumour formation.

Tumours often express tumour associated antigens (TAAs) encoded by cellular oncogenes. These antigens are also present in normal cells encoded by the corresponding proto-oncogene. Viral integration into normal cellular proto-oncogenes can result in the production of oncogenic proteins. These molecules are often processed and presented as peptides in association with MHC I molecules and can act as tumour antigens. As mutated proteins are generally identified as foreign by the immune system, it is long been assumed that all tumour antigens are mutated. However, in many cases there is no difference between the oncogene and proto-oncogene, and it is purely the increased levels of the oncogene product that result in an immunological response.

As many oncogene and tumour suppressor gene sequences have been characterized and are widespread among tumours, they have become worthy targets for immunotherapy. Some of the well documented genetic events leading to the development of cancer cells are mutations in the p53 tumour suppressor gene, the K-Ras oncogene and abnormalities in the retinoblastoma gene pathway.

Research has demonstrated a crucial role for wild-type p53 in intrinsic tumour suppression. In normal cells p53 is expressed at very low levels, with a very short half-life. However, in response to stress p53 expression is stabilized and binds to target DNA, resulting in cell cycle arrest or apoptosis. In fact, it is reported that the high incidence of tumours in p53-deficient animals is highly attributed to the loss of p53-induced apoptosis. Recent studies suggest that cytosolic p53 directly interacts with the BCL-2 family of proteins, which regulate apoptosis, and trigger mitochondrial outer membrane permeabilization and apoptosis.

p53 mutations are found in up to 50% of human malignancies and therefore p53 is currently the most popular molecule in cell biology. However, it still unknown whether intracellular p53 is presented at the tumour cell surface or in the extracellular cancer environment, although in many human cancers the accumulation of wild-type p53 in the cytosol is observed.

p53 represents a specific target for anticancer drug design. In fact, recent reports have indicated that it is possible to influence the mutant form of p53 in tumour cells, so it regains its wild-type form. These investigations may be the significant breakthrough required in our fight against mutated p53-induced cancer (Brachmann et al. 1998).

The Ras genes are a family of related proteins that have strong transforming potential. Although mutations in Ras genes are commonly found in human disease, they are not distributed evenly between the different Ras members, but are predominantly in K-Ras. K-Ras is one of the best characterized tumour-related genes, which somatically mutates in several types of human cancers. K-Ras mutations involve single amino acid substitutions, mainly at positions 12, 13, and 61. As these mutations are frequently detected and well characterized in colorectal, pancreas, and lung cancers, molecular diagnosis using K-ras mutations are being developed. Mutations of K-Ras are found in 50% of colorectal cancers and up to 87% of pancreatic cancers and 48% of lung cancers (Minamoto et al. 2000).

MUM (melanoma-ubiquitous mutated)-1 is a lymphocyte-specific member of the IFN regulatory factor family, expressed by late centrocytes and post-germinal centre B cells. MUM-1 is an antigen whose mutated form is only recognized by T cells and whose expression levels may be a significant marker for Hodgkin's lymphoma (Carbone et al. 2002).

The retinoblastoma protein (pRb) pathway regulates cellular processes of the cell cycle. Derailments of this pathway are implicated in the deregulation of the cell cycle machinery, resulting in uncontrolled cell proliferation, tumour cell formation, invasion, and metastasis. Cyclin-dependent kinase 4 (CDK4), is an enzyme involved in cell cycle control, which can be often be found in a mutated form. The CDK4 protein usually forms a complex with cyclin D1 and phosphorylates pRb, thus promoting cell cycle progression from G_1 to S phase, which is inhibited by a protein called p16. However, p16 cannot bind to mutated CDK4 and thus fails to inhibit the kinase activity of CDK4/cyclin D, resulting in a loss of cell cycle control. Data currently suggest that CDK4 may be used as a marker for a number of tumour types, including melanomas (Wolfel et al. 1995).

The mutated β-catenin gene product was also identified in melanomas and colon cancer and may be a reliable tumour marker. β-catenin is a cytoplasmic protein that interacts with the cellular adhesion protein e-cadherin. A loss of cell adhesion is thought to enhance the metastatic process and this may be mediated, at least in part, by the mutations found in β-catenin (Robbins et al. 1996).

The CASP-8 gene codes for the caspase-8 protease and its mutated form has been used to identify human squamous tumours of the oral cavity. Caspase-8 is required for apoptosis through the Fas and tumour necrosis factor pathways and the mutation, which is only found in tumour cells, may therefore block cell death (Mandruzzato *et al.* 1997). Thus CASP-8 mutations may be important tumour markers for squamous cell carcinomas.

Melanoma-associated tumour antigens

A number of TAAs have been characterized on human melanomas. Melanoma antigen genes (MAGE)-1, MAGE-3, B melanoma antigen gene (BAGE), G melanoma antigen gene (GAGE)-1 and GAGE-2 are oncofetal-type antigens expressed on a significant proportion of human melanoma tumours and other tumour types (Van der Bruggen *et al.* 1991). These antigens are not normally present on healthy tissue, except the placenta and testis, and are therefore often designated 'cancer testis' antigens. It is postulated that these are immunologically privileged sites, where T cells do not respond effectively to antigens, so the antigens are ignored.

Recently a new cancer testis antigen, NY-ESO-1, was cloned from oesophageal cancer. As NY-ESO-1 and other members of the MAGE gene family are often expressed in tumours of different histological type, they are important targets for antigen-specific immunotherapy (Korangy *et al.* 2004).

A second group of antigens is expressed during melanocyte differentiation and act as targets for CTLs in melanomas. These include tyrosinase, glycoprotein (gp)100, Melan-A/MART-1, and gp75, which are present on normal melanocytes, but act as TAAs when overexpressed on melanoma cells. Phase I clinical trials in melanoma patients have shown that intradermal injections of these antigenic peptides improved response rates in patients with melanomas (Maeurer *et al.* 1996).

Often the human melanoma tumour antigens are shared by other tumours, for example MAGE-1–3 are often found on melanoma cells, but they can also be expressed by a significant number of other tumour types, including breast, hepatocellular, ovarian, and head or neck carcinomas. In fact, MAGE-1 is expressed on up to 48% of melanomas and 31% of breast carcinomas (Brasseur *et al.* 1995).

Tumour-associated mucins

Change in glycosylation of proteins appears to be a constant phenomenon associated with oncogenic transformation in all types of human cancers. Mucins are large glycoproteins (>200 kDa) with high carbohydrate content and are expressed by a variety of normal and malignant epithelial cells. Each mucin molecule bears several hundred carbohydrate antigens, which act as binding sites for antibodies.

There are at least 14 mucin tumour marker antibodies that are used in diagnosing pancreatic cancer. CA19-9 was the first reliable tumour marker antibody for pancreatic cancer. It is a monoclonal antibody that has as its epitope the carbohydrate antigen siayl Lewis. In pancreatic cancer patients CA19-9 detects the epitope expressed on circulating mucins. Mucins activate clotting factor 10 and may therefore be responsible for the increased thrombotic tendency in patients with pancreatic cancer. Mucins also inhibit nature killer cell activity (NK activity) and may thus be significant in tumour resistance to natural immunity (Ogata *et al.* 1992).

MUC-1 is a membrane bound mucin that reduces cell–cell interaction, thereby facilitating tumour invasion. Its expression has been associated with breast and pancreatic adenocarcinoma. MUC-1 is expressed on epithelial cells, fibroblasts, and B cells, and can act as a target for T-cell recognition. Recent investigations using dendritic cells pulsed with peptides from the MUC-1 protein, induced CTLs that were able to induce lysis of tumour cells expressing MUC-1. These results demonstrate that immunotherapy in patients with advanced malignancies, using MUC-1 derived peptides, can induce significant immunological and clinical responses.

Other tumour antigens used in the clinic

There are a number of tumour antigens used in our clinics to diagnose and monitor tumours. A spectrum of tumour markers are often used in tumour analysis, thus providing more accurate detection. The most significant antigens that have not already been mentioned in this chapter are detailed below:

- The tissue-specific expression of thyroglobulin is used in the diagnosis and follow-up of thyroid cancer (Rosai 2003).

- CA15.3, CEA, and cytokeratins are used to monitor the treatment of patients with breast cancer and to monitor recurrence of the disease (Dimas *et al.* 2001). The MUC-1-associated antigen CA27.29 may also be used to detect the relapse of breast cancer and detect whether treatment has succeeded (Gion *et al.* 2001).

- The oestrogen receptor is routinely used as a breast cancer tumour marker in helping decide on adjuvant hormone treatment (American Society of Clinical Oncology 1998).

- In relation to ovarian cancer, CA125 is a tumour marker used to monitor postoperative cancer. An increase in CA125 serum concentrations may indicate recurrent disease or serious adenocarcinomas (Bast *et al.* 1998).

◆ The CA19.9/CA72.4 marker has been used experimentally to follow-up patients with a number carcinomas, such as ovarian and pancreatic (Gao et al. 1996).

Conclusions

As we have discussed in this section, tumour markers are potentially useful in screening for early malignancy, aiding diagnosis, assessing prognosis, determining the likely response to therapy and monitoring patients with diagnosed disease. Over the last 30 years many tumour markers have become commonplace in clinical use, and measurement of certain cancer markers can clearly result in improved patient management. Tumour markers have also become significant targets for immunotherapy and are proving to be reliable and specific targets in vaccination studies. Therefore, with tumour antigen-related research having already progressed to clinical trials, subsequent years will certainly provide a wealth of knowledge and hopefully answers in our fight against cancer.

References

1997 American Society of clinical oncology. (1998). 1997 update of recommendations for the use of tumour markers in breast and colorectal cancer. *J clin oncology* **16**: 793–5

Abelev GI, Perova SD, Khramkova NI, *et al.* (1963). Production of embryonal alpha-globulin by transplantable mouse hepatomas. *Transplantation*. **1**: 174–80.

Bast RC Jr, Xu FJ, Yu YH, *et al.* (1998). CA 125: the past and the future. *Int J Biol Markers*. **13**(4): 179–87

Beetham R. (2000). Detection of Bence-Jones protein in practice. *Ann Clin Biochem*. **37** (Pt 5): 563–70

Bewick M, Conlon M, Gerard S, *et al.* (2001). HER-2 expression is a prognostic factor in patients with metastatic breast cancer treated with a combination of high-dose cyclophosphamide, mitoxantrone, paclitaxel and autologous blood stem cell support. *Bone Marrow Transplant*. **27**(8): 847–53.

Boon T, Coulie PG, and Van den Eynde B. (1997) Tumor antigens recognized by T- cells. *Immunol Today* **18** (6): 267–8.

Brachmann RK, Yu K, Eby Y, *et al.* (1998). Genetic selection of intragenic suppressor mutations that reverse the effect of common p53 cancer mutations. *EMBO J*. **17**(7): 1847–59.

Brasseur F, Rimoldi D, Lienard D, *et al.* (1995). Expression of MAGE genes in primary and metastatic cutaneous melanoma. *Int J Cancer*. **63**(3): 375–80.

Bunting PS. (2002). Screening for prostate cancer with prostate-specific antigen: beware the biases. *Clin Chim Acta*. **315**(1-2): 71–97.

Carbone A, Gloghini A, Aldinucci D, *et al.* (2002). Expression pattern of MUM1/IRF4 in the spectrum of pathology of Hodgkin's disease. *Br J Haematol*. **117**(2): 366–72.

Chang MH, Chen CJ, Lai MS, *et al.* (1997) Universal hepatitis B vaccination in Taiwan and the incidence of hepatocellular carcinoma in children. Taiwan Childhood Hepatoma Study Group. *N Engl J Med* **336**:1855–9.

Chiplunkar SV. (2001). The immune system and cancer. *Current science* **81**; 5: 542–548

Daniel D, Meyer-Morse N, Bergsland EK, et al. (2003). Immune Enhancement of Skin Carcinogenesis by CD4+ T Cells. *J. Exp. Med.* **197**: 1017–18.

de Visser KE, Korets LV and Coussens LM. (2005). De novo carcinogenesis promoted by chronic inflammation is B lymphocyte dependent. *Cancer Cell* **7**: 411?423.

Dimas C, Fragos-Plemenos M, Gennatas C, et al. (2001). Prognostic significance of tissue DF3 antigen and CA15-3 tumor marker in primary breast cancer. *Eur J Gynaecol Oncol.* **21**(3): 278–81.

Duffy MJ. (2001). Carcinoembryonic antigen as a marker for colorectal cancer: is it clinically useful? *Clin Chem.* **47**(4): 624–30

Gao G, Peng Z, and He B. (1996). The value of urine cystein proteinase and serum CA125 measurement in monitoring the treatment of malignant ovarian tumor. *Hua Xi Yi Ke Da Xue Xue Bao.* **27**(3): 291–4

Gion M, Mione R, Leon AE, et al. (2001). CA27.29: a valuable marker for breast cancer management. A confirmatory multicentric study on 603 cases. *Eur J Cancer.* **37**(3): 355–63.

Gold P, and Freedman SO. (1965). Specific carcinoembryonic antigens of the human digestive system. *J Exp Med.* **122**(3): 467–81.

Hanke P, Serwe M, Dombrowski F, et al. (2002). DNA vaccination with AFP-encoding plasmid DNA prevents growth of subcutaneous AFP-expressing tumors and does not interfere with liver regeneration in mice. *Cancer Gene Ther.* **9**(4): 346–55

Hirsch FR, and Witta S. (2005). Biomarkers for prediction of sensitivity to EGFR inhibitors in non-small cell lung cancer. *Curr Opin Oncol.* **17**(2): 118–22.

Karin M, and Greten FR. (2005). NF-kappaB: linking inflammation and immunity to cancer development and progression. *Nat Rev Immunol.* **5**(10):749–59.

Korangy F, Ormandy LA, Bleck JS, et al. (2004). Spontaneous tumor-specific humoral and cellular immune responses to NY-ESO-1 in hepatocellular carcinoma. *Clin Cancer Res.* **10**(13): 4332–41.

Lin EY, Nguyen AV, Russell RG, et al. (2001). Colony-stimulating Factor 1 Promotes Progression of Mammary Tumors to Malignancy. *J. Exp. Med.* **193**: 727–740.

Maeurer MJ, Storkus WJ, Kirkwood JM, et al. (1996). New treatment options for patients with melanoma: review of melanoma-derived T-cell epitope-based peptide vaccines. *Melanoma Res.* **6**(1): 11–24

Mandruzzato S, Brasseur F, Andry G, et al. (1997). A CASP-8 mutation recognized by cytolytic T lymphocytes on a human head and neck carcinoma. *J Exp Med.* **186**(5): 785–93.

Marshall BJ. (1989). History of the discovery of C. pylori. In Blaser MJ, editor. Campylobacter pylori in gastritis and peptic ulcer disease. New York: Igaku-Shoin: 7–23.

Minamoto T, Mai M and Ronai Z. (2000). K-ras mutation: early detection in molecular diagnosis and risk assessment of colorectal, pancreas, and lung cancers—a review. *Cancer Detect Prev.* **24**(1): 1–12

Ogata S, Maimonis PJ & Itzkowitz SH. (1992). Mucins bearing the cancer-associated sialosyl-Tn antigen mediate inhibition of natural killer cell cytotoxicity. *Cancer Res.* **52**(17): 4741–6

Paik S, Shak S, Tang G, et al. (2004). A multigene assay to predict recurrence of tamoxifen-treated, node-negative breast cancer. *N. Engl. J. Med.* **351**, 2817–2826.

Robbins PF, EL-Gamil M, Li YF, *et al.* (1996). A mutated beta-catenin gene encodes a melanoma-specific antigen recognized by tumor infiltrating lymphocytes. *J Exp Med.* **183**(3): 1185–92.

Rosai J. (2003). Immunohistochemical markers of thyroid tumors: significance and diagnostic applications. *Tumori.* **89**(5): 517–9.

Rotzschke O, Falk K, Deres K, *et al.* (1990) Isolation and analysis of naturally processed viral peptides as recognized by cytotoxic T cells. *Nature* **348** (6298): 252–4.

Sjoegen HO. (1964). Studies on specific transplantation resistance to polyoma-virus-induced tumors. Transplantation resistance to genetically compatible polyoma tumors induced by polyoma tumor homografts. *J Natl Cancer Inst.* **32**: 645–59.

Van der Bruggen P, Traversari C, Chomez P, *et al.* (1991). A gene encoding an antigen recognized by cytolytic T lymphocytes on a human melanoma. *Science* **254**(5038): 1643–7.

Wolfel T, Hauer M, Schneider J, *et al.* (1995). A p16ink4a-insensitive CDK4 mutant targeted by cytolytic T lymphocytes in a human melanoma. *Science.* **269**(5228): 1281–4

Yamamoto S, Tomita Y, Hoshida Y, *et al.* (2003). Expression level of valosin-containing protein is strongly associated with progression and prognosis of gastric carcinoma. *J Clin Oncol.* **21**(13): 2537–44

Zavros Y, Eaton KA, Kang W, *et al.* (2005) Chronic gastritis in the hypochlorhydric gastrin-deficient mouse progresses to adenocarcinoma. *Oncogene,* **24**: 2354–2366.

Chapter 3

Head and neck/ear, nose, and throat

V.J. Lund, J. Powles, and D.J. Howard

Introduction

There are many aspects in which infection plays a part in malignant tumours of the head and neck. As the ears, nose, and throat represent collectively one of the main portals to the body, they are subject to continual assault from outside organisms. Under normal circumstances they provide a more than adequate defence through structures such as the lymphoid tissue comprising the ring of Waldeyer and physiological mechanisms such as mucociliary clearance and secretion content. However, under circumstances of genetic predisposition, immune compromise, and/or social habits such as smoking or drinking, resistance may be lowered, enabling infective agents to contribute to the development of cancer in the upper aerodigestive tract (Table 3.1). Furthermore, once malignancy has developed, a combination of malnutrition, age, and co-morbidities make these patients susceptible to secondary infection, which complicates difficult treatment, contributing to morbidity and mortality. The importance of infection in the overall prognosis of these patients cannot be overestimated.

Infection as a cause of cancer

Viruses

Human immunodeficiency virus and head and neck cancer

HIV infection may present to ENT surgeons in many guises, in the seroconversion and latent phases and during the pre-AIDS and AIDS syndrome. However, it is only in the latter where an association between HIV-1 and head and neck malignancy is manifest. An increased incidence of squamous cell carcinoma and lymphoma is seen in the head and neck in addition to the classical Kaposi's sarcoma, which predominantly occurs on the palate, gingiva, and tongue. These manifestations form part of the diagnostic criteria for the

Table 3.1 Infective agents in head and neck cancer

Virus
Human immunodeficiency virus (HIV)
  Kaposi's sarcoma
  Squamous cell carcinoma lymphoma

Epstein–Barr virus (EBV)
  Nasopharyngeal carcinoma
  Burkitt's lymphoma
  T-cell lymphoma

Human papillomavirus (HPV)
  Squamous cell carcinoma

Prions
Variant Creutzfeld–Jacob disease (vCJD)

Bacteria
Aerobes
  Helicobacter pylori
  Streptococcus anginosus
  Methicillin-resistant staphylococcus (MRSA)

Anaerobes
  Bacteroides fragilis

Mycoplasma
  Mycoplasma tuberculosis

Fungus

Aspergillus

Candida

Rhizopus oryzae (Mucor)

---

full-blown AIDS syndrome. In an age-matched study, head and neck cancer occurred more frequently in HIV-positive individuals than in controls (1.66 versus 0.55/10 000 patient years respectively) (Powles *et al.* 2004). These tumours also appear to behave more aggressively, with all but one patient dying of their tumour with a median survival of 28 months.

There also appears to be an association with Epstein–Barr virus (EBV), which was found in all head and neck tumours occurring in a cohort of HIV-positive patients (Powles *et al.* 2004).

In any surgical procedure, there is a risk of cross-contamination between surgeon and patient and the 'usual' precautions are required. In one USA series, 60% of HIV carriers were also hepatitis B positive.

Epstein–Barr virus

The exact role of EBV in the development of tumours is unclear but it has been implicated in both nasopharyngeal cancer (NPC) and Burkitt's lymphoma (Zur-Hausen *et al.* 1970; Henle *et al.* 1977; de-Thé *et al.* 1982; Henle and Henle 1985) both of which have defined geographical distributions. EBV is a double-stranded DNA virus classified as a member of the herpes family. It was first described by Epstein *et al.* (1964) from electron microscopic studies of cultured cells from Burkitt's lymphoma. Approximately 10% of these cultured lymphoma cells would spontaneously produce infectious virus and human B lymphocytes were found to be the only susceptible cells for EBV infection *in vitro* (Jondal and Klein 1973). This may lead to two outcomes, either transformation of the B cells into lymphoblastoid lines or activation of the latent virus into its lytic growth cycle in some cells leading to cell death with, or without, the production of infectious virions.

Nasopharyngeal carcinoma is a unique head and neck cancer in its epidemiology and aetiology. In most parts of the world the incidence is <1/100 000 (Mallen and Shandro 1974; Waterhouse *et al.* 1976; Lanier 1977; Hirayama 1978; Simmons and Shanmugaratanam 1982; Hu 1985; Muir *et al.* 1987), but in specific populations the rate rises to >30/100 000 (Liang 1964; Ho 1972; Ho 1975; Simmons and Shanmugaratanam 1982; Hu 1985; Muir *et al.* 1987). These areas include China, particularly in eastern Guangxi province, Africa, Canada, Alaska, and among Greenland Eskimos (Nielsen *et al.* 1977). This predilection is seen in Chinese populations who have emigrated to South-east Asia and California. The tumour is generally twice as common in men than women. Many possible explanations have been sought, including genetically determined susceptibility, environmental factors, such as diet and infection with EBV.

EBV is ubiquitous and spreads horizontally probably during childhood usually without major clinical manifestations. This is accompanied by seroconversion and permanent immunity to future infection. The virus may be shed in saliva, resulting in the horizontal transmission. Virtually all Chinese children have serological evidence of EBV infection before the age of 15 years, whereas in Western populations, this occurs later and presents with infectious mononucleosis.

The relationship between NPC and EBV was first described by Old in 1966 (Old *et al.* 1966). In contrast to controls, higher levels of EBV antibodies are consistently found in NPC, especially of the IgA class and these are seen to rise with increasing tumour burden (Henle *et al.* 1973, 1977). This is true of both undifferentiated and well-differentiated tumours (Klein *et al.* 1974; Desgranges *et al.* 1975, Andersson-Anvret *et al.* 1977; Raab-Traub *et al.* 1987).

Studies have shown genetic variants of EBV between those viruses found in the USA and those in south China (Lung *et al.* 1988, 1989, 1990). This combined with possible genetic predispositions of certain human populations, suggests a causal relationship, although this is as yet unproven.

The IgA response is particularly marked against the viral capsid antigen and early intracellular antigen and notwithstanding the possible aetiological relationship, this serological profile is now utilized routinely in diagnosis. Furthermore long-term studies of IgA-viral capsid antigen levels correlate with response to treatment (Lynn *et al.* 1985; de-Vathaire *et al.* 1988). The profile also shows certain geographical variations (Tam 1991). Furthermore, antibody profiles against other antigens such as lymphocyte-detected membrane antigen, latent membrane protein, and late membrane antigen have prognostic significance. Other EBV serological markers may have a role in mass-screening for NPC in high-risk populations such as undertaken by Zheng (1985) in over 195 000 people in south China, which identified 106 new cases.

Sinonasal T/natural killer cell lymphoma may present as an aggressive destructive lesion of the mid-face. Current evidence shows that this lymphoma is an EBV-associated angiocentric neoplasm with T-cell or natural killer cell phenotypic and genotypic features. Necrosis of the lymphoma cells and normal tissues is almost always seen (Guinee *et al.* 1994). This is thought to occur due to occlusion of vessels or the overexpression of tumour necrosis factor and other cytokines possibly induced by EBV (Jaffe *et al.* 1996).

Human papillomavirus

Epidemiological and molecular pathology studies have suggested that human papillomavirus (HPV) infection may be associated with head and neck cancer. When alcohol and tobacco exposure are taken into account, certain sexual behaviour increases this risk in keeping with known modes of transmission in cancers of the cervix and anogenital tract (Gillison 2004) An HPV prevalence of between 20 and 30% for oropharyngeal, hypopharyngeal, and laryngeal squamous cell carcinoma and >50% for squamous cell carcinoma of the tonsil has been found (Hoffman *et al.* 2005). However, the frequency of HPV positivity in oral samples from healthy individuals varies from 1 to 60% and prevalence varies depending on the detection methodology. When the most sensitive method, polymerase chain reaction was utilized, the overall prevalence of HPV in 1205 head and neck tumours was 34.5% (McKaig *et al.* 1998). There is currently sufficient evidence that HPV plays a role in the pathogenesis of a distinct subset of tumours, particularly in the tonsil (Gillison 2004), probably due to an interaction between HPV oncoproteins and genes important in cell cycle control. High-, intermediate, and low-risk genotypes of HPV have been defined depending on their presence in carcinoma or precursor lesions. One high-risk type, HPV16 has been associated with an increased risk for subsequent development of oropharyngeal cancer. Various phylogenic groups can be correlated with different types of malignant tumour (Szentirmay et al. 2005). For example, groups A6, A7, and A9 are associated with basaloid and verrucous squamous cell carcinoma. This opens up the possibility of prophylactic and therapeutic vaccines.

Better survival was shown in patients with tumours that were HPV-positive compared with those that were HPV-negative and the HPV-positive patients also showed increased radiocurability. The HPV-positive patients had no or light alcohol consumption and the majority were female in contrast to the 'normal' patient profile (Szentirmay et al. 2005). Improved survival was also demonstrated when HPV-positive head and neck cancer patients with lymph node metastases were compared with HPV-negative patients and this was largely attributed to a better radiation response (Hoffman et al. 2005).

Prions

There has been no suggestion of an aetiological role for prions in the development of head and neck cancer but the debate on the likely societal impact of bovine spongiform encephalopathy and variant Creutzfeld–Jacob disease will rumble on for some time. ENT has been rather at the 'sharp end' of this debate through the discussion around tonsillectomy and the chances of transference of infection on surgical instruments. Similarly, in head and neck cancer, neck dissection of cervical lymphoid tissue may potentially pose problems, as yet unresolved. This has also resulted in an embargo on the use of autogenic materials such as lyophilized dura for anterior skull base repair.

Bacteria

Heliobacter pylori and other bacteria

The association between H. pylori and stomach cancer in a number of epidemiological studies has led to interest in its aetiological role in upper aerodigestive tract tumours. This possible relationship, however, was not supported by a study of 21 patients with matched controls (Grandis 1997). By contrast, a study from Japan, found DNA evidence of Streptococcus anginosus in 100% of 217 cases of oesophageal cancer, which may be of significance (Tateda et al. 2000).

Chronic otitis media in carcinoma of the ear

Infection in the upper respiratory tract is common, but only in the middle ear cleft is there a significant correlation with the development of carcinoma. In over three-quarters of cases of squamous cell carcinoma of the middle ear, there is a history of chronic otorrhoea leading to the assumption that chronic irritation is responsible for this rare and unpleasant tumour, an association recognized by Politzer in 1883 (Maran *et al.* 1983). However, the exact mechanism is unknown.

Chronic rhinosinusitis

By contrast, chronic rhinosinusitis, which is one of the most common chronic inflammatory conditions, does not appear to increase significantly the risk of developing nasal cancer, which fortunately remains extremely rare (<1/100 000 population).

Sepsis in oral cancer

The old addage of the five 'Ss' includes sepsis and syphilis together with smoking, spirits, spices are among the causes of tumours in the oral cavity. As dental hygiene has improved and syphilis declined, the incidence of oral cancer, and in particular tongue cancer has also fallen though the male to female ratio has also changed from 9:1 to 1.5:1, possibly reflecting the alteration in smoking habits among women.

Tuberculosis

Mycoplasma are not thought to have a casual role in head and neck cancer but head and neck patients are often debilitated and elderly, with a degree of immunosuppression. Thus, reactivation of previous infection remains a possibility and should be borne in mind in this patient population. Thus, interpretation of chest imaging to exclude metastatic disease should include tuberculosis (TB) in the differential diagnosis. Furthermore, there are many case reports in the literature where TB has mimicked head and neck malignancy either at a primary site or in the cervical lymph nodes. In 202 consecutive patients with a pre-operative diagnosis of squamous cell carcinoma who underwent 307 neck dissections, subsequent histology confirmed TB in two patients rather than the presumptive diagnosis (Sheahan *et al.* 2005). There are also a number of reports documenting coexisting TB with malignant tumours in the head and neck as well as granulomatous reactions after radiation. For example in nasopharyngeal carcinoma, abnormal tissue post-therapy may prove to be TB masquerading as residual or recurrent disease (Chan *et al.* 2004). Other causes of severe cervical lymphadenopathy such as toxoplasmosis can also catch out the unwary.

Fungi

Fungi are increasingly recognized as possible factors in the development of upper aerodigestive inflammation. They are not specifically implicated in the development of head and neck malignancy but may complicate the course of the disease, especially in those who may be immunosuppressed while receiving chemoradiation. Menzin *et al.* (2005) found 52 patients with squamous cell carcinoma of the head and neck who had experienced a serious fungal infection during the course of their treatment, which led to significantly increased mortality (40% versus 14%, $P = 0.002$) relative to matched controls and had experienced significantly longer index hospitalizations.

Pre-operative implications

Infection in the debilitated patient with poor nutrition, pre-existing MRSA

Many patients with cancer of the upper aerodigestive tract suffer from progressive dysphagia resulting in severe malnourishment. This makes them susceptible to infection and in particular nosocomial pathogens such as methicillin-resistant *Staphylococcus aureus* (MRSA). The morbidity and cost of MRSA in head and neck cancer was estimated over a 1-year period (Watters *et al.* 2004) and affected 45% (25 of 55) of patients who underwent major head and neck procedures, resulting in cellulitis, osteomyelitis, and MRSA pneumonia. Over 50% of this group required further surgery including new flaps and wound debridement and in-patient hospital stay was almost three times longer as compared with patients without MRSA. Inevitably this resulted in significantly increased costs including antibiotics, extra days in intensive care, and additional medical and nursing care.

Aspiration pneumonia

Malignancy of the upper aerodigestive tract may be associated with aspiration of food and saliva, either due to the mass effect of the tumour and/or functional disability from cranial nerve palsies and a depressed cough reflex. This combined with a history of cigarette smoking in the majority of patients, renders them highly susceptible to chest infections. A small prospective study of 27 patients with advanced head and neck cancer showed that clinicians underestimated the presence of aspiration as compared with videofluoroscopy (Rosen *et al.* 2001). Assessment of swallowing is therefore an important part of the therapeutic work-up and pre- and postoperative physiotherapy should be undertaken in these individuals.

The use of a percutaneous endoscopic gastrostomy will reduce the risks of aspiration while improving the nutritional state of the patient but obviously still leave the patient exposed to aspiration of their own saliva.

It should also be remembered that aspiration pneumonia can also occur after chemoradiation, leading to acute respiratory failure or more chronic insidious pulmonary problems (Nguyen *et al.* 2004).

Consequence of infection: immediate and long term

Risk factors

A number of risk factors for postoperative infective complications can be identified (de Melo *et al.* 2001). In a retrospective study of 110 patients undergoing major resection for oral squamous cell carcinoma, dehiscence, and infection rates of 21% and 23%, respectively, were reported. A regression analysis not surprisingly found extent of disease, extent of surgery and reconstruction to be most important. This corroborated a univariate analysis from the MD Anderson Cancer Center (Robbins *et al.* 1990) prospectively performed on 400 cases during an 18-month period. A logistic regression analysis of the group in addition highlighted the presence of concomitant disease and choice of antibiotic in addition to the type of surgery and N stage as predictors of wound infection.

In the early 1990s it was suggested that a postoperative wound infection might actually have a favourable effect on prognosis when other factors were taken into account, presumably due to some form of immune stimulation (Ramadan and Wetmore 1992), although this was challenged by other authors (Grandis *et al.* 1992). More recent studies support the latter view. A study of 158 patients with supraglottic cancer, a recurrence rate of 57% was found in those who had infection versus 27% for those without ($P = 0.041$), although it is unclear whether the relationship is causal or consequent upon factors such as those detailed above (Rodrigo and Suarez 1998). In a recent study from Belgium (Penel *et al.* 2004) also failed to show any effect on local or distant recurrence or overall prognosis from wound infections. However, they did confirm the heavy postoperative morbidity from infection, which was surprisingly high, affecting 50.5% of patients despite prophylactic antibiotics. Curiously, the same group identified the presence of a post-laryngectomy tracheostomy as the most important factor in developing a wound infection from a multivariate analysis of 260 patients (Penel *et al.* 2005).

Wound infection and breakdown (Figures 3.1 and 3.2)

In 'clean' head and neck surgery where the digestive tract is not opened, postoperative infection rates are <1% but where oral, pharyngeal, or oesophageal contamination occurs, rates of between 18 and 78% have been reported in the literature (Shapiro 1991). The major postoperative problem in the past was

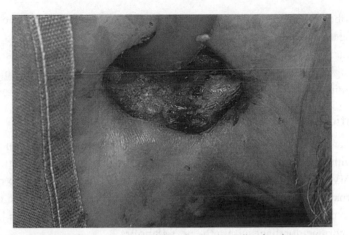

Fig. 3.1 Wound breakdown around tracheostomy site following laryngectomy. See colour plate section.

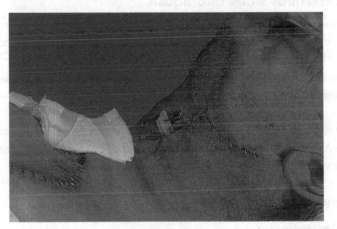

Fig. 3.2 Salivary fistula following pharyngolaryngectomy. See colour plate section.

the development of salivary fistulas following repair of the upper digestive tract, which often led to patients spending many weeks in hospital, undergoing further reparative procedures and delaying adjunctive therapy. Similarly infections of wounds and flaps used in reconstruction produced significant morbidity though interestingly a study using an experimental animal model together with a prospective clinical study failed to show a strong association between salivary fistula and free flap failure (Huang *et al.* 2005).

While many factors contribute to their development, including poor nutrition and previous radiotherapy, a major breakthrough in reducing postoperative fistulas and wound infections came in the 1970s with the recognition that anaerobes as well as Gram-positive and -negative bacteria were responsible, leading to effective prophylaxis (Becker *et al.* 1978).

Occasionally actinomycosis can occur following head and neck surgery, although rather rarely given that this organism is a common potential contaminant of the pharynx and oral cavity (Zitsch *et al.* 1999).

Carotid artery blow out

The catastrophic complication of carotid artery blow-out is most often associated with wound breakdown and infection. Although fortunately rare, there are few survivors and once exposure of the great vessels occurs, steps to redress the situation should be undertaken promptly, usually by bringing in a muscle graft to protect them. There is often a smaller prodromal bleed, which heralds the major haemorrhage within the next 48 hours.

Meningitis, extradural and cerebral abscess, sagittal and cavernous sinus thrombosis

Skull base surgery for malignancy carries the additional risk of intracranial infection due to exposure and resection of dura. This may take a number of forms, of which meningitis is probably the commonest. The frequency with which this occurs varies from series to series, ranging from <1% in a cohort of 309 craniofacial resections (Howard *et al.*) to 4.8% in 107 skull base procedures for malignancy (Donald 1999). This latter series also reported a 15% incidence of wound breakdown (and 6.5% frequency of pneumonia). Notwithstanding these risks, perioperative mortality is generally low in most major series due to appropriate skull base repair and the use of prophylactic antibiotics.

Prophylaxis

Antibiotic cover

The use of prophylactic broad-spectrum antibiotics such as amoxicillin-clavulanate or a second-generation cephalosporin and metronidazole have drastically reduced the frequency of salivary fistula and wound infection in head and neck cancer surgery (Innes *et al.* 1980; Sawyer *et al.* 1990). Since their introduction, many other antibiotic combinations and regimens have been proposed (Dominici *et al*, 1992; Phan *et al.* 1992; Callender 1999; Rodrigo *et al.* 2004). It would appear that 24 hours therapy is as effective as 5 days or longer (Shapiro 1991; Bhathena and Kavarana 1998) and as a consequence current UK practice usually involves up to three doses of amoxicillin-clavulanate during the 24-hour perioperative period for cases in which the digestive mucosa is opened.

In skull base surgery where there is a risk of intracranial infection and where packing is often left in place for some days, the same broad spectrum antibiotic cover is normally given until the pack is removed (Howard *et al.* in press).

Other measures

Some surgeons have advocated wound irrigation to reduce metastatic seeding of tumour and reduce infection. In a postal survey of members of a national ENT society, 203 of 301 undertook head and neck procedures of whom 68% routinely performed wound irrigation (McGahey and Gallagher 2000). Sterile water and saline were the most popular though there are no randomized controlled studies to support this practise.

Infection in chemoradiation for head and neck malignancy

Patients with head and neck malignancy often undergo radiation ± chemotherapy, either in combination with surgery or *ab initio*. By adding to the debility and immunosuppression of these individuals, it is not surprising that the potential complications of medical oncology are significant and can be life-threatening.

Oral *Candida*

Oral *Candida* is a frequent occurrence in patients undergoing radiotherapy and chemotherapy for tumours in this region. This results in pain and/or a burning sensation. In a study of 39 patients undergoing radiotherapy, 30 of 39 developed candidiasis (colony-forming units 35—>60/lesion), most often due to *Candida albicans*, which responded to oral itraconazole (200 mg/day) (Belazi *et al.* 2004) replicating similar findings by Redding *et al.* (1999). Non-albicans *Candida* is emerging as a relatively common source of oropharyngeal candidiasis in head and neck cancer patients (Dahiya 2003). Prophylactic treatment of *Candida*, for example with amifostine cytoprotection may be of value (Nicolatou-Galitis *et al.* 2003).

Osteoradionecrosis

Osteoradionecrosis means death of irradiated bone. Clinically, the term is normally associated with dead bone losing its mucosal covering to become exposed. Irradiation lethally damages osteoclasts and osteoblasts leading to a slow loss of bone with a slowing down of the remodelling process together with a reduced vascularity of the periosteum. The mandible is more affected than the maxilla, largely due to it being more compact bone with greater radiation absorption. However, with modern supervoltage, the incidence is lower and dose-dependent. The incidence of necrosis of healthy uninvolved mandible at varying doses of supervoltage irradiation using daily fractions of 2 Gy was studied. No cases of osteoradionecrosis were recorded with doses under 60 Gy, was 1.8% in those receiving up to 70 Gy and increased to 9% above 70 Gy (Bedwinek *et al.* 1976).

Osteoradionecrosis is at least three times higher in dentate compared with edentulous patients largely due to periodontal disease (Hinds 1971). There is a high risk of necrosis when extraction is performed after radiotherapy due to damage to osteoblasts and devascularization. This risk is less if extraction is performed before radiotherapy, the earlier the better. However, notwithstanding this, infection can gain entry to the bone via trauma, tooth extraction, pulpal infection, or ulceration of overlying mucosa (Bragg *et al.* 1970). Once bone death occurs, additional opportunistic infection by organisms will occur, which may delay recovery. Actinomycosis was found in 12% of 50 patients with osteoradionecrosis in a retrospective study, which led to significantly longer treatment in those affected (29.7 months versus 13.4 months) (Curi *et al.* 2000).

Clinically, the condition may be recognized by brownish looking bone at the base of mucosal ulceration. This may be associated with secondary infection, which can be painful though the condition itself is rarely so even when pathological fractures through the area occur. Prevention is obviously better than therapy so prophylactic measures such as mouthwashes and irrigation with solutions such as 0.01% chlorhexidine or hydrogen peroxide are of value. To minimize oral sepsis during radiotherapy, patients should be assessed by an oral hygienist and where dental condition is poor, extraction is offered prior to commencing the radiotherapy (Epstein and Stevenson-More 2001). The exact timing of the extractions is open to debate particularly for combined therapy though one retrospective study supported pre- versus postoperative intervention (Doerr and Marunick 1997). Fewer postoperative wound complications and shorter postoperative hospitalization occurred in those undergoing pre-operative extraction.

Sequestrated bone should be removed but it is recommended to restrict surgery as much as possible until the full extent of the process has declared itself as the surgery itself may exacerbate the process. Long-term antibiotics may be of value but penetration of bone is poor under the best of circumstances. Tetracyclines are the most effective but will be required over many months in combination with metronidazole. Hyperbaric oxygen has also been used with some success but no randomized controlled trials have been undertaken.

Oral zinc supplements have been used as a prophylaxis against oropharyngeal infection, which seem to have some benefit in reducing colonization with *Candida* and staphylococci (Ertekin *et al.* 2003). However, no effect was observed against group A β-haemolytic streptococci or *Streptococcus pneumoniae*.

Soft tissue necrosis

Other tissues in addition to bone may be adversely affected by radiotherapy. Cartilage in the larynx may necrose, exacerbated by secondary infection and has sometimes necessitated total laryngectomy in the absence of residual tumour.

These problems can occur irrespective of the type of radiation delivery, including brachytherapy. Infection and tissue breakdown comprised a significant proportion of the complications experienced by 14 of 28 (50%) of patients undergoing this form of treatment (Righi *et al.* 1997).

Palliative care

Up to two-thirds of patients with head and neck cancer ultimately succumb either as a direct or indirect result of their disease and as in all terminal situations, infection plays a significant role. Local or nodal recurrence may produce a fungating mass with secondary infection of necrotic tumour or patients may be overwhelmed by a chest infection. In either case, the decision to treat actively will depend upon many factors, most important of which will be the wishes of the patient and their family.

References

Andersson-Anvret M, Forsby N, Klein G, and Henle W. (1977). Relationship between Epstein-Barr virus and undifferentiated nasopharyngeal carcinoma: correlated nucleic acid hybridisation and histopathological examination. *International Journal of Cancer*, **20**, 486–494.

Becker GD, Parell J, Busch DF, Finegold SM, and Acquarelli MJ. (1978). Anaerobic and aerobic bacteriology in head and neck cancer surgery. *Archives of Otolaryngology*, **104**, 591–594.

Bedwinek JM, Shukovsky LJ, Fletcher GH, and Daley TE. (1976). Osteonecrosis in patients treated with definitive radiotherapy for squamous cell carcinomas of the oral cavity and naso- and oropharynx. *Radiology*, **119**, 665–667.

Belazi M, Velegraki A, Koussidou-Eremondi T, *et al.* (2004). Oral Candida isolates in patients undergoing radiotherapy for head and neck cancer: prevalence, azole susceptibility profiles and response to antifungal treatment. *Oral Microbiology and Immunology* **19**, 347–351.

Bhathena HM and Kavarana NM. (1998). Prophylactic antibiotics administration head and neck cancer surgery with major flap reconstruction: 1-day cefoperazone versus 5-day cefotaxime. *Acta Chirurgiae Plasticae*, **40**, 36–40.

Bragg DG, Shidnia H, Chu F, and Higginbotham NL. (1970). Clinical and radiographic aspects of radiation osteitis. *Radiology*, **97**, 103–111.

Callender DL. (1999). Antibiotic prophylaxis in head and neck oncologic surgery: the role of gram-negative coverage. *International Journal of Antimicrobial Agents*, **12**, s21–25, s26–27.

Chan AB, Ma TK, Yu BK, King AD, Ho FN, and Tse GM. (2004). Nasopharyngeal granulomatous inflammation and tuberculosis complicating undifferentiated carcinoma. *Otolaryngology Head and Neck Surgery*, **130**, 125–130.

Curi MM, Dib LL, Kowalski LP, Landman G, and Mangini C. (2000). Opportunistic actinomycosis in osteoradionecrosis of the jaws in patients affected by head and neck cancer: incidence and clinical significance. *Oral Oncology*, **36**, 294–299.

Dahiya MC. (2003). Oropharyngeal candidiasis caused by non-albicans yeast in patients receiving external beam radiotherapy for head and neck cancer. *International Journal of Radiation Oncology, Biology, Physics*, **57**, 79–83.

Desgranges C, Wolf H, de-Thé G, *et al.* (1975). Nasopharyngeal carcinoma, X. Presence of Epstein-Barr genomes in separate epithelial cells of tumours in patients from Singapore, Tunisia and Kenya. *International Journal of Cancer*, **16**, 7–11.

Doerr TD and Marunick MT. (1997). Timing of edentulation and extraction in the management of oral cavity and oropharyngeal malignancies. *Head and Neck*, **19**, 426–430.

Dominici L, Gondret R, Broc V, Dubos S, Viallard M, and Deligne P. (1992). Antimicrobial prophylaxis for major head and neck cancer surgery with piperacillin and ornidazole. *Journal of Laryngology and Otology*, **106**, 409–411.

Donald PJ. (1999). Complications in skull base surgery for malignancy. *Laryngoscope*, **109**, 1959–1966.

Epstein JB and Stevenson-More P. (2001). Periodontal disease and periodontal management in patients with cancer. *Oral Oncology*, **37**, 613–619.

Epstein MA, Achong BG, and Barr YM. (1964). Virus particules in cultured lymphoblasts from Burkitt's lymphoma. *Lancet*, **i**, 702–703.

Ertekin MV, Uslu H, Harslioglu I, Ozbek E, and Ozbek A. (2003). Effect of oral zinc supplementation on agents or oropharyngeal infection in patients receiving radiotherapy for head and neck cancer. *Journal of International Medical Research*, **31**, 253–266.

Gillison ML. (2004). Human papillomavirus associated head and neck cancer is a distinct epidemiologic, clinical, and molecular entity. *Seminars in Oncology*, **31**, 744–754.

Grandis JR, Snyderman CH, Johnson JT, Yu VL, and D'Amico F. (1992). Postoperative wound infection. A poor prognostic sign for patients with head and neck cancer. **70**, 2166–2170.

Grandis JR, Perez-Perez GI, Yu VL, Johnson JT, and Blaser MJ. (1997). Lack of serologic evidence for Helicobacter pylori infection in head and neck cancer. *Head and Neck*, **19**, 216–218.

Guinee D Jr, Jaffe E, Kingma D, *et al.* (1994). Pulmonary lymphomatoid granulomatosis. Evidence of Epstein-Barr virus infected B-lymphocytes with a predominant T-cell component and vasculitis. *American Journal of Surgical Pathology*, **18**, 753–764.

Henle W and Henle G. (1985). Epstein-Barr virus and human malignancies. In: *Advances in Viral Oncology* (ed. G Klein), pp. 201–238. New York: Raven Press.

Henle W, Ho JHC, Henle G, and Kwan HC. (1973). Antibodies to Epstein-Barr virus related antigens in nasopharyngeal carcinoma. Comparison of active cases and long-term survivors. *Journal of the National Cancer Institute*, 51, 361–369.

Henle W, Ho JHC, Henle G, Chau JCW, and Kwan HC. (1977). Nasopharyngeal carcinoma: siginificance of changes in Epstein-Barr virus related antibody positives following therapy. *International Journal of Cancer*, 20, 663–672.

Hinds EC. (1971). Dental care and oral hygiene before and after treatment. *JAMA*, 215, 964–966.

Hirayama T. (1978). Descriptive and analytical epidemiology of nasopharyngeal carcinoma. In: *Nasopharyngeal Carcinoma: etiology and control* (eds G de-Thé and YU Ito), pp. 167–189. Lyon: IARC Scientific Publications No. 20.

Ho JHC. (1972). Nasopharyngeal carcinoma (NPC). *Advanced Cancer Research*, 15, 57–62.

Ho HC. (1975). Epidemiology of nasopharyngeal carcinoma. *Journal of the Royal College of Surgeons Edinburgh*, 20, 223–235.

Hoffman M, Gorough T, Gottschlich S, *et al.* (2005). Human papillomaviruses in head and neck cancer: 8 year survival—analysis of 73 patients. *Cancer Letters*, 218, 199–206.

Howard DJ, Lund VJ, and Wei WI. Craniofacial resection for sinonasal neoplasia—a twenty-five year experience. *Head and Neck*, published ahead of print Jul 5, 2006.

Hu M. (1985). Epidemiology of Nasopharyngeal Carcinoma. In: *Etiology and Pathogenesis of Nasopharyngeal Carcinoma* (eds Y Zeng and O Baoxiang), pp. 1–17. People's Republic of China: Chinese Academy of Science Press.

Huang RY, Sercarz JA, Smith J, and Blackwell KE. (2005). Effect of salivary fistulas on free flap failure: a laboratory and clinical investigation. *Laryngoscope*, 115, 517–521.

Innes AJ, Windle-Taylor PC, and Harrison DF. (1980). The role of metronidazole in the prevention of fistulae following total laryngectomy. *Clinical Oncology*, 6, 71–77.

Jaffe ES, Chan JK, Su IJ, *et al.* (1996). Report of the workshop on nasal and related extranodal angiocentric T/natural killer cell lymphomas. Definitions, differential diagnosis, and epidemiology. *American Journal of Surgical Pathology*, 20, 103–111.

Jondal M and Klein G. (1973). Surface markers on human B and T lymphocytes. II. Presence of Epstein-Barr virus receptors on B lymphocytes. *Journal of Experimental Medicine*, 138, 1365–1378.

Klein G, Giovanella BC, Lindahl T, Fiakow PJ, Singh S, and Stehlin JS. (1974). Direct evidence for the presence of Epstein-Barr virus DNA and nuclear antigen in malignant epithelial cells from patients with poorly differentiated carcinoma of the nasopharynx. *Proceedings of the National Academy of Sciences USA*, 71, 4737–4741.

Lanier AP. (1977). Surgery of cancer incidence in Alaskan natives. *National Cancer Institute monograph*, 47, 87–88.

Liang PC. (1964). Studies on nasopharyngeal carcinoma in the Chinese: statistical and laboratory investigations. *Chinese Medical Journal*, 83, 373–390.

Lung ML, Chang RS, and Jones JH. (1988). Genetic polymorphism of natural Epstein-Barr virus isolates from infectious mononucleosis patients and healthy carriers. *Journal of Virology*, 62, 3862–3866.

Lung ML, Chang RS, Huang ML, *et al.* (1989). Natural Epstein-Barr virus isolates from Southern China and California differ in the Bam HI I region. In: *Epstein-Barr Virus and Human Diseases* (eds DV Ablashi *et al.*), pp. 369–74. The Humana Press.

Lung ML, Chang RS, and Huang ML. (1990). Epstein-Barr virus genotypes associated with nasopharyngeal carcinoma in Southern China. *Virology,* **176**, 44–53.

Lynn TC, Tu S-M, and Kawamma A. (1985). Long-term follow-up of IgG and IgA antibodies against viral capsid antigens of Epstein-Barr virus in nasopharyngeal carcinoma. *Journal of Laryngology and Otology,* **99**, 567–572.

Mallen RW and Shandro WG. (1974). Nasopharyngeal carcinoma in Eskimos. *Canadian Journal of Otolaryngology,* **3**, 175–179.

Maran AGD, Gaze M, and Wilson JA (1993). *Stell and Maran's Head and Neck Surgery,* p. 203. Oxford: Butterworth Heinemann.

McGahey D and Gallagher G. (2000). A survey of current wound irrigation practice in head and neck tumour surgery. *Revue de Laryngologie Otologie Rhinologie,* **121**, 103–106.

McKaig RG, Baric RS, and Olshan AF. (1998). Human papillomavirus and head and neck cancer: epidemiology and molecular biology. *Head and Neck,* **20**, 250–265.

de Melo GM, Ribeiro KC, Kowalski LP, and Deheinzelin D. (2001). Risk factors for postoperative complications in oral cancer and their prognostic implications. *Archives of Otolaryngology Head and Neck Surgery,* **127**, 828–833.

Menzin J, Lang KM, Friedman M, Dixon D, Marton JP, and Wilson J. (2005). Excess mortality, length of stay, and costs associated with serious fungal infections among elderly cancer patients: findings from linked SEER-Medicare data. *Value Health,* **8**, 140–148.

Muir C, Waterhouse J, Mack T, Powell J, and Whelan S. (1987). *Cancer Incidence in Five Continents.* Lyon: IARC Scientific Publication No. 88.

Nguyen NP, Moltz CC, and Frank C. (2004). Dysphagia following chemoradiation for locally advanced head and neck cancer. *Annals of Oncology,* **15**, 383–388.

Nicolatou-Galitis O, Sotiropoulou-Lontou A, Velegraki A, *et al.* (2003). Oral candidiasis in head and neck cancer patients receiving radiotherapy with amifostine cytoprotection. *Oral Oncology,* **39**, 397–401.

Nielsen NH, Mikkelsen F, and Hansen JP. (1977). Nasopharyngeal carcinoma in Greenland: The incidence in an arctic Eskimo population. *Acta Pathologica et Microbiologica Scandinavica A,* **85**, 850–858.

Old LJ, Boyes Ea, and Oettgen HF. (1966). Precipitating antibody in human serum to an antigen present in cultured Burkitt's lymphoma cells. *Proceedings of the National Academy of Sciences USA,* **56**, 1699–1704.

Penel N, Fournier C, Roussel-Delvallez M, *et al.* (2004). Prognostic significance of wound infections following major head and neck cancer surgery: an open non-comparative prospective study. *Support Care Cancer,* **12**, 634–639.

Penel N, Fournier C, Lefebvre D, and Lefebvre JL. (2005). Multivariation analysis of risk factors for wound infection in head and neck squamous cell carcinoma surgery with opening of mucosa. Study of 260 surgical procedures. *Oral Oncology,* **41**, 294–303.

Phan M, Van-der-Auwera P, Andry G, *et al.* (1992). Antimicrobial prophylaxis for major head and neck cancer patients. *Antimicrobial Agents and Chemotherapy,* **36**, 2014–2019.

Powles T, Powles J, Nelson M, *et al.* (2004). Head and neck cancer in patients with human immunodeficiency virus-1 infection: incidence, outcome and association with Epstein-Barr virus. *Journal of Laryngology and Otology,* **118**, 207–212.

Raab-Traub N, Flynn K, and Pearson G. (1987). The differentiated form of nasopharyngeal carcinoma contains Epstein-Barr virus DNA. *International Journal of Cancer,* **39**, 25–29.

Ramadan HH and Wetmore SJ. (1992). Effect of wound infections on head and neck cancer. *Archives of Otolaryngology—Head and Neck Surgery*, 118, 486–487.

Redding SW, Zellars RC, Kirkpatrick WR, *et al.* (1999). Epidemiology of oropharyngeal Candida colonization and infection in patients receiving radiation for head and neck cancer. *Journal of Clinical Microbiology*, 37, 3896–3900.

Righi PD, Weisberger EC, Krakovits PR, Timmerman RD, Wynne MK, and Shidnia H. (1997). Wound complications associated with brachytherapy for primary or salvage treatment of head and neck cancer. *Laryngoscope*, 107, 1464–1468.

Robbins KT, Favrot S, Hanna D, and Cole R. (1990). Risk of wound infection in patients with head and neck cancer. *Head and Neck*, 12, 143–148.

Rodrigo JP and Suarez C. (1998). Prognostic significance of postoperative wound infection on head and neck cancer. *Otolaryngology Head and Neck Surgery*, 118, 272–275.

Rodrigo JP, Suarez C, Bernaldez R, and Collado D. (2004). Efficacy of piperacillin-tazobactam in the treatment of surgical wound infection after clean-contaminated head and neck oncologic surgery. *Head and Neck*, 26, 823–828.

Rosen A, Rhee TH, and Kaufman R, (2001). Prediction of aspiration in patients with newly diagnosed untreated advanced head and neck cancer. *Archives of Otolaryngology—Head and Neck Surgery*, 127, 975–979.

Sawyer R, Cozzi L, Rosenthal DI, and Maniglia AJ. (1990). Metronidazole in head and neck surgery—the effect of lengthened prophylaxis. *Otolaryngology—Head and Neck Surgery*, 103, 1009–1011.

Shapiro M. (1991). Prophylaxis in otolaryngologic surgery and neurosurgery: a critical review. *Reviews of Infectious Diseases*, 13, 858–868.

Sheahan P, Hafidh M, Toner, M, and Timon C. (2005). Unexpected findings in neck dissection for squamous cell carcinoma: incidence and implications. *Head and Neck*, 27, 28–35.

Shiga K, Tateda M, Saijo S, *et al.* (2001). Presence of Streptococcus infection in extra-oropharyngeal head and neck squamous cell carcinoma and its implication in carcinogenesis. *Oncology Report*, 8, 245–248.

Simmons MJ and Shanmugaratanam K. (1982). Epidemiology of nasopharyngeal carcinoma. In: *The Biology of Nasopharyngeal Carcinoma* (eds MJ Simmons and K Shanmugaratman), pp. 10–16. UICC Technical Reports Series, Vol. 71. Geneva: International Union Against Cancer.

Szentirmay Z, Polus K, Tamas L, *et al.* (2005). Human papillomavirus in head and neck cancer: Molecular biology and clinicopathological correlations. *Cancer and Metastasis Reviews*, 24, 19–34.

Tam JS. (1991). Epstein-Barr Virus Serological Markers. In: *Nasopharyngeal Carcinoma* (eds CA van Hasselt and AG Gibb), pp. 145–156. Hong Kong: The Chinese University Press, The Chinese University of Hong Kong Shatin N.T.

Tateda M, Shiga K, Saijo S, *et al.* (2000). Streptococcus anginosus in head and neck squamous cell carcinoma. *International Journal of Molecular Medicine*, 6, 699–703.

de-Thé G. (1982). Epidemiology of Epstein-Barr virus and associated diseases in man. In: *Herpesviruses* (ed. B Roizman), pp. 25–87. Plenum Press.

de-Vathaire F, Sancho-Grarnier H, de Thé H, *et al.* (1988). Prognostic value of Epstein-Barr virus makers in the clinical management of nasopharyngeal carcinoma (NPC): a multi center follow-up study. *International Journal of Cancer*, 42, 176–181.

Waterhouse J, Muri C, Correa P, and Powell J. (1976). *Cancer Incidence in Five Continents*. Scientific Publication No. 15. Lyon: IARC.

Watters K, O'Dwyer TP, and Rowley H. (2004). Cost and morbidity of MRSA in head and neck cancer patients: What are the consequences? *Journal of Laryngology and Otology*, **118**, 694–699.

Zheng Y. (1985). Seroepidemiologial studies on nasopharyngeal carcinoma in China. *Advances in Cancer Research*, **14**, 121–138.

Zitsch RP and Bothwell M. (1999). Actinomycosis: a potential complication of head and neck surgery. *American Journal of Otolaryngology*, **20**, 260–262.

Zur Hausen H, Schulte-Holthausen H, Klein G, *et al.* (1970). EB virus DNA in biopsies of Burkitt tumours and anaplastic carcinomas of the nasopharynx. *Nature*, **228**, 1056–1058.

Chapter 4

Gastrointestinal infections

Vicky Coyle, Ronan McMullan, and
Patrick G. Johnston

Introduction

Gastrointestinal (GI) infections are a significant cause of morbidity and
mortality in patients with cancer. As with other categories of infection,
susceptibility is contributed to by immunodeficiency secondary to underlying disease, but most significantly is attributable to toxicity from anticancer
therapy. The range of GI infection syndromes observed in this population is
perhaps more variable than that seen in any other system. These range from
gastroenteritis-like illnesses attributable to primary pathogens that commonly
affect the competent host, to severe intra-abdominal and visceral infections
attributable to opportunistic pathogens and commensal organisms.

This chapter is structured by syndrome rather than pathogen as this best
reflects the manner in which clinical problems present to physicians and
oncologists caring for cancer patients. We also suggest some measures to
prevent GI infections in this group.

Spectrum of pathogens

The spectrum of pathogens responsible for GI infection in patients with
cancer is best thought of in terms of the conventional classification of micro-
organisms into bacterial, viral, fungal, and parasitic. While bacteria are the
most common pathogens, the other categories are responsible for some
characteristic GI infection syndromes.

Bacteria

The spectrum of bacteria involved may be broadly categorized as either exogenous, as in most diarrhoeal illness, or endogenous, reflecting the composition
of the intestinal microbiota when the mucosal barrier is disturbed. Exogenous
pathogens include those responsible for food-borne infection (e.g.
Salmonellae) and nosocomial diarrhoeal illness (e.g. *Clostridium difficile*).

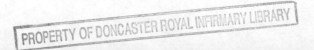

Endogenous pathogens include a broad range of anaerobes (e.g. *Bacteroides fragilis*), Gram-negative aerobes (e.g. *Escherichia coli*) and Gram-positive aerobes (e.g. enterococci) responsible for a wide spectrum of intra-abdominal infections.

Fungi

Candida spp. represent the most important group of fungi in this context. These exist as a component of the normal microbiota in many individuals but *Candida* spp. are present in greater numbers in hospitalized patients, especially those receiving antibiotics and cytotoxic agents. They are capable of causing ulceration in any part of the GI tract and are a putative cause of diarrhoea when present in high numbers. *Candida* spp. are responsible for severe invasive or disseminated disease in some individuals with a defective mucosal barrier; this is especially true in cancer patients.

When other unusual fungi involve the GI tract, this is usually only as a constituent of disseminated infection.

Viruses

The herpesviruses, herpes simplex virus (HSV) and cytomegalovirus (CMV), are the most relevant in this population as both may cause oesophagitis, a particular problem in this patient group; CMV is also a cause of colitis in the immunosuppressed patient. Norovirus is also of interest as it is capable of causing outbreaks in hospitals, as it survives for long periods in the environment, has a low infective dose, and spreads between individuals with relative ease.

Parasites

This group is not particularly associated with cancer patients in developed countries as they are not typically exposed to high-risk environments. However, *Cryptosporidium* spp. can be a major problem in the compromised host; these may cause a severe prolonged illness, in contrast to the transient illness typical in the competent host.

Mucositis and typhlitis

Mucositis

Mucositis is a common complication of cytotoxic chemotherapy, and one that has increased both in frequency and severity in recent years as a result of the high doses of chemotherapy delivered with haemopoietic growth factors and bone marrow transplant support. In addition, radiotherapy can cause direct mucosal injury in treatment fields or a severe generalized mucositis if total body irradiation is administered as part of a conditioning regimen for bone marrow transplantation.

Breakdown of the mucosal epithelium can occur anywhere along the GI tract, predisposing to bacterial or fungal infection, or reactivation of latent viral infection. This risk of infection is proportional to both the severity and duration of the mucosal insult, and the situation is often aggravated by frequently accompanying neutropenia, with risk of life-threatening systemic infection (Bow 1998). Among patients with neutropenia, the relative risk of septicaemia is about four times higher in those with mucositis.

Oral mucositis is extremely common, occurring in 40% of patients receiving chemotherapy and up to 85% of patients receiving treatment for leukaemia (Pico *et al.* 1998). The frequency depends on a number of factors including patient age, diagnosis, pre-existing periodontal disease, or poor oral hygiene, and the type and dose of administered drug. Use of chlorhexidine mouthwash has been shown to reduce the rate of associated bacterial and *Candida* infections. Infection with HSV is common with 40–70% of specimens from oral lesions in patients with mucositis demonstrating the virus. This can be difficult to diagnose clinically, as the usual cutaneous or mucous membrane vesicles may be absent. Polymerase chain reaction of swabs from oral lesions is a rapid and reliable method to confirm the diagnosis. Treatment is with aciclovir 5 mg/kg i.v. t.d.s. for 7 days or 400 mg orally five times daily if oral medication can be tolerated.

Bacterial infection can be caused by a number of organisms. Previously, Gram-negative organisms were dominant, but with increasing antibiotic use, there are an increasing number of infections from Gram-positive cocci, especially the viridans group of streptococci. A number of multidrug-resistant organisms have also been recognized in association with mucosal damage including *Stenotrophomonas maltophila* and vancomycin-resistant enterococcus. In addition, the abnormal bacterial overgrowth that occurs after mucosal injury can result in usual gut pathogens, such as *Clostridium* spp., causing bacteraemia.

Fungal infection secondary to mucositis affecting the small and large intestines is also recognized; although less commonly than secondary bacterial infection. *Candida* and, occasionally, *Aspergillus* species are the most frequent causes. As in the upper GI tract, diagnosis is difficult with variable appearances at endoscopy, often resembling pseudomembranous colitis.

Standard management of mucositis is essentially supportive, ensuring that oral hygiene and analgesia are adequate, prompt treatment of any secondary infection, and regular assessment of nutritional status, including consideration of parenteral nutrition if necessary. New targeted therapeutic agents that increase mucosal healing such as fibroblast and keratinocyte growth factors are under evaluation at present.

Typhlitis

Typhlitis (necrotizing enterocolitis) describes a particular inflammation of the caecum occurring in severe neutropenia. Although first described in patients with prolonged neutropenia after treatment for acute leukaemia, any neutropenic patient is at risk, particularly when broad-spectrum antibiotics have been used. The taxanes, paclitaxel and docetaxel, are particularly associated (Ibrahim et al. 2000).

The common clinical findings are pyrexia, abdominal pain, diarrhoea, and right iliac fossa tenderness and rebound, often preceding development of an acute abdomen. Typically the bowel wall is thickened and oedematous, often with evidence of ulceration, transmural inflammation, and necrosis. It is postulated that severe neutropenia facilitates the opportunistic invasion of ulcerated mucosa by normal gut bacteria, which then proliferate and cause local destruction by endotoxin release. Bacteraemia due to Gram-negative bacteria, in particular *Pseudomonas* spp., is a significant risk; less frequently *Clostridia* may cause this. Abdominal imaging may show the thickened or possibly gas-filled caecal wall; however, direct visualization or contrast enemas should be avoided. There is evidence that the degree of bowel wall thickening is of prognostic significance, with mural thickness greater than 10 mm on ultrasound scanning associated with poorer outcomes (Cartoni et al. 2001).

Management is conservative, with intravenous fluid replacement, broad-spectrum antimicrobial treatment with activity against anaerobes and pseudomonas, haematological support, and parenteral nutrition as necessary. Surgery should be reserved for specific situations; these include ongoing GI bleeding despite correction of haematological abnormalities, bowel perforation and peritonitis, resection of necrotic bowel, drainage of abscesses, or clinical deterioration in keeping with uncontrolled sepsis. Imaging with computed tomography allows early detection of, and therefore early intervention for, these problems. Despite aggressive management, mortality rates of 30–50% are reported.

Oesophagitis

Oesophagitis is a significant problem among cancer patients, and often is difficult to differentiate from mucositis induced by chemotherapy or radiotherapy; patients typically complain of retrosternal chest pain or epigastric pain, odynophagia, or nausea and vomiting.

The commonest causes are *Candida* and herpes simplex virus (HSV). Clinically, these infections are often difficult to distinguish and often coexist. CMV is also a recognized cause of oesophagitis in bone marrow transplant patients. Definitive diagnosis requires endoscopy and biopsy of lesions; laboratory confirmation principally relies on histological examination as detecting HSV, CMV, or *Candida* from specimens has limited diagnostic meaning without compatible findings from histology. However, endoscopy is not universally feasible in this often severely ill group of patients. Moreover it may be poorly tolerated and also carries a significant bleeding risk. Therefore, in some circumstances, detecting HSV from oral lesions by polymerase chain reaction may help to support the diagnosis of herpetic infection, but is not definitive.

Treatment of oesophagitis depends on the causative organism; however, given the diagnostic difficulties encountered and frequency of co-infection, empirical antifungal and antiviral agents are often given. For HSV oesophagitis, appropriate treatment is aciclovir 5 mg/kg intravenously 8-hourly for 7–14 days. Alternatively aciclovir 400 mg five times daily orally for 14–21 days or famciclovir 250 mg orally b.d. can be considered if oral medications can be tolerated or in less severe cases. Aciclovir resistance can occur and is suggested by lesions that fail to respond, in which case foscarnet is the treatment of choice. Finally, in the case of CMV oesophagitis, ganciclovir 5 mg/kg per day or 6 mg/kg five times weekly is the usual treatment.

For *Candida* oesophagitis, therapy is usually with oral or intravenous fluconazole 100–400 mg once daily for 14–21 days, although neutropenic patients with fever are often given amphotericin as a component of empirical therapy. Preliminary reports of caspofungin, a newer broad-spectrum antifungal agent, have suggested that it is as effective as amphotericin and better tolerated. However, at this stage data are lacking, and its use is limited to patients who are unresponsive to, or intolerant of, conventional therapy. Similarly, experience with both voriconazole (a novel triazole with broader spectrum than fluconazole) and caspofungin is limited. Both of these agents have demonstrated non-inferiority when compared with fluconazole; caspofungin has also been shown to be of similar efficacy to amphotericin B for the treatment of oesophageal candidiasis (Ally *et al.* 2001; Villaneuva *et al.* 2002). Therefore, these agents are likely to have a defined role in therapy for this disease in the near future.

Intra-abdominal sepsis (Figure 4.1)

Intra-abdominal sepsis (IAS) typically presents as secondary peritonitis, abscess formation, or both and can also result in bacteraemia. In the context of the cancer patient it will usually arise either as a postoperative complication

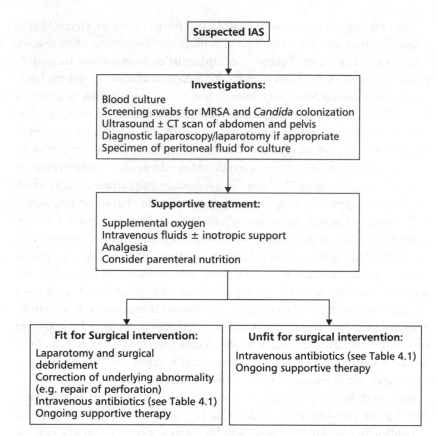

Suspected IAS

Investigations:
Blood culture
Screening swabs for MRSA and *Candida* colonization
Ultrasound ± CT scan of abdomen and pelvis
Diagnostic laparoscopy/laparotomy if appropriate
Specimen of peritoneal fluid for culture

Supportive treatment:
Supplemental oxygen
Intravenous fluids ± inotropic support
Analgesia
Consider parenteral nutrition

Fit for Surgical intervention:
Laparotomy and surgical debridement
Correction of underlying abnormality (e.g. repair of perforation)
Intravenous antibiotics (see Table 4.1)
Ongoing supportive therapy

Unfit for surgical intervention:
Intravenous antibiotics (see Table 4.1)
Ongoing supportive therapy

Fig. 4.1 Management algorithm for Intra-abdominal sepsis (IAS).

such as anastomotic dehiscence or as a result of perforation or obstruction (including strangulation) of a viscus. However, loss of integrity of the urinary tract barrier or suppurative infection of the hepatobiliary tract are also important causes of IAS.

As a result, such infections are usually attributable to endogenous organisms associated with the mucous membranes of various intra-abdominal organs. This is especially true of the GI tract, when a defect of the mucosal barrier (either anatomical or functional) leads to translocation of commensal organisms to a sterile site, such as the peritoneal cavity or bloodstream, where an inflammatory process is initiated.

The variety and density of organisms implicated varies according to the point along the gut at which mucosal disruption occurs. For example, in the stomach, the normal flora consists of streptococci, lactobacilli, and *Candida*, but the number and constituents are influenced by factors such as stasis or achlorhydria. The microbioica of the upper small intestine in health is usually scant, but increases in disease states and with achlorhydria; in the distal small intestine there are Gram-negative aerobes and enterococci, which are approximately matched in number by obligate anaerobic organisms. This is in sharp contrast to the large intestine, where almost all organisms are obligate anaerobes, with comparatively few Gram-negative aerobes and streptococci.

It is therefore unsurprising that in various studies, where careful anaerobic cultures are performed, anaerobes recurrently emerge as the most frequently isolated class of organism in IAS, reflecting their predominance on the intestinal mucosa. However, an important feature of IAS is polymicrobial infection. Indeed, the recovery of two or more pathogens from blood culture should prompt clinicians to consider possible intra-abdominal sources of infection.

As it is impossible to exclude any of the major groups of pathogens discussed, empirical therapy for IAS will almost always include coverage of anaerobes and Gram-negative aerobes; this is extended to streptococci and enterococci in proximal small bowel disease. Antifungal therapy is often incorporated in complicated cases, patients requiring emergency re-operations, and in most upper GI perforations (Table 4.1). Clinical studies have shown that inadequate initial therapy has an adverse impact on outcomes, including mortality.

Even when culture results become available, it is difficult to de-escalate to narrow-spectrum therapy given the polymicrobial nature of IAS and the variable sensitivity of microbiological sampling and processing. However, some data have suggested that not all pathogens involved need to be targeted to achieve an adequate outcome; this is especially true of enterococci. It seems that the necessary antimicrobial spectrum for empirical therapy is not well defined, but should probably be guided by severity of illness.

As with most infections, in patients who develop IAS while hospitalized, more resistant pathogens are implicated; this obviously impacts on empirical therapy. Organisms such as *Enterobacter, Pseudomonas, Acinetobacter*, and non-albicans *Candida* are more often isolated in this group.

A further consideration of great importance when selecting therapy for IAS is penetration to and activity at the site of infection. For example, when targeting Gram-negative aerobes, aminoglycosides penetrate poorly into intra-abdominal collections and are minimally active in the low redox potential milieu of an abscess; however, they may be useful adjunctive therapy when trying to manage an associated bacteraemia. By comparison, ciprofloxacin penetrates well into collections and suffers no substantial loss of activity. As illustrated in Table 4.1, there are many potential single and

Table 4.1 Suggested regimens for treatment of intra-abdominal sepsis

Regimen	Comments
Ampicillin/Sulbactam OR Amoxycillin/Clavulanic acid Cefuroxime or Cefotaxime AND Metronidazole Cefoxitin	Most suited to patients with community-acquired infection, without history of life-threatening β-lactam allergy
Piperacillin/Tazobactam Ampicillin AND Ciprofloxacin AND Metronidazole Carbapenem (e.g. imipenem, meropenem, ertepenem)	Suitable for patients who develop intra-abdominal sepsis while hospitalized May not be appropriate in patients with life-threatening β-lactam allergy
Aztreonam or Ciprofloxacin AND Clindamycin	Suitable for patients with serious β-lactam allergy and either community-acquired or nosocomial infection

Consider addition of:	Comments
Glycopeptide (vancomycin/teicoplanin)	May be added to any of the above regimens when MRSA infection is proven or suspected
Linezolid	May be added to any of the above regimens when VRE or MRSA infection is proven or suspected
Antifungal agents (fluconazole amphotericin B caspofungin voriconazole)	Addition of an antifungal agent should be considered in patients undergoing emergency reoperations and those with upper GI perforation. Also among patients with a yeast isolated from blood or peritoneal fluid as well as those heavily colonized with yeasts. Caspofungin, voriconazole and amphotericin are most appropriate for patients infected (or heavily colonized) with fluconazole-resistant species

VRE, vancomycin-resistant enterococci; MRSA, methicillin-resistant staphylococcus.

combination therapies for IAS; however, optimal therapy should be intravenous because of both the severity of infection and the need to deliver high tissue levels, which would be impossible with oral therapy, especially when absorptive function is likely to be substantially impaired.

Apart from antimicrobial therapy, supportive measures to maintain physiological functions are critical and in almost all cases, surgical debridement to achieve adequate primary source control is of paramount importance. Indeed, when good surgical clearance is achieved, dramatic clinical improvement is usually observed. However, in instances when surgical drainage is impossible, antimicrobial therapy is heavily relied upon and in such cases its optimization becomes essential.

Hepatosplenic candidiasis (Figure 4.2)

This is an emerging problem in immunocompromised patients, and presents a major diagnostic and therapeutic challenge. It mainly occurs in patients receiving treatment for leukaemia occurring in 3–6% of this group, and tends to present after the neutrophil count has recovered from cytotoxic chemotherapy. Classically, patients develop pyrexia, abdominal pain, and hepatosplenomegaly with an elevated serum alkaline phosphatase. However, commonly, the classical constellation of clinical findings is not apparent.

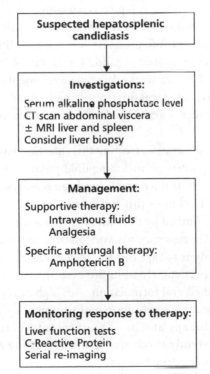

Fig. 4.2 Management algorithm for hepatosplenic candidiasis.

Abdominal imaging with ultrasound or computed tomography reveals multiple hepatic abscesses, typically with a 'bulls-eye' appearance, which are usually not detectable while the patient remains neutropenic. MRI is extremely sensitive (approaching 100%) and has high specificity; it can be especially helpful in characterizing small lesions, but may not be accessible to all patients in whom this diagnosis is a possibility. Definitive diagnosis is made with positive histology from a biopsy specimen. The diagnostic challenge is twofold. First, one must have a high index of suspicion of this clinical syndrome for which there are few specific clinical findings. Secondly, diagnosis is limited by difficulty in obtaining biopsies from patients who are often severely thrombocytopenic. Furthermore, these are frequently culture-negative with non-specific histology and normally there are no preceding or concurrent positive blood cultures for *Candida* spp. In view of the diagnostic difficulty associated with this infection, international consensus guidelines have been published with a view to standardizing the diagnosis of this and other invasive fungal infections in cancer patients (Ascioglu *et al.* 2002). However, these may be somewhat laborious when applied routinely and are of greatest benefit in the context of a clinical trial.

Clinical management involves a prolonged course of antifungal treatment, although the ideal duration of treatment remains unclear. Ongoing measurement of liver enzymes, inflammatory indices, and clinical state as well as repeated imaging are required to guide the length of treatment, which is typically between 12 and 25 weeks. When conventional amphotericin B has been chosen, the average total dose resulting in good outcomes has been reported to be between 3 and 5 g administered over many weeks (Sallah *et al.* 1999).

Although most experience in treating this infection has been with various formulations of amphotericin, including lipid preparations, other antifungal drugs may be used. While fluconazole has been reported to be effective, one would be unlikely to choose this unless *in vitro* susceptibility had been confirmed, which is limited by the difficulty in isolating the organism from clinical specimens. The newer agents, voriconazole and caspofungin, although currently used mainly as salvage therapy, may have a more prominent role in the future. This is particularly so in the case of voriconazole, as resistant isolates are rare and an oral formulation with high bioavailability facilitates outpatient management towards the end of treatment.

Further chemotherapy and bone marrow transplantation have been reported after apparently successful resolution of the primary infection, with ongoing antifungal drug therapy.

Antibiotic-associated diarrhoea

As a result of the frequency and severity of infections there is substantial use of antibiotics in cancer patients. Diarrhoea is the most frequent adverse effect of antibiotic therapy and is worse in patients with serious comorbidities, elderly patients, those who have undergone recent surgery, and those who have had exposure to antimotility drugs.

Although *Clostridium difficile* disease represents only a small minority of antibiotic-associated diarrhoea, when it occurs it is usually associated with prior antibiotic exposure; it has been seen to prolong inpatient stay, and increase hospitalization costs as well as mortality. Furthermore, it is the commonest cause of nosocomial diarrhoeal illness; moreover, it is much more common among hospitalized patients receiving antibiotics than those in the community. This is presumably because three steps appear to precede infection: (1) the organism is acquired, which is much more likely in hospital; (2) it must reach significant numbers, which is facilitated by antibiotic exposure; and (3) a host trigger factor sufficient to precipitate clinical infection is usually present.

While up to 20% of hospitalized patients may be colonized with toxin-producing *C. difficile*, only a minority develop symptoms. Adequate numbers of organisms may be achieved when the normal 'background' intestinal commensals are diminished in number as these provide a degree of protection against pathogens, often referred to as *colonization resistance*. Loss of colonization resistance is associated with various antibiotics and some cytotoxic agents, including doxorubicin, cisplatin, cyclophosphamide, 5-fluorouracil, and methotrexate. Table 4.2 classifies some common antibiotics associated with *C. difficile* infection. It is important to note that the onset of clinical illness, which usually occurs after 5–10 days of antibiotic therapy, may also begin several weeks after cessation of antibiotics.

Host factors that facilitate infection in colonized individuals include age, severity of comorbidities, underlying malignancy (especially intestinal), recent GI surgery and use of enemas, bowel stimulants, and stool softeners.

Table 4.2 Common antibiotics and relative risk of *Clostridium difficile* infection

Low risk	Intermediate risk	High risk
Aminoglycosides	Quinolones (e.g. ciprofloxacin)	Ampicillin
Glycopeptides	Carbapenems	Amoxycillin/clavulanate
Metronidazole		Cephalosporins
Piperacillin/tazobactam		Clindamycin

The spectrum of *C. difficile* disease is broad, ranging from minimal inflammatory diarrhoea to fulminant, relapsing colitis sometimes with formation of a pseudomembrane, which may, occasionally, be fatal. Most patients fall somewhere between these extremes, skewed towards milder disease, with commonly observed features, including diarrhoea, fever, leucocytosis, and abdominal pain. Overall, the most frequently observed complication of this infection is recurrence.

In some cases of more severe disease diarrhoea may be absent; this may confound the diagnosis initially. For example, individuals may present with fever and abdominal pain in the setting of extremely high peripheral blood white cell counts ($>30\,000/mm^3$). This should prompt the clinician to consider severe *C. difficile* infection and intra-abdominal abscess formation, both of which may present in this manner. Such severe infection may be associated with toxic megacolon, a surgical emergency, which can be complicated by perforation.

In most diagnostic laboratories, *C. difficile* infection is routinely diagnosed by an enzyme immunoassay on faecal specimens as culture is much more laborious, slower, and provides similar diagnostic performance. Molecular assays have not been fully evaluated in this context. Although endoscopy is very specific for disease when a pseudomembrane is visualized, its poor sensitivity and invasive nature limits its utility.

Treating *C. difficile* disease should firstly involve general supportive measures such as fluid replacement and avoidance of antiperistaltic drugs; cessation of the antibiotic driving the proliferation of this pathogen is a desirable goal and if necessary, it could be replaced by an alternative that exerts less adverse selective pressure at the mucosal surface. In the presence of toxic megacolon or colonic perforation surgical intervention is essential. Of paramount importance are strict infection-control precautions as this pathogen can easily spread to other susceptible individuals in the nearby environment.

Typically, first-line antibiotic therapy involves metronidazole, preferably administered orally, for 10 days; a second course can be initiated if the primary course is inadequate or recurrence arises. In cases where the disease remains refractory or recurrent, vancomycin can be introduced; only oral vancomycin is appropriate in view of poor tissue levels at the site of infection when administered systemically. Vancomycin is not recommended as first-line therapy as it is a significant risk factor for colonization with vancomycin-resistant enterococci, which can present a major therapeutic challenge. Its main indications are failure or intolerance of primary therapy, pregnancy, or very severe disease. There are several other antimicrobial and probiotic options for persistent or multiply-recurring disease; however, probiotics (especially *Saccharomyces* spp.) are not universally suitable for patients with bowel tumours because of the risk of bloodstream infection.

Prevention of *C. difficile* disease is of great importance; the main strategies for this are twofold. First, implementation of antibiotic policies favouring those drugs that do not promote the infection sequence described above in susceptible populations, such as cancer patients. Secondly, improved hand decontamination of healthcare workers and rigorous environmental cleaning of healthcare facilities are aimed towards limiting spread and acquisition of the organism.

Food-borne illness

An almost identical spectrum of pathogens causing food-borne (and water-borne) illness is seen in cancer patients as in competent hosts; the principal difference is the severity of illness attributed to these. In general terms, cancer patients are susceptible to more severe, more invasive, and more prolonged infections. For example, while *Campylobacter* spp. usually cause a self-limiting diarrhoeal illness requiring no specific treatment, immunosuppressed individuals are known to be at risk of sustained bloodstream infection, without necessarily showing evidence of severe enteritis; this population also has a higher mortality associated with such infection. For these reasons, cancer patients who are substantially immunocompromised will often receive antimicrobial therapy for *Campylobacter* enteritis with erythromycin or a quinolone.

Two enteric pathogens deserve particular mention as they may be associated with some specific clinical problems in the most susceptible hosts: *Samonella* spp. and *Cryptosporidium* spp.

Salmonella

The vast majority of samonellosis in developed countries is non-typhoidal; typhoid fever is now rare in such populations, except when acquired abroad. Eggs or poultry are the usual food vehicles for salmonellae in Western societies; however, contamination of other prepared food by these sources is also important.

Host defence relies heavily on cell-mediated immunity, which is defective in patients with lymphoproliferative disorders. Other factors that predispose cancer patients to salmonellosis include diminished gastric acidity, GI surgery, and altered endogenous flora.

The most commonly observed clinical syndrome is a gastroenteritis-like illness; vomiting and diarrhoea usually arise within 48 hours of consuming the contaminated foodstuff. This may be accompanied by fevers, abdominal pain, and sometimes headaches and myalgia. In the competent host, it is usually a self-limiting illness that resolves without specific therapy within 3–7 days; however, bacteraemia may complicate the illness in 1–4% of otherwise healthy persons. In immunosuppressed cancer patients, the duration of the illness is typically longer and the risk of bacteraemia is increased significantly. Indeed, high-grade bacteraemia is a risk marker for invasive vascular infection, as these organisms may seed vascular tissue such as atherosclerotic plaques or aneurysms.

Severe salmonella infection in cancer patients may be represented by acute enterocolitis, perhaps including rectal ulceration. Extra-intestinal infection may complicate the illness in this population, which may manifest as osteomyelitis, lung abscess, or renal abscess/pyelonephritis, especially in patients with bone metastases, lung cancer, or renal tumours, respectively.

Because of the severity of salmonellosis in the immunosuppressed individual, patients presenting with even limited GI infection are often given antimicrobial therapy. Oral quinolones represent suitable empirical treatment. Typically, a short course of about 72 hours, or until defervescence occurs, is preferred as longer courses have been associated with chronic carriage.

Bacteraemic patients require longer courses (7–14 days) of intravenous antibiotic; either a quinolone or a third-generation cephalosporin is suitable. Of note, those with multiple positive blood cultures are more likely to have vascular infection and attempts to exclude this by imaging should be made. If such a complication is presumed or confirmed, a long course (about 6 weeks) of intravenous antibiotics, such as a third-generation cephalosporin, would be appropriate as well as resection of the infected structures where possible. Where resection is impossible, lifetime suppressive therapy with oral antibiotics may be an option. Similar therapeutic principles extend to bone infection.

Cryptosporidium

This ubiquitous protozoan parasite, which is largely refractory to most disinfectants, has several environmental reservoirs; although most clinical infections (including outbreaks) are linked with contaminated water, food, and other infected persons are also sources. Very low doses of this pathogen, perhaps as little as one organism, may be enough to cause clinical infection. Diagnosis may be hampered by both intermittent shedding of organisms in the faeces and the need to examine specimens specifically and carefully for oocysts.

While it is difficult to derive data from cancer populations, mortality in HIV-positive groups has been reported to be as high as 61%. Furthermore, some reported outbreaks appear to correlate with immunosuppressed populations. The main problem with this infection in the most immunosuppressed cancer patients is difficulty with clearing the organisms leading to chronic, severe diarrhoeal illness. Disseminated disease appears not to occur, but affected individuals may have persistent, high volume watery diarrhoea. However, even within any relatively homogeneous susceptible population, the spectrum of clinical illness may be very broad.

The mainstay of treatment is restoration of immune function, as no antimicrobial drugs are clearly effective. When immune restoration is impossible, attempts at pharmacological control become more important. Antimotility drugs can help to alleviate symptoms; however, fluid replacement and perhaps parenteral nutrition may be required. Many drugs targeted towards killing the pathogen have been reported, but few have been thoroughly evaluated and none appear to be ideal. The most frequently discussed agent is spiramycin, with which most experience has been described.

For this reason, prevention of infection in susceptible persons is critical. Advice should be given regarding limiting pet exposure and excluding strays and pets with intestinal illness. Avoidance of foods in which a major constituent is water (e.g. ice cream) is a valuable strategy, especially in the setting of a waterborne outbreak or in the minority of very high-risk patients. For this high-risk subpopulation, use of boiled, cooled water is recommended and applies to both bottled mineral water and tap water (Bouchier Report; Department of the Environment, Transport and the Regions and Department of Health, London 1998). This presents substantial logistic and safety issues, particularly in hospital wards, where facilities for such practices may not be adequate.

Prevention of gastrointestinal infections in cancer patients

In addition to developing clear diagnostic and therapeutic strategies for GI infections in cancer patients, attention must also be paid to their prevention. In the hospital environment, general measures include maintaining good hand hygiene among healthcare workers, safe food preparation, isolation, and barrier nursing of patients with documented infection or diarrhoeal illness, and policies not permitting flowers or cooked food to be given to patients by visitors; advising visitors with infective illnesses not to attend hospitals is also prudent. For patients in the community, common sense advice about safe food preparation, or drinking bottled water, and avoiding unwashed food when travelling abroad should be given.

In addition to these general measures, a number of more specific measures can be taken. Careful oral hygiene, often with the use of chlorhexidine mouthwash, aims to minimize infective complications arising as a result of oral mucosal damage. The GI tract is the major anatomical reservoir of *Candida*, and may be a source of disseminated infection following mucosal damage and immunosuppression from cytotoxic treatment. There is evidence that oral fluconazole is effective in preventing superficial and deep *Candida* infection in bone marrow transplant patients, and a smaller body of evidence demonstrating a survival advantage from this. Prophylaxis with fluconazole is commonly given to patients receiving an allogeneic bone marrow transplant. Other antifungal agents are given to a wider group of patients, principally to reduce the risk of *Aspergillus* infection, although this has an impact on *Candida* also.

Although prophylactic antifungal agents have a proven role, there is no clear role for attempting to reduce potential sources of infection from the GI tract with prophylactic antibiotics (Momin and Chandrasekar, 1995). Previously, a number of strategies have been used to attempt to reduce the number of gut bacteria on either a non-selective or selective basis, including systemic prophylaxis, decontamination, and selective decontamination of the GI tract. Although the latter strategy appeared promising initially, it has not demonstrated a reduction in GI infection or associated mortality, while the other methods have been associated with poor compliance and emergence of resistant strains of bacteria. Allogeneic bone marrow transplant recipients frequently also receive prophylactic antiviral agents.

Finally, poor nutritional status is often encountered in cancer patients, and this further impairs immune defences. Maintenance of nutritional status is therefore important; however, this should ideally be achieved by oral intake. In some situations this is not possible, and in this setting enteral feeding should be considered for those with a functioning gut, using parenteral nutrition only if unavoidable.

Further reading

DeVita VT, Hellman S, and Rosenberg SA. (2004). *Cancer, Principles and Practice of Oncology*, 7th edn. Lippincott-Raven.

Johnston PG, Spence RAJ. (2002). *Oncologic Emergencies*, 1st edn. Oxford University Press.

Mandell GL, Bennett JE and Dolin R. (2000). *Principles and Practice of Infectious Disease*, 5th edn. Churchill Livingstone.

Souhami RL, Tannock I, Hohenberger P and Horiot J-C. (2002). *Oxford Textbook of Oncology*, 2nd edn. Oxford University Press.

References

Ally R, Schurmann D, Kreisel W, et al. (2001). Esophageal Candidiasis Study Group. A randomised, double-blind, double-dummy, multicenter trial of voriconazole and fluconazole in the treatment of esophageal candidiasis in immunocompromised patients. *Clinical Infectious Diseases*, **33**, 1447–1454.

Ascioglu, S, Rex, JH, de Pauw, B, et al. Invasive Fungal Infections Cooperative Group of the European Organisation for Research and Treatment of Cancer, Mycoses Study Group of the National Institute of Allergy and Infectious Diseases (2002). Defining opportunistic invasive fungal infections in immunocompromised patients with cancer and haematopoietic stem cell transplants: an international consensus. *Clinical Infectious Diseases*, **34**, 7–14.

Bow EJ. (1998). Infection risk and cancer chemotherapy: the impact of the chemotherapeutic regimen in patients with lymphoma and solid tissue malignancies. *Journal of Antimicrobial Chemotherapy*, **41** (Suppl. D), 1–5.

Cartoni, C, Dragoni, F, Micozzi, A, et al. (2001). Neutropenic enterocolitis in patients with acute leukaemia: prognostic significance of bowel wall thickening detected by ultrasonography. *Journal of Clinical Oncology*, **19**(3), 756–61.

Department of the Environment, Transport and the Regions and Department of Health, London (1998). *Cryptosporidium and Water Supplies* (The 'Bouchier Report'), Available at http://www.dwi.gov.uk/pubs/bouchier/index.htm

Ibrahim NK, Sahin AA, Dubrow RA, et al. (2000). Colitis associated with docetaxel-based chemotherapy in patients with metastatic breast cancer. *Lancet*, **355**, 281–283.

Momin F and Chandrasekar PH. (1995). Antimicrobial prophylaxis in bone marrow transplantation. *Annals of Internal Medicine*, **123**, 205–215.

Pico J, Avila-Garavito A, and Naccache P. (1998). Mucositis: its occurrence, consequences, and treatment in the oncology setting. *The Oncologist*, **3**, 446–451.

Sallah S, Semelka RC, Wehbie R, Sallah W, Nguyen NP, and Vos P. (1999). Hepatosplenic candidiasis in patients with acute leukaemia. *British Journal of Haematology*, **106**, 697–701.

Villanueva A, Gotuzzo E, Noriega LM, et al. (2002). Randomised, double blind, multicenter study of caspofungin versus amphotericin B for treatment of oropharyngeal and esophageal candidiases. *Antimicrobial Agents and Chemotherapy*, **46**, 451–457.

Chapter 5

Pulmonary infections in cancer patients: diagnosis, aetiology, and principles of treatment

Lionel Karlin, Aurelie Lefebvre, and
Elie Azoulay

Introduction

Pulmonary complications are a major cause of morbidity and mortality in patients with cancer and particularly in those with haematological malignancies (Hilbert *et al.* 2001). Nearly one-third of these patients are affected, with a mortality rate of up to 50% (Wardman *et al.* 1984). Pulmonary complications account for most of the intensive care unit (ICU) admissions in critically ill cancer patients (Kress *et al.* 1961; Blot *et al.* 1997). Mortality in the ICU is extremely high, particularly in bone marrow recipients and when mechanical ventilation is required (Ewig *et al.* 1998; Rabe *et al.* 2004).

Many disorders can lead to respiratory symptoms in cancer patients. Several interlinked disorders may occur in combination in the individual patient. Infections are the leading causes of respiratory symptoms (Azoulay *et al.* 2004), not only because the respiratory tract is the main route of entry for many microbial agents, but also because host defences are impaired by the underlying disease (e.g. hypogammaglobulinaemia in chronic lymphocytic leukaemia and multiple myeloma) and anticancer treatments, which can induce neutropenia and immune dysfunction. Other causes include chemotherapy or radiation-induced pulmonary toxicity, leukaemic infiltration (Cordonnier *et al.* 1994), and intra-alveolar haemorrhage.

Early aetiological treatment improves the chances of survival (Von Eiff *et al.* 1995). This, together with the large number of possible causes, requires a rapid and orderly diagnostic evaluation. The most likely causes should be identified based on the underlying disease (e.g. *Legionella pneumophila* pneumoniae is common in hairy cell leukaemia) and previous treatments (e.g. fludarabine therapy is associated with pneumocystis jiroveci pneumoniae (PCP). Once pulmonary oedema due to congestive heart failure is ruled out, fibreoptic bronchoscopy and bronchoalveolar lavage (FB-BAL) constitute a crucial diagnostic tool. In addition to an aetiological evaluation, a prompt evaluation of disease severity should be conducted in order to determine whether ICU admission is required.

This chapter is a review of the bacterial, fungal, parasitic, and viral infections seen in critically ill cancer patients. It is organized under two subheadings: diagnostic procedures and diagnostic criteria. The principles of treatment are also discussed. The management of patients with malignancies often requires close co-operation among haematologists/oncologists, infectious disease physicians, internists, and intensivists.

Diagnostic investigations

Clinical, radiological, and laboratory test features of pulmonary infections may be atypical in patients with malignancies. For example, systemic symptoms such as fever may be blunted or absent, most notably when antimicrobials or steroids have been given. In neutropenic patients with pneumoniae, suggestive pulmonary symptoms are usually lacking. Pulmonary symptoms are often more noticeable at the onset of neutropenia recovery, as a result of neutrophil migration to the infected site (Maunder et al. 1986), and radiological changes often become apparent during the same period (Heussel et al. 1999). Microbiological documentation is obtained in only 30–40% of cases (Cordonnier et al. 2002). Moreover, the causative organisms in immunocompromised patients with malignancy differ markedly from those in other populations, due to the high rate of opportunistic infections.

Four points should be considered when selecting diagnostic investigations.

1 The underlying characteristics of the patient (Table 5.1):
- type of malignancy
- previous stem cell transplantation
- previous cancer chemotherapy and/or radiation therapy
- neutropenia (grade and duration), lymphopenia, hypogammaglobuli-naemia
- antimicrobial prophylaxis
- prognosis of the underlying disease, most notably when transfer to the ICU is required.

2 Clinical data from a detailed physical examination for infectious risk factors, possible portals of entry, and indicators of disease severity.

3 Results of previous laboratory tests and imaging studies.

4 Evidence pointing to:

- specific infectious agents
- non-infectious aetiologies, including:
  - pulmonary involvement by the underlying malignancy (leukaemic infiltration or leucostasis) (Azoulay *et al.* 2003)
  - pulmonary toxicity of chemotherapy (bleomycin, methotrexate, ara-cytine) and/or radiation therapy
  - alveolar haemorrhage
  - alveolar proteinosis.

FB-BAL deserves special attention as an investigation with a well-proven role in the aetiological diagnosis of respiratory distress in cancer patients (Von Eiff *et al.* 1995; Pagano *et al.* 1997). FB-BAL should be performed in

Table 5.1 Main pathogens according to underlying conditions and laboratory test results

Underlying conditions	Lab results	Main pathogens
Intensive chemotherapy BMT	Prolonged neutropenia	Gram-positive pathogens Gram-negative pathogens Aspergillus
Corticosteroids (GVHD, ALL, NHL)	Lymphopenia Impaired cell-mediated immunity	Nocardiosis Aspergillus, mucormycosis *Pneumocystis jiroveci*, Strongyloides stercoralis
Multiple myeloma CLL Asplenia	Hypogammaglobulinaemia Impaired humoral immunity	Encapsulated bacteria (*Streptococcus pneumoniae*, *Haemophilus influenzae*) Gram-negative bacteria
Allogeneic BMT	Impaired T-cell-mediated immunity	Mycobacteria Toxoplasmosis viruses (CMV, RSV)
Corticosteroids Purine analogues (fludarabine)	Lymphopenia Impaired cell-mediated immunity	*Pneumocystis jiroveci* Cryptococcosis
Hairy cell leukaemia	Monocytopenia	*Legionella pneumophila*

GVHD, graft-versus-host disease; ALL, acute lymphoblastic leukaemia; NHL, non-Hodgkin lymphoma; CLL, chronic lymphocytic leukaemia; BMT, bone marrow transplantation; CMV, cytomegalovirus; RSV, respiratory syncytial virus.

patients who have diffuse or focal pulmonary infiltrates without suggestive clinical characteristics, without microbiological documentation, and without evidence of congestive heart failure, as well as in patients whose symptoms persist after several days of empirical antimicrobial treatment (Danés et al. 2002). In a prospective trial by Jain et al. (2004), the diagnostic yield was 50% overall and 70% in the subset of patients investigated by transbronchial lung biopsy. Procedure-related morbidity was low. However, transbronchial lung biopsy could be hazardous in patients with thrombocytopenia, and in other studies it increased the diagnostic yeild only for non-infectious pulmonary diseases but not for infections (Mulabecirovic et al. 2004). FB-BAL is performed to assist in the diagnosis of bacterial, fungal, parasitic, and viral infections. Protected distal samples have a lower diagnostic yield than FB-BAL. Either the lobe containing a focal infiltrate or the middle lobe in patients with diffuse infiltrates is explored. If necessary, the procedure is done in the ICU. BAL specimens must be sent rapidly to laboratories for microbiological studies (bacteria, mycobacteria, fungi, parasites, and viruses) and cytological studies (which assist in ruling out differential diagnoses such as alveolar haemorrhage, toxic pneumoniae, and neoplastic cell infiltration). In patients with focal lesions, fine-needle aspiration may be useful, particularly for the diagnosis of fungal infections, although the yield is operator-dependent (Wong et al. 2002).

Aetiology, manifestations, and principles of treatment

Bacterial pneumoniae

Common pyogens

Pneumonia due to common bacterial pathogens is the leading pulmonary complication in patients with cancer (Rossini et al. 2000; Azoulay et al. 2003). Few epidemiological data on the relative frequencies of causative bacteria are available. Gram-negative pathogens, most notably Gram-negative bacilli, predominate (Carratala et al. 1998; Ewig et al. 1998; Offidani et al. 2004) (Table 5.2). Among them, Pseudomonas aeruginosa, often acquired from exogenous sources, is the most frequent pathogen, followed by Escherichia coli and Klebsiella pneumoniae, both of which are present in the normal gastrointestinal flora. Other Gram-negative pathogens such as Stenotrophomonas maltophila may be found. Gram-positive pathogens constitute the second most common group of causative agents. They include Streptococcus pneumoniae, non-haemolytic streptococci from the oral cavity, and Staphylococcus aureus.

Table 5.2 Distribution of causative pathogens in patients with haematological malignancies and bacterial pneumoniae

	Carratala et al. 1998	Ewig et al. 1998	Rossini et al. 2000	Offidani et al. 2004
Gram-negative	25 (58%)	9 (41%)	13 (50%)	24 (70%)
P. aeruginosa	17	4	4	11
E. coli	5	2	3	7
M. catarrhalis	1			
H. influenzae	1			
K. pneumoniae	1		3	1
Enterobacter		2		
Acinetobacter		1	3	
Stenotrophomonas				5
Gram-positive	18 (42%)	13 (59%)	13 (50%)	10 (30%)
S. pneumoniae	12	1		
Streptococci sp	3	7	3	2
S. non-aureus	2	4		
S. aureus	1	1	4	1
Enterococcus sp		3	2	7
Bacillus sp		1		

A dramatic increase in Gram-positive pathogens has occurred over the last few years, and both pneumoniae and bacteraemia due to Gram-positive cocci are becoming the most common infectious diseases in neutropenic patients (Torres et al. 2003). Possible contributing causes include the introduction of high-dose aracytine, rising incidence of high-grade mucositis, and increasing use of central venous catheters (Kern et al. 1990; Elting et al. 1992). Studies of patients with Streptococcus viridans infections identified mucositis and antacids as risk factors (Cordonnier et al. 2003).

Neutropenia is the main biological risk factor for pneumoniae due to common pathogen bacteria. Hypogammaglobulinaemia, commonly seen during the course of malignancies such as multiple myeloma, chronic lymphocytic leukaemia, lymphoma, or asplenia, increases the risk of infection with encapsulated organisms (S. pneumoniae, Haemophilus influenzae) and Gram-negative bacilli. Monocytopenia, which is encountered in hairy cell leukaemia, is a risk factor for Legionnaires' disease.

Although pneumoniae is usually focal initially, rapid extension is common, so that chest radiographs show diffuse confluent lesions. Pulmonary oedema may be difficult to rule out. In patients with neutropenia, hypogammaglobuli-naemia, or asplenia, antibacterial therapy should be started promptly. The results of microbiological studies may require changes in the antimicrobial regimen. In the absence of microbiological documentation, empirical antibi-otics are selected based on epidemiological and clinical data, laboratory tests, previous documented infections or colonizations, risk factors for *P. aerugi-nosa*, and contraindications to antibiotics (e.g. renal insufficiency for amino-glycosides and glycopeptides). Patients with neutropenia should be given antibiotics

that are effective against a broad array of pathogens. Human granulocyte colony-stimulating factor, which is widely used in cancer patients to curtail chemothera-py-induced neutropenia, should be used with caution given the risk of acute respiratory deterioration at the onset of neutropenia recovery (Rinaldo and Borovetz 1985; Karlin *et al.* 2005). In patients with hypogammaglobulinaemia, antibiotics that are active against encapsulated pathogens should be used.

The mortality rate for neutropenic cancer patients with severe pneumoniae is high and is similar for Gram-negative and Gram-positive pneumoniae. However, in afebrile neutropenic patients free of respiratory symptoms, antibiotic prophylaxis is not helpful and may select antibiotic-resistant strains (Hughes *et al.* 2002). In patients with multiple myeloma, trimethoprime–sul-phamethoxazole prophylaxis significantly decreases the number of pul-monary infections, but this effect is confined to the first 2 months of chemotherapy.

Finally, although vaccines directed against encapsulated pathogens usually afford protection to patients with asplenia, they have not proven effective in patients with multiple myeloma or chronic lymphocytic leukaemia. The effectiveness of intravenous immunoglobulins in these lymphoproliferative disorders is also a matter of debate.

Legionella pneumophila pneumoniae

Deficiencies in cell-mediated immunity can lead to *Legionella pneumophila* infection. Instead of neutropenia, monocyte function impairment is the main risk factor. This is the case in hairy cell leukaemia, a lymphoproliferative disorder that often presents with profound monocytopenia. Allogeneic bone marrow recipients and patients receiving prolonged steroid therapy are also at risk; in these populations, nosocomial acquisition is common.

Clinical manifestations and radiological features are not different from those classically described in immunocompetent patients (Tkatch *et al.* 1998). However, cases presenting with chest radiograph findings suggestive of invas-ive pulmonary aspergillosis (IPA) have been reported. Diagnostic procedures and treatment are not different from immunocompetent patients. An active and synergic antibacterial regimen containing a quinolone is recommended.

Mycobacterial infections

Mycobacterial infections usually occur in patients with impaired T-cell-mediated immunity. Proof is lacking that the risk of tuberculosis is increased in patients with haematological malignancies, except in bone marrow recipients. In the only published study, a cohort of cancer patients was monitored for 10 years (De La Rosa *et al.* 2004); only 19 cases of tuberculosis occurred in the subset with haematological malignancies, and the occurrence rate for tuberculosis was 1.3 cases for 1000 new acute leukaemia cases. The risk of tuberculosis in bone marrow recipients has been found to vary widely across geographic areas, from 0.5% to 15%. Use of allogeneic (not autologous) and matched unrelated donor transplants, conditioning with total body irradiation, graft-versus-host disease (GVHD), and steroid therapy are strongly associated with tuberculosis (Ip *et al.* 1998). In stem-cell transplant recipients, tuberculosis develops several months after transplantation and is confined to the lungs in 80% of cases. Clinical manifestations and radiological features share many similarities with those observed in non-cancer patients.

However, steroid therapy, concomitant pulmonary disorders (infectious or non-infectious), and the frequently negative tuberculin test results may make the diagnosis difficult. Anti-tuberculous treatment for 12 months, with four agents initially, has been recommended. In patients taking cyclosporin, *rifampicin* should be used only when absolutely necessary and with great caution, as it decreases cyclosporin levels by inducing hepatic metabolism of the drug. Serum cyclosporin levels should be monitored very closely. Tuberculosis is fatal in 25% of stem-cell transplant recipients and concomitant steroid therapy is associated with higher mortality. Prophylaxis should be discussed in patients previously exposed to tuberculosis, but no guidelines have been developed as yet.

Few cases of pulmonary infections due to atypical mycobacteria have been reported in patients with malignancies (Castor *et al.* 1994); however, they are more common in patients with HIV infection. The most common species seen in patients with cancer (especially acute leukaemia) and in bone marrow recipients are *Mycobacterium kansasii*, *M. fortuitum*, and *M. chelonae*. These last two agents belong to the group of rapidly growing mycobacteria (Rolston *et al.* 1985). Systemic or pulmonary symptoms and radiological changes can help to differentiate pulmonary colonization from infection. In this last case, specific treatment should be initiated promptly given the risk of severe extensive disease, particularly with rapidly growing mycobacteria. A combination of two effective drugs (anti-tuberculous agents, macrolides, quinolones, or aminoglycosides) is required to reduce the risk of selecting resistant pathogens (Jacobson *et al.* 1998).

Pulmonary nocardiosis

Nocardia spp. are ubiquitous aerobic Gram-positive bacteria belonging to the Actinomycetales order. In humans, *N. asteroides* is the predominant pathogen, although several other species occur. Penetration is usually via the respiratory tract. Most patients have immunodeficiencies, particularly impaired cell-mediated immunity (lymphopenia). Neutropenia does not seem to be a major risk factor (Watkins *et al.* 1999). Thus, most of the reported cases occurred in patients with acute leukaemia or lymphoma, in allogeneic bone marrow recipients, or in patients receiving steroid therapy or immunosuppressive drugs (fludarabine, cyclosporin).

The lungs are the most common site of infection with *Nocardia* spp. Haematogenous dissemination to the central nervous system or skin is rare (Berkey and Bodey 1989). Onset is abrupt or gradual. The pulmonary manifestations are non-specific. Chest radiographs may show unilateral or bilateral infiltrates, solitary nodules, pleural effusions, or pulmonary abscesses. The diagnosis rests on examination of sputum specimens, transtracheal aspirates, BAL fluid, fine-needle aspiration specimens, or lung biopsies.

Trimethoprime–sulphamethoxazole is the cornerstone of therapy and can be used in combination with amikacin, a third-generation cephalosporin, or tetracycline. The optimal treatment duration is unknown and mortality is high.

Pulmonary fungal infections

Pulmonary fungal infections, which are dominated by invasive pulmonary apergillosis (IPA), require special attention in patients with cancer and are most frequent in those with haematological malignancies and those receiving prolonged high-dose chemotherapy. Moreover, their frequency is increasing, particularly in transplant recipients and in patients receiving intensive cancer treatment responsible for prolonged and profound neutropenia and immunosuppression (Patterson *et al.* 2000). In addition the mortality is high despite the introduction of new treatments. We will review fungal infections due to filamentous moulds then those due to yeasts.

Filamentous moulds

Invasive pulmonary aspergillosis   Of the approximately 200 species of *Aspergillus*, *A. fumigatus* is the main cause of disease in humans (Soubani and

Chandrasekar 2002). These ubiquitous organisms are found in air ventilation systems, flowers, and food (e.g. fruits, cereals, and pepper) and in demolition and construction sites. Transmission to humans occurs chiefly via inhalation. Humans have a remarkable capacity to eliminate *Aspergillus* spores, which undergo phagocytosis by neutrophils and alveolar macrophages. Thus, invasive aspergillosis is rare in immunocompetent individuals. The two main risk factors are profound and prolonged neutropenia (neutrophil count <500/μl for more than 3 weeks, the risk of IPA being estimated at 4% each day) and prolonged steroid therapy. Acute leukaemia, myelodysplastic syndromes, aplastic anaemia, and allogeneic bone marrow transplantation are the main underlying diseases associated with IPA. In bone marrow recipients, the risk is greatest during the first week after transplantation and during GVHD onset (Denning *et al.* 1998).

Hyphal invasion of blood vessels causing infarction and necrosis is the hallmark of invasive aspergillosis. Fever, cough, sputum production, and dyspnoea are non-specific symptoms. Two other symptoms that should suggest IPA are pleuritic chest pain (due to small pulmonary infarctions secondary to vascular invasion) and haemoptysis (rarely massive). However, the symptoms may be limited, and in patients with risk factors the diagnosis of IPA should be considered when fever persists despite antibacterial therapy. Minor haemoptysis should be taken as a warning signal that may herald massive haemoptysis at the onset of neutropenia recovery. Therefore, mild haemoptysis should prompt intensive supportive care (ventilation, blood, and platelet transfusions) and imaging studies capable of localizing fungal infiltrates in the lung and determining their proximity to large pulmonary vessels. Surgical treatment is required in some patients.

Chest radiographs often show non-specific changes. Lesions consistent with IPA include round densities, pleural-based infiltrates suggestive of pulmonary infarctions, and cavitations. Computed tomography (CT) of the chest is far more helpful, typically showing multiple nodules, sometimes with the very early halo sign seen as a zone of low attenuation due to haemorrhage surrounding the pulmonary nodule (Franquet *et al.* 2004). This sign is very specific, although it can be found in other pulmonary fungal infections. As it is often fleeting, CT of the chest should be obtained as soon as IPA is suspected. The air crescent sign, which suggests necrosis of the lesions after neutropenia recovery, develops late (after 2 weeks) and is less specific. CT of the chest may show that a lesion is located near a large vessel, a situation that may require surgery to prevent massive haemoptysis. CT of the sinuses is useful to look for concomitant sinus aspergillosis. CT of the brain should be performed if dissemination to the central nervous system is suspected.

A high fibrinogen level (8–10 g/l) suggests fungal infection, and IPA should be suspected in patients with risk factors. Early detection of circulating galactomannan by enzyme-linked immunosorbent assay is an important advance in the non-microbiological diagnosis of IPA and is now widely used throughout the world. Galactomannan is a polysaccharide cell-wall component released by growing hyphae during the dissemination phase. Specificity and sensitivity of the assay are good, despite variations across studies. In a recent study, sensitivity ranged from 67% to 100% and specificity from 86% to 98%, sometimes with very early positivity. However, false-negative results can occur in patients with a history of antifungal therapy, and false-positive results were recently reported in patients who had a history of treatment with β-lactams, particularly piperacillin-tazobactam (Walsh *et al.* 2004). Nevertheless, the galactomannan test is useful for diagnosing IPA, and serial monitoring of galactomannan levels provides a reliable index of the course under treatment. Moreover, galactomannan tests in other specimens, such as BAL fluids, has produced promising results. Finally, detection of *Aspergillus* DNA by quantitative polymerase chain reaction (PCR) in serum, BAL, and tissues holds promise as a diagnostic tool for IPA used as an adjunct to galactomannan testing.

FB-BAL is a major tool for diagnosing IPA, although its sensitivity has been less than 50% in most studies. Sputum specimen examination is an easy and cost-effective tool that can give good results. Fine-needle aspiration holds promise but has not been thoroughly evaluated (Nosari *et al.* 2003). Finally, lung biopsy is the diagnostic procedure of choice for IPA but is rarely performed, given the risk of adverse events associated with neutropenia, coagulation disorders, and a precarious respiratory status.

Data from the physical examination, laboratory tests, and imaging studies should be used to differentiate colonization from IPA. The European Organization for Research and Treatment of Cancer (EORTC) and the Mycoses Study Group of the National Institute of Allergy and Infectious Diseases have developed criteria for the diagnosis of proven, probable, or possible IPA (Table 5.3).

Because of the high mortality rate associated with IPA in immunocompromised hosts, antifungal therapy should be started promptly when the diagnosis is suspected, without waiting for definitive microbiological results. In haematological patients, antifungal therapy is often initiated when fever persists despite broad-spectrum antibacterials. Amphotericin *B* in a daily dosage of 1 mg/kg was the treatment of choice for several years, but the response rate

Table 5.3 EORTC criteria for invasive pulmonary apergillosis (Ascioglu *et al.* 2002)

Level of proof	Description
Proven IPA	Histopathological or cytopathical showing hyphae from needle aspiration or biopsy specimen with evidence of associated tissue damage
Probable IPA	**1 host factor criterion** (neutropenia, persistent fever refractory to broad-spectrum antibacterial treatment, severe GVHD, or prolonged use of corticosteroids) **and 1 microbiological criterion** (positive result of culture or microscopic evaluation from sputum or BAL, or positive result for *Aspergillus* antigen in specimens of bronchoalveolar lavage fluid or ≥ two bold samples) **and one major clinical criterion** (halo sign, air-crescent sign, or cavity) **or 2 minor clinical criteria** (any other infiltrate, cough, chest pain, haemoptysis, dyspnoea, pleural rub or pleural effusion)
Possible IPA	**One host factor criterion and one microbiological or 1major (or 2 minor) clinical criterion**

IPA: invasive pulmonary aspergillosis; GVHD: graft versus host disease

was less than 40% (Denning 1998) and renal toxicity was common. Moreover, many patients experienced immediate infusion-related reactions such as fever and chills. Antihistamine drugs and antipyretics can attenuate these reactions. Administration of steroids to combat infusion-related reactions is not recommended in this group of patients. Renal toxicity of amphotericin B manifests as decreased glomerular filtration with tubulopathy causing metabolic acidosis, profound hypokalemia, and hypomagnesaemia. These abnormalities occur after a few days of treatment and can persist long after the discontinuation of amphotericin B. Liposomal amphotericin B is associated with significantly less renal toxicity and sometimes with fewer infusion-related side-effects for an equivalent antifungal effect. It is indicated in patients with renal toxicity due to conventional amphotericin B and as first-line antifungal therapy in patients receiving other nephrotoxic drugs or having pre-existing renal failure. Voriconazole is a new broad-spectrum triazole that is active *in vitro* against various yeasts and moulds, including *Aspergillus* spp. In a randomized trial, initial voriconazole therapy was associated with better responses, improved survival, and fewer severe side-effects than initial therapy with amphotericin B. The main toxic effects are liver function abnormalities and reversible visual disturbances (altered colour perception, hallucinations). The spectrum of echinocandin antifungals is limited to *Candida* and *Aspergillus* (Denning 2003). Among these agents, caspofungin was as effective as liposomal amphotericin B in terms of survival and responses and may therefore be an alternative to other antifungal regimens. Studies are needed to evaluate the effectiveness of combinations such as voriconazole + caspofungin and caspo-fungin + liposomal amphotericin B. An exhaustive review published in 2003 discussed antifungal drug combinations (Steinbach *et al.* 2003). Care should be taken to avoid combining drugs with antagonistic effects. The optimal duration of therapy is unknown but depends on the extent of invasive aspergillosis, response to therapy, underlying disease, and future modalities of cancer treatment (chemotherapy, allogeneic transplantation). Neutropenia duration is a major prognostic factor, and neutropenia recovery is necessary to achieve a cure.

Because the overall mortality rate in patients with IPA remains very high (30–60%), surgical treatment combined with antifungal drugs has been evalu-ated. Although the numbers of patients are small, the results are promising in terms of survival and safety. This approach may be particularly interesting in patients with focal lesions (most notably threatening infiltrates) and in those who require further chemotherapy and/or bone marrow transplantation in the short term. No medications have been found effective in protecting against IPA. Laminar flow in hospital rooms, elimination of hyphae-containing material (including foods), and careful closing of windows reduce the risk of IPA.

Mucormycosis (**zygomycosis**)   Although rare, this infection is the second leading cause of invasive filamentous-mould infections, after aspergillosis. The lungs are the most common site of infection in cancer patients (most notably those with acute leukaemia). Pulmonary manifestations are similar to those found in IPA. There are a number of differences with aspergillosis: glycaemic disorders (often due to steroid therapy) and unstable diabetes mellitus are risk factors in addition to prolonged neutropenia, facial involvement (nose, sinuses, orbits) and cerebral involvement are common, and mortality is higher. Patients with other cancers are seldom complicated by this infection

Miscellaneous fungal infections   Pulmonary histoplasmosis, due to *Histoplasma capsulatum*, is exceedingly rare in Europe. This disease is endemic in North America, where it occurs chiefly in HIV-positive patients. It is often asymptomatic, and the diagnosis is usually made upon evaluation of cuta-neous or mucosal involvement or in patients with disseminated infection (Medeiros *et al.* 2004). Amphotericin B is the cornerstone of treatment.

Coccidioidomycosis is uncommon in patients with cancer. The manifesta-tions of pulmonary involvement range from flu-like symptoms to pneumoniae.

Yeasts

Candidiasis Invasive candidiasis, together with IPA, is the most common fungal infection observed in cancer patients. *Candida albicans* is the main pathogen; other species are *C. parapsilosis, C. tropicalis, C. glabrata,* and *C. krusei.* Secondary pulmonary involvement complicating systemic candidiasis with positive blood cultures leads to disseminated micro-abscesses. This situation should be differentiated from 'primary *Candida* pneumoniae', which is controversial as it cannot be distinguished from simple colonization or contamination of the respiratory tract.

Patients with secondary pulmonary candidiasis should receive *fluconazole* or amphotericin B, according to the susceptibility of the causative species. If pneumoniae is suspected, the need for antifungal therapy should be evaluated according to the severity of immunosuppression, clinical manifestations, and response to previous antibacterial agents.

Cryptococcosis Although the respiratory tract is the main route of entry for *Cryptococcus neoformans*, pulmonary involvement is second in frequency after neuromeningeal involvement (Saag *et al.* 2000). Risk factors consist of HIV infection and other causes of impaired cell-mediated immunity (haematological malignancies, treatment with steroids, fludarabine). In the past, patients treated for Hodgkin's disease were at high risk for cryptococcosis. As a result of changes in chemotherapy regimens, the risk is lower now, but cryptococcosis is also seen in patients with acute leukaemia. Among patients with pulmonary cryptococcosis, 25% present with limited clinical symptoms; the most common respiratory signs are a cough (60%) and dyspnoea (50%). Imaging studies show 5–20-mm solitary or multiple nodules, sometimes with parenchymal masses. Ground-glass opacities are less common but a halo sign may be present. Diagnostic investigations range from FB-BAL to pulmonary biopsy, depending on the desired level of proof and respiratory status. Cerebrospinal fluid should be obtained for an India ink test and antigen detection, which is also performed on a serum sample. Mortality rates in patients with pulmonary cryptococcosis are lower than in those with cryptococcal meningitis, and fluconazole is effective.

***Pneumocystis jiroveci* pneumoniae** The incidence of *Pneumocystis jiroveci* pneumoniae (PCP) is increasing in HIV-negative immunocompromised patients (Pagano *et al.* 2002). Given that impairment of cell-mediated immunity (alterations in the number and function of CD4 lymphocytes) is the usual underlying condition, the growing use of allogeneic bone marrow transplantation and the increasing intensity of chemotherapy regimens may explain this phenomenon. The main risk factors in patients with haematological malignancies are allogeneic transplantation (particularly when GVHD requires high doses of immunosuppressants); prolonged or high-dose steroid therapy; treatment with purine analogs (fludarabine, 2-cda); and treatment with alemtuzumab (*CamPath*), a recently developed monoclonal antibody directed against lymphocytes and used chiefly to treat chronic lymphocytic leukaemia.

The presentation of PCP in the immunocompromised patients differs substantially from that in HIV-positive patients. First, symptom onset in HIV-negative patients is abrupt and the symptoms worsen at a faster pace than in HIV-positive patients. However, the symptom triad (fever, dyspnoea, cough) is present in only one-third of HIV-negative immunocompromised patients (Pareja *et al.* 1998; Zahar *et al.* 2002). Second, the number of *P. jiroveci* organisms recovered from BAL fluid is smaller in HIV-negative patients, so that sputum examination has a far lower yield. *P. jiroveci* detection by PCR in BAL may be useful in this situation, but reliable data are lacking. Third, the use of adjunctive corticosteroids in HIV-negative patients with PCP is less well established than in HIV-positive patients.

Trimethoprim–sulphamethoxazole prophylaxis is essential in cancer patients receiving prolonged steroid therapy (>20 mg/day for >1 month) or repeated high doses of steroids (multiple myeloma, GVHD) and is also recommended for patients treated by purine analogues and alemtuzumab. Because of its haematological toxicity, prophylactic use of trimethoprim–sulfamethoxazole must be very prudent, and the drug should be stopped in patients with prolonged chemotherapy-related neutropenia or delayed neutropenia recovery. Because trimethoprim–sulphamethoxazole may antagonize folate metabolism, it should be temporarily discontinued when high-dose methotrexate is given.

Pulmonary parasitic infections

Toxoplasmosis

Toxoplasmosis is extremely serious in immunocompromised patients. Compared with HIV-positive patients, toxoplasmosis is far less common in cancer patients and occurs chiefly in bone marrow recipients. However, the incidence is not well known and varies across geographical areas, from 0.3% in the USA to 5% in France. Toxoplasmosis may be underestimated because of diagnostic difficulties related to the paucity of clinical manifestations. Thus, autopsy diagnoses of toxoplasmosis are not infrequent. Toxoplasmosis usually occurs 60–150 days after bone marrow transplantation, although cases starting as early as 9 days or as late as 1 year post-transplantation have been reported. Most cases occur in seropositive recipients as a result of reactivation of latent infection, often in association with profound immunosuppression due to GVHD and its treatment. The central nervous system is the most common target in immunocompromised patients. Pulmonary involvement may occur in recipients of allogeneic bone marrow transplants, usually as part of disseminated infection with myocarditis and liver involvement (Small *et al.* 2000). Diffuse bilateral interstitial infiltrates are visible on chest radiographs. The best diagnostic tool is FB-BAL to look for *Toxoplasma gondii* cysts. PCR detection of parasite DNA in BAL, serum, and cerebrospinal fluid holds promise. Because of the immunodeficiency, antibody detection does not carry promise as a diagnostic tool. The overall mortality rate is 60%. Chemoprophylaxis should be considered in high-risk patients. Pyrimethamine–sulfadoxine is effective, whereas *cotrimoxazole* fails to afford complete protection against *T. gondii* infection.

Other parasitic infections

Strongyloides stercoralis is an endemic nematode in tropical and subtropical areas world-wide and in the southeastern USA. *S. stercoralis* can cause pulmonary disease in immunocompromised patients (Wehner and Kirsch 1997). Two clinical variants exist, hyperinfection syndrome corresponding to accelerated autoinfection and disseminated infection with larval migration to other organs than those usually involved (lungs and gastrointestinal tract). Both variants develop in patients with deficiencies in eosinophilic and T-helper 2 responses, which are usually due to prolonged and/or high-dose steroid therapy. Diminished intestinal motility secondary to alkaloid treatment has been incriminated also. Alkaloids are widely used to treat non-Hodgkin's lymphoma and acute lymphoblastic leukaemia. Clinical manifestations range from isolated cough or chest pain to haemoptysis, dyspnoea, and acute respiratory distress syndrome. Accompanying gastrointestinal symptoms are inconsistent and non-specific. Skin lesions suggesting larva currens syndrome are common in patients with hyperinfection syndrome. The parasitological diagnosis can be made by stool or sputum examination, by FB-BAL, and by serological testing. Bacteraemia from a gastrointestinal source is often present concomitantly. Thiabendazole is effective. Finally, ivermectin chemoprophylaxis must be started before steroid therapy in patients from endemic areas.

A few cases of pulmonary infection with microsporidia after allogeneic bone marrow transplantation have been reported. Microsporidia are obligate, intracellular protozoal parasites belonging to the phylum *Microspora*. Lung involvement is far less common than involvement of the gastrointestinal tract and bile ducts.

Viral infections

Although pulmonary viral infections are not as common as infections due to common pyogens or to fungi, they are severe in critically ill cancer patients, most notably bone marrow transplant recipients. Causative agents fall into two groups: herpes viruses (chiefly cytomegalovirus or CMV) and community respiratory viruses.

Herpes viruses

Cytomegalovirus pneumoniae   Among herpes viruses, CMV is the main cause of pulmonary infections. In haematology patients, CMV pneumoniae occurs chiefly as a complication of bone marrow transplantation, with a very high mortality rate, most notably when mechanical ventilation is required. CMV-positive status of the recipient before allografting is the main risk factor. Other risk factors consist of CMV-positive status in the donor, matched unrelated donor transplant, severe GVHD, and T-cell-depleted marrow transplant. Most cases of CMV infection develop within 100 days after the transplant, although very late CMV pneumoniae (>1 year) may occur, particularly in patients using prophylactic ganciclovir.

Clinical manifestations consist of fever, dyspnoea, and hypoxia (Tamm *et al.* 2001). Gastrointestinal symptoms, mild liver function abnormalities, and splenomegaly are often present also. Imaging studies of the chest usually disclose bilateral lesions that may be seen as alveolar-interstitial infiltrates with ground-glass opacities, nodules or, less often, consolidation. Diagnostic tools include histopathological examination (with, or without, immunofluorescence) of a lung biopsy. In transplant recipients, necrotizing inflammation predominates, with relatively few CMV-infected cells (Kim *et al.* 2002). Lung biopsy is rarely performed in patients with thrombocytopenia. CMV pp65 antigen detection in serum is rapid, sensitive, and specific. This test is useless, however, in patients with neutropenia. Viraemia or viruria can be measured instead in this situation, although neither test is as specific as the antigen assay. Antigen detection in BAL may yield good results. Quantitative PCR can be used to detect CMV genetic material in blood and/or BAL samples. Culturing to look for a cytopathic effect is much longer. Antibody assays are not effective diagnostic tools in patients with immunodeficiency. Finally, the distinction between CMV infection and CMV disease should be made by an ophthalmological examination. The curative treatment is based on ganciclovir.

Herpes simplex virus (HSV) pneumoniae   HSV pneumoniae is rare and occurs chiefly in bone marrow transplant recipients. HSV1 is responsible for the majority of cases. HSV2 pneumoniae is exceedingly rare. The clinical and radiological features are not very different from those seen in other viral pneumonias. Treatment is based on intravenous aciclovir.

Varicella-zoster virus pneumoniae   This usually occurs in patients with no history of varicella in childhood. Symptoms of pneumoniae develop within a few days after the appearance of a skin rash and include fever, cough, dyspnoea, and tachypnoea (Frangides and Pneumotikes 2004). Chest radiographs typically show ill-defined nodular or reticular densities scattered throughout both lung fields. Rapid extension of these lesions is common. Treatment is based on intravenous aciclovir.

Human herpes virus 6 (HHV6)   A recent prospective study in 228 stem-cell recipients (most of whom received allogeneic cells) showed viral reactivation in the peripheral blood and other specimens in about half the patients. HHV6 reactivation was significantly associated with the occurrence of GVHD. However, HHV6 was considered a causal agent in only a minority of cases. Interstitial or alveolar pneumoniae occurred in association with HHV6 reactivation in some patients.

Community respiratory viruses

Respiratory syncytial virus pneumoniae   This causes about 50% of community-acquired respiratory virus infections in immunocompromised patients. Respiratory syncytial virus is also the most common viral cause of both upper and lower respiratory tract infections in children and can be transmitted to healthy adults, who then experience unremarkable upper respiratory tract infections. However, respiratory syncytial virus causes lethal infections in haematological patients, most notably bone marrow recipients (Whimbey *et al.* 1995). Pulmonary signs may be combined with rhinopharyngitis and sinus congestion. Radiological features are non-specific. The diagnosis relies on viral cultures, immunofluorescence techniques, and PCR on pulmonary, nasal, and pharyngeal samples. Because no effective treatment is available, the mortality rate is high (60–80%).

Other community respiratory viruses   These viruses are less common. They include influenza viruses, parainfluenza viruses, enteroviruses belonging to the *Picornaviridae* family, and adenoviruses. The influenza vaccine shows low immunogenicity within the first 6 months after transplantation and is therefore not recommended during this period. Adenovirus infection usually causes multiorgan failure in patients with severe immunodeficiencies. *Ribavirine* and cidofovir may be effective (Gavin and Katz 2002). Concomitant infection with more than one virus is not uncommon. The prognosis is usually poor (Martino *et al.* 2003).

Conclusions

Patients with cancer who are receiving treatments such as chemotherapy and bone marrow transplantation are extremely fragile and require close monitoring. Infectious diseases, heart failure, and metabolic disorders are the most common complications. Pulmonary infections constitute a major source of morbidity during haematological diseases. Many microbial agents can be involved. All forms of pulmonary infection can be life-threatening in critically ill cancer patients. Because increasingly intensive cancer chemotherapy regimens are being used, the frequency of opportunistic infections is rising in this patient population.

Although documented infection is rare, a detailed evaluation of underlying conditions, previous treatments, and clinical features often suggests a specific pathogen, thus helping to select the antimicrobial agents.

References

Ascioglu S, Rex JH, de Pauw, *et al.* (2002). Defining opportunistic invasive fungal infections in immunocompromised patients with cancer and hematopoietic stem cell transplants: an international consensus. *Clinical Infectious Disease*, **34**, 7–14.

Azoulay E, Fieux F, Moreau D, *et al.* (2003). Acute monocytic leukaemia presenting as acute respiratory failure. *American Journal of Respiratory and Critical Care Medicine*, **167**, 1329–1333.

Azoulay E, Thiéry G, Chevret S, *et al.* (2004). The prognosis of acute respiratory failure in critically ill cancer patients. *Medicine*, **83**, 1–11.

Berkey P and Bodey GP. (1989). Nocardial infection in patients with neoplastic disease. *Reviews of Infectious Diseases*, **11**, 407–412.

Blot F, Guiguet M, Nitenberg G, Leclercq, Gachot B, and Escudier B. (1997). Prognostic factors for neutropenic patients in an intensive care unit: respective roles of underlying malignancies and acute organ failures. *European Journal of Cancer*, **33**, 1031–1037.

Carratala J, Roson B, Fernandez-Sevilla A, Alcaide F, and Gudiol F. (1998). Bacteremic pneumoniae in neutropenic patients with cancer. *Archives of Internal Medicine*, **158**, 868–872.

Castor B, Juhlin I, and Henriques B. (1994). Septic cutaneous lesions caused by Mycobacterium malmoense in a patient with hairy cell leukaemia. *European Journal of Clinical Microbiology and Infectious Diseases*, **13**, 145–148.

Cordonnier C, Fleury-Feith J, Escudier E, Atassi K, and Bernaudin JF. (1994). Secondary alveolar proteinosis is a reversible cause of respiratory failure in leukaemic patients *American Journal of Respiratory and Critical Care Medicine*, **149**, 788–794.

Cordonnier C, Blot F, Yakouben K, and Pautas C. (2002). Neutropénies fébriles. In: *Pathologies infectieuses en réanimation*, pp. 452–476. Paris: Elsevier.

Cordonnier C, Buzyn A, Leverger G, *et al.* (2003). Epidemiology and risk factors for gram-positive coccal infections in neutropenia: toward a more targeted antibiotic strategy. *Clinical Infectious Diseases*, **36**, 149–158.

Danés C, Gonzalez-Martin J, Pumarola T, *et al.* (2002). Pulmonary infiltrates in immunosuppressed patients: analysis of a diagnostic protocol. *Journal of Clinical Microbiology*, **40**, 2134–2140.

De La Rosa GR, Jacobson KL, Rolston KV, Raad II, Kontoyiannis DP, and Safdar A. (2004). Mycobacterium tuberculosis at a comprehensive cancer centre: active disease in patients with underlying malignancy during 1990–2000. *Clinical Microbiology and Infection*, 10, 749–752.

Denning DW. (1998). Invasive aspergillosis. *Clinical Infectious Diseases*, 26, 781–803.

Denning DW. (2003). Echinocandin antifungal drugs. *Lancet*, 362, 1442–1151.

Denning DW, Marinus A, Cohen J, et al. (1998). An EORTC multicentre prospective survey of invasive aspergillosis in haematological patients: diagnosis and therapeutic outcome. EORTC Invasive Fungal Infections Cooperative group. *Journal of Infection*, 37, 173–180.

Elting LS, Bodey GP, and Keefe BH. (1992). Septicemia and shock syndrome due to viridans streptococci: a case-control study of predisposing factors. *Clinical Infectious Diseases*, 14, 1201–1207.

Ewig S, Glasmacher A, Ulrich B, Wilhelm K, Schäfer H, and Nachtsheim K. (1998a). Pulmonary infiltrates in neutropenic patients with acute leukaemia during chemotherapy. *Chest*, 114, 444–451.

Ewig S, Torres A, Riquelme R, et al. (1998b). Pulmonary complications in patients with haematological malignancies treated at a respiratory ICU. *European Respiratory Journal*, 12, 116–122.

Frangides CY and Pneumotikos I. (2004). Varicella-zoster virus pneumoniae in adults: report of 14 cases and review of the literature. *European Journal of Internal Medicine*, 15, 364–370.

Franquet T. (2004). Respiratory infection in the AIDS and immunocompromised patient. *European Radiology*, 14, E21–E33.

Gavin PJ and Katz BZ. (2002). Intravenous ribavirin treatment for severe adenovirus disease in immunocompromised children. *Pediatrics*, 110, 1–8.

Heussel CP, Kauczor HU, Heussel GE, et al. (1999). Pneumonia in febrile neutropenic patients and in bone marrow and blood stem-cell transplant recipients: use of high resolution computed tomography. *Journal of Clinical Oncology*, 17, 796–805.

Hilbert G, Gruson D, Vargas F, et al. (2001). Noninvasive ventilation in immunosuppressed patients with pulmonary infiltrates, fever, and acute respiratory failure. *New England Journal of Medicine*, 344, 481–487.

Hughes WT, Armstrong D, Bodey GP, et al. (2002). 2002 guidelines for the use of antimicrobial agents in neutropenic patients with cancer. *Clinical Infectious Diseases*, 34, 730–751.

Ip MS, Yuen KY, Woo PC, et al. (1998). Risk factors for pulmonary tuberculosis in bone marrow transplant recipients. *American Journal of Respiratory and Critical Care Medicine*, 158, 1173–1177.

Jacobson K, Garcia R, Libshitz H, et al. (1998). Clinical and radiological features of pulmonary disease caused by rapidly growing mycobacteria in cancer patients. *European Journal of Clinical Microbiology and Infectious Diseases*, 17, 615–621.

Jain P, Sandur S, Meli Y, Arroliga AC, Stoller JK, and Mehta AC. (2004). Role of flexible bronchoscopy in immunocompromised patients with lung infiltrates. *Chest*, 125, 712–722.

Karlin L, Darmon M, Thiery G, et al. (2005). Respiratory status deterioration during G-CSF-induced neutropenia recovery. *Bone Marrow Transplant*, 36, 245–250

Kern W, Kurrle E, and Schmeiser T. (1990). Streptococcal bacteremia in adult patients with leukaemia undergoing aggressive chemotherapy: a review of 55 cases. *Infection*, 18, 138–145.

Kim EA, Lee KS, Primack SL, *et al.* (2002). Viral pneumonias in adults: radiologic and pathologic findings. *Radiographics*, **22**, S137–S149.

Kress JP, Christenson J, Pohlman AS, Linkin DR, and Hall JB. (1999). Outcomes of critically ill cancer patients in a University Hospital Setting. *American Journal of Respiratory and Critical Care Medicine*, **160**, 1957–1961.

Martino R, Ramila E, Rabella N, *et al.* (2003). Respiratory virus infections in adults with haematological malignancies: a prospective study. *Clinical Infectious Diseases*, **36**, 1–8.

Maunder RJ, Hackman RC, Riff E, Albert RK, and Springmeyer SC. (1986). Occurrence of the adult respiratory distress syndrome in neutropenic patients. *American Review of Respiratory Disease*, **133**, 313–316.

Medeiros AI, Sa-Nunes A, Soares EG, Peres CM, Silva CL, and Faccioli LH. (2004). Blockade of endogenous leukotrienes exacerbates pulmonary histoplasmosis. *Infection and immunity*, **72**, 1637–1644.

Mulabecirovic A, Gaulhofer P, Auner HW, *et al.* (2004). Pulmonary infiltrates in patients with haematologic malignancies: transbronchial lung biopsy increases the diagnostic yield with respect to neoplastic infiltrates and toxic pneumonitis. *Annals of Hematology*, **83**, 420–422.

Nosari A, Anghilieri M, Carrafiello G, *et al.* (2003). Utility of percutaneous lung biopsy for diagnosing filamentous fungal infections in haematological malignancies. *Haematologica*, **88**, 1405–1409.

Offidani M, Corvatta L, Malerba L, *et al.* (2004). Risk assessment of patients with haematological malignancies who develop fever accompanied by pulmonary infiltrates. *Cancer*, **101**, 567–577.

Pagano L, Pagliari G, Basso A, *et al.* (1997). The role of bronchoalveloar lavage in the microbiological diagnosis of pneumoniae in patients with haematological malignancies. *Annals of Medicine*, **29**, 535–540.

Pagano L, Fianchi L, Mele L, *et al.* (2002). Pneumocystis jiroveci pneumoniae in patients with malignant haematological diseases: 10 years' experience of infection in GIMEMA centres. *British Journal of Haematology*, **117**, 379–386.

Pareja JG, Garland R, and Koziel H. (1998) Use of adjunctive corticosteroids in severe adult non-HIV *Pneumocystis carinii* pneumoniae. *Chest*, **113**, 1215–1224.

Patterson TF, Kirkpatrick WR, White M, *et al.* (2000). Invasive aspergillosis. Disease spectrum, treatment practices, and outcomes. I3 Aspergillus Study Group. *Medicine (Baltimore)*, **79**, 250–260.

Rabe C, Mey U, Paashaus M, *et al.* (2004). Outcome of patients with acute myeloid leukaemia and pulmonary infiltrates requiring invasive mechanical ventilation—a retrospective analysis. *Journal of Critical Care*, **19**, 29–35.

Rinaldo JE and Borovetz H. (1985). Deterioration of oxygenation and abnormal lung microvascular permeability during resolution of leukopenia in patients with diffuse lung injury. *American Review of Respiratory Disease*, **131**, 579–583.

Rolston KV, Jones PG, Fainstein V, and Bodey GP. (1985). Pulmonary disease caused by rapidly growing mycobacteria in patients with cancer. *Chest*, **87**, 503–506.

Rossini F, Verga M, Pioltelli P, *et al.* (2000). Incidence and outcome of pneumoniae in patients with acute leukaemia receiving first induction therapy with anthracycline-containing regimens. *Haematologica*, **85**, 1255–1260.

Saag MS, Graybill RJ, Larsen RA, *et al.* (2000). Practice guidelines for the management of cryptococcal disease. *Clinical Infectious Diseases*, 30, 710–718.

Small TN, Leung L, Stiles J, *et al.* (2000). Disseminated toxoplasmosis following T cell-depleted related and unrelated bone marrow transplantation. *Bone Marrow Transplantation*, 25, 969–973.

Soubani AO and Chandrasekar PH. (2002). The clinical spectrum of pulmonary aspergillosis. *Chest*, 121, 1988–1999.

Steinbach WJ, Stevens DA, and Denning DW. (2003). Combination and sequential antifungal therapy for invasive aspergillosis: review of published in vitro and in vivo interactions and 6281 clinical cases from 1966 to 2001. *Clinical Infectious Diseases*, 37, S188–S224.

Tamm M, Traenkle P, Grilli B, *et al.* (2001). Pulmonary cytomegalovirus infection in immunocompromised patients. *Chest*, 119, 838–843.

Tkatch LS, Kusne S, Irish WD, Krystofiak S, and Wing E. (1998). Epidemiology of legionella pneumonia and factors associated with legionella-related mortality at a tertiary care center. *Clinical Infectious Diseases*, 27, 1479–1486.

Torres HA, Bodey GP, Rolston KVI, Kantarjian HM, Raad II, and Kontoyiannis DP. (2003). Infections in patients with aplastic anemia. *Cancer*, 98, 86–93.

Von Eiff M, Zuhlsdorf M, Roos N, *et al.* (1995a). Pulmonary infiltrates in patients with non-invasive bronchoscopic procedures. *European Journal of Haematology*, 54, 157–162.

Von Eiff M, Zuhlsdorf M, Roos N, Hesse M, Schulten R, and Van de Loo J. (1995b). Pulmonary fungal infections in patients with haematological malignancies—diagnostic approaches. *Annals of Hematology*, 70, 135–141.

Walsh TJ, Shoham S, Petraitiene R, *et al.* (2004). Detection of galactomannan antigenemia in patients receiving piperacillin-tazobactam and correlations between in vitro, in vivo, and clinical properties of the drug-antigen interaction. *Journal of Clinical Microbiology*, 42, 4744–4748.

Wardman AG, Milligan DW, Child JA, Delamore IW, and Cooke NJ. (1984). Pulmonary infiltrates and adult acute leukaemia: empirical treatment and survival related to the extent of pulmonary disease. *Thorax*, 39, 568–571.

Watkins A, Greene JN, Vincent AL, and Sandin RL. (1999). Nocardial infections in cancer patients: our experience and a review of the literature. *Infectious Diseases in Clinical Practice*, 8, 294–300.

Wehner JH and Kirsch CM. (1997). Pulmonary manifestations of strongyloidiasis. *Seminars in Respiratory Infections*, 12, 122–129.

Whimbey E, Couch RB, Englund JA, *et al.* (1995). Respiratory syncitial virus pneumoniae in hospitalized adult patients with leukaemia. *Clinical Infectious Diseases*, 21, 376–379.

Wong PW, Stefanec T, Brown K, and White DA. (2002). Role of fine-needle aspirates of focal lung lesions in patients with haematological malignancies. *Chest*, 121, 527–532.

Zahar JR, Robin M, Azoulay E, Fieux, Nitenberg G, and Schlemmer B. (2002). *Pneumocystis carinii* pneumoniae in critically ill patients with malignancy: a descriptive study. *Clinical Infectious Diseases*, 35, 929–934.

Chapter 6

Genitourinary tract infections in cancer patients

T. Nambirajan and Joe M. O'Sullivan

Introduction

Infections of the genitourinary (GU) tract are a relatively uncommon complication of cancer treatment; however, they can be very debilitating and difficult to treat. In patients with cancer, susceptibility to urinary tract infection (UTI) is contributed to by immunodeficiency secondary to underlying disease, damage to the urothelium from the tumour itself, blockage of normal urinary flow by tumour, and most significantly to toxicity from anticancer therapy. There is a relatively wide spectrum of possible infections of the GU tract in this group of patients. A source of difficulty in the diagnosis and treatment of GU syndromes in the cancer patient is that some cancer therapies, in particular pelvic radiotherapy, and certain chemotherapeutic agents, e.g. cyclophosphamide, can mimic the symptoms of bladder infection leading to unnecessary antibiotic therapy. In this chapter we will discuss the spectrum of common pathogens as well as the spectrum of syndromes they cause. This chapter will address some of the common GU infection syndromes that can be complicated by a cancer diagnosis or cancer therapy. The specific management of neutropenic fever and sepsis caused by UTI is discussed in greater detail elsewhere in this text. The clinical syndromes discussed here are pyelonephritis, cystitis, prostatitis, sexually transmitted urethritis, and epididymo-orchitis.

Pathogens

The spectrum of pathogens responsible for GU infection in patients with cancer is best thought of in terms of the conventional classification of micro-organisms into bacterial, viral, fungal, and parasitic. Bacteria are the most common pathogens, responsible for the characteristic GU infection syndromes, including cystitis, pyelonephritis, prostatitis, epididymo-orchitis, and urethritis.

Pathogenesis

It is important to recognize the normal defence mechanisms against infections to understand how these are impaired in cancer patients. These natural defence mechanisms include flow of urine, voiding, and the presence of a normal epithelial lining, mucopolysaccharides coating uroepithelium, a normal perineal/vaginal flora, polymorphonuclear leucocytes, cytokines such as interleukins 6 and 8, and possibly immunoglobulins IgG and IgA (Korzeniowski 1991). The epithelial lining of the bladder and a layer of mucopolysaccharide form a protective barrier against bacterial colonization and invasion. Injury to the bladder mucosa by cytotoxic agents increases the risk of infection. In dogs, stripping of the bladder mucinous layer leads to increased colonization of the bladder mucosa by bacteria (Parsons *et al.* 1977). Radiotherapy and chemotherapy can interfere with the protective mucopolysaccharides on the surface of the urothelium and hence predispose to UTI.

Obstruction to urinary flow and stasis promotes bacterial multiplication and can lead to serious sepsis. In patients with cancer, obstruction may result from tumours originating within, and outside, of the GU tract (e.g. retroperitoneal tumours). Poor bladder emptying can be secondary to pelvic tumours obstructing the bladder outlet (e.g. prostatic, urethral, vaginal tumours) or neurogenic dysfunction (e.g. spinal metastasis and cord compression, radiation myelopathy). Instrumentation or indwelling catheters (Foley catheter, nephrostomy tubes) predispose to colonization from native flora and UTI especially in the presence of neutropenia from chemotherapy. Occasionally, urinary stones can predispose to infection in cancer patients. Stone formation in cancer patients can be related to hypercalcuria from hormonal abnormalities, bony metastases, or impaired mobility.

Various forms of urinary diversion after ablative surgery for pelvic cancers incorporate bowel in the urinary tract and these patients have permanent bacteriuria, which make them prone to UTI. Apart from the above-mentioned defects in local defence mechanisms, the general defence mechanisms can be compromised in cancer patients. These include neutropenia related to chemotherapy, defective T-cell immunity (hairy-cell leukaemia, lymphoma, steroid therapy) and defective humoral immunity (multiple myeloma, lymphatic leukaemia). Most uropathogens reach the urinary tract through the ascending route greatly enhanced by the bacterial pili, which aid the adhesion of bacteria to the uroepithelium. Haematogenous or lymphatic routes of spread are rare.

Signs and symptoms

Patients with compromised immunity secondary to cancer therapy can present without the classical symptoms of UTIs such as dysuria, frequency, and suprapubic pain. Another problem in the cancer patient is that these symptoms may also be misinterpreted as side-effects of radiotherapy or chemotherapy. The value of urine culture in these patients in differentiating infective from non-infective cystitis has been substantiated by various studies (Roberts *et al.* 1990; Prasad *et al.* 1995). Patients with neutropenia can develop frank sepsis in the absence of classical symptoms such as dysuria and frequency. In the neutropenic patient a bacteraemia of $>10^5$ colonies/ml is not necessary to trigger the instigation of appropriate antibiotic therapy.

Clinical syndromes (Table 6.1)

Pyelonephritis

Pyelonephritis is infection of the parenchyma and pelvis of the kidney. Acute pyelonephritis is most commonly caused by *Escherichia coli* (commonest), *Proteus* spp., *Klebsiella* spp., and *Staphylococcus saprophyticus*. It is usually an ascending infection from the urethra, or lower GU tract, and is rarely haematogenous in origin. Pyelonephritis commonly presents with the abrupt onset of chills, fever, loin pain, and tenderness over costo-vertebral angle, although it may also present as an episode of acute confusion. Investigations reveal pyuria and haematuria, as well as leucocytosis. Organisms can be cultured from the urine. Treatment with broad-spectrum antibiotics should commence immediately. These are usually administered intravenously initially, switching to the oral route after 2–3 days and then completing 2 weeks therapy. Antibiotics should be changed according to culture and sensitivity results from the urine culture. All patients should have complete imaging of urinary tract to rule out anatomical abnormalities, particularly those patients with the potential for obstruction to urine flow. While infection itself can be life threatening in cancer patients; infection superadded to obstruction (infected hydronephrosis or pyonephrosis) is more sinister, unless intervened urgently. Often these patients require urgent nephrostomy or double JJ stent to relive obstruction in addition to broad-spectrum antibiotics.

Cystitis

The usual causative organisms of bladder infection are Gram-negative bacteria. After obtaining urine for culture, broad-spectrum antibiotic therapy

Table 6.1 Commonly used antibiotics in genitourinary tract infection

Antibiotic	Spectrum of activity	Comments
Amoxycillin/ampicillin	*Streptococcus*, *Enteroccoccus*, *Escherichia coli*, and *Proteus*	Resistance due to β-lactamase activity is common all *staphylococcus*, 50% of *E. coli* and *Klebsiella*
Co-amoxiclav	Additionally covers β-lactamase producing organisms	Side-effects include hypersensitivity, hepatitis and cholestatic jaundice
Anti-pseudomonal penicillin—	Broad spectrum particularly	Shows synergistic action with aminoglycosides
Piperacillin, ticarcillin	against *Pseudomonas* and *Serratia* spp.	
Doxycycline	Chlamydia	Gastrointestinal upset
Cephalosporins 1st, 2nd, and 3rd generation	*Streptococcus*, *E. coli*, *Proteus*, and *Klebsiella*	3rd generation acts against pseudomonas in addition caution in patients with penicillin allergy
Trimethoprim	Covers 70% common pathogens—*E. coli*, *Enterobacter*, *Klebsiella*, *Proteus*, and *Serratia*	May act against some strains of MRSA
Aminoglycosides	Some Gram-negative and most Gram-positive organisms	Caution in renal impairment and in conjunction with other ototoxic agents, e.g. cisplatin, frusemide
Quinilones	Covers *Staphylococcus*, most Gram-negative organisms. Less effective against *Streptococcus*	Avoid in children. Caution in those with history of seizures, and renal impairment. Increases Warfarin levels
Nitrofurantoin	*Staphylococcus*, *Streptococcus* and most Gram-negative organisms	Gastrointestinal upset and rarely neuropathy

is commenced. The common antibiotics used include trimethoprim, nitrofurantoin, cephalosporins, and fluoroquinolone. The aminoglycosides are often used in patients with sepsis. The fluoroquinolones have broad spectrum of activity that makes them ideal for the empirical treatment of UTI. The use of ampicillin and amoxycillin has declined with the increase in the resistant strains (up to 30% of organisms). The potential nephrotoxicity of the aminoglycosides and fluoroquinolones should be considered before making the choice and dose may need to be adjusted according to renal function. Symptomatic cystitis should be treated with antibiotics for at least 7 days instead of usual 3 days course in the non-cancer patient population.

Catheter-associated infections (Table 6.2)

Though not unique to cancer patients, catheter-associated infections are a common source of Gram-negative sepsis. The following measures can be used to minimize the chances of UTI caused by catheterization. In the first instance, catheters should only be used when absolutely necessary. The catheter should be inserted by experienced staff under strict aseptic conditions in order to prevent the introduction of bacteria. Once the catheter has been inserted, a closed system of drainage should be maintained and patients should be adequately hydrated in order to maintain a good urine flow. It is important that gravity drainage is maintained by keeping the catheter bag below the bladder. Patients requiring long-term catheterization should have a change of catheter every 3 months. Once a catheter has been removed, urine should be analysed for culture and sensitivity and symptomatic or persistent bacteriuria should be treated.

When bacteriuria is identified in a catheterized patient (Table 6.3), antibiotic irrigation of the catheter may be tried; however, this technique does not appear to be as effective as closed drainage. In most circumstances asymptomatic bacteriuria does not need to be treated unless the patient is neutropenic. Patients with fever, systemic signs should be treated with broad-spectrum antibiotics and after obtaining urine and blood cultures, the catheter should be replaced. Removal of the catheter should be performed under antibiotic cover in order to prevent further infection by bacteria sequestered in the biofilm on the surface of the catheter.

Table 6.2 Prevention and treatment of urinary catheter related infection

- Catheter should be used only when absolutely needed
- Insertion should be under strict aseptic precautions
- Maintain closed system of drainage
- Maintain good urine flow by adequately hydrating patients
- Maintain gravity drainage
- After catheter is removed, obtain urine culture. Symptomatic or persistent bacteriuria should be treated.

Table 6.3 Management of catheter associated bacteriuria

- Antibiotic irrigation of catheter or bladder does not appear to be as effective as closed drainage.
- Asymptomatic bacteriuria should not be treated unless patients is neutropenic.
- Patients with fever, systemic signs and indwelling catheter should be treated with broad-spectrum antibiotics.
- Obtain urine and blood cultures.
- Replace catheter under antibiotic cover to allow for possible bacteria sequestered in the biofilm on the surface of the catheter.

Viral cystitis

Viral cystitis should be considered in immunocompromised patients with persistent symptoms of cystitis despite antibiotic therapy or negative urine culture. The viral agents involved include adenovirus, polyomavirus BK and rarely cytomegalovirus. Adenovirus has been associated with haemorrhagic cystitis (HC) in bone marrow transplant recipients. There is an increasing recognition of the role of adenovirus shedding in the urine in this clinical scenario due to widespread availability of polymerase chain reaction. Polyomavirus hominis 1, better known as BK virus (BKV) infects up to 90% of the general population. Owing to high prevalence and frequent reactivation, the role of BKV in the causation of HC has been difficult to define. The virus has been incriminated in HC and ureteric stenosis. Infection is diagnosed by urine cytology, polymerase chain reaction, and electron microscopy. The majority of viral cystitis episodes are mild and respond to conservative treatment with hydration. Intractable haematuria, needs bladder irrigation, washouts and occasionally, surgical intervention. Various surgical measures including diathermy or laser ablation have been tried without promising results. Isolated case reports of successful use of antiviral agent cidofovir have been reported (Hirsch and Steiger 2003).

Fungal cystitis

While these infections can occur in any cancer patients, those with diabetes, haematological malignancy, indwelling catheters, corticosteroid therapy, or prolonged antibiotic therapy are particularly vulnerable. Malignancy accounted for 22.2% of candiduria episodes in one multicentre study (Kauffman *et al.*

2000). The majority of these patients were asymptomatic and only 4% of patients had symptoms. Recurrent fever in these patients may be due to fungal infection and diagnosis often clinched by a high index of suspicion. *Candida albicans* is the commonest fungus encountered. The rare fungal organisms include *Candida glabrata, Aspergillus* spp., *Cryptococcus neoformans, Blastomyces dermatitidis*, and rarely other mould fungi. Urine and blood culture are essential for diagnosis. It is often difficult to differentiate colonization from infection in the presence of indwelling catheters. Total clinical assessment of the patient is needed before deciding on the need for antifungal treatment. Consideration should be given to remove the catheter, stent and stop antibiotic treatment when feasible. Local antifungal irrigant (e.g. amphotericin 50 mg in 1 litre of water administered at 42 ml/h) has been found to be effective for candiduria. Amphotericin B (6 mg/kg) is the gold standard agent for systemic candidiasis. Fluconazole and voriconazole both penetrate urine in therapeutic concentrations and can be used for treating infection.

Non-infective cystitis in the cancer patient

There a number of causes of non-infective cystitis in the cancer patient that can be mistaken for UTIs and merit some discussion here. The three most significant causes are alkylating chemotherapy agents, pelvic radiotherapy, and intravesical chemotherapy.

Radiation cystitis

Radiation cystitis is an uncommon side-effect of pelvic radiotherapy. It results from radiation-induced damage to the urothelium of the bladder. Radiation cystitis can occur during or shortly after a course of pelvic radiotherapy (acute) or more than 6 months after the completion of therapy (late). The symptoms of radiation cystitis are very similar to those of infective cystitis namely increased urinary frequency, dysuria, nocturia, abdominal pain, and haematuria. Urine culture should be taken to rule out an infective cause.

The symptoms of acute radiation cystitis usually subside in the weeks following the course of radiotherapy. A minority of patients require treatment for acute radiation cystitis. Dysuria can usually be helped by mild to moderate analgesia. Patients anecdotally seem to benefit from cranberry juice for the relief of dysuria; however, the mechanism of action is unclear. Previous work has suggested a potential role for cranberry juice in the prevention of UTIs (Reid *et al.* 2001). Alpha blockers such as alfuzosin hydrochloride, tamsulosin hydrochloride, and terazosin, can used to good effect in the management of frequency and nocturia particularly in men receiving radiotherapy for prostate cancer (Elshaikh *et al.* 2005).

Late radiation cystitis is a more serious complication of pelvic irradiation, which can again mimic UTI. The principal features of late radiation cystitis are haematuria and dysuria as well as reduced bladder capacity.

Chemotherapy-induced cystitis

A severe form of HC can be caused by oxazaphosphorine alkylating agents, particularly cyclophosphamide and isophosphamide (Pedersen-Bjergaard *et al.* 1988). Urothelial damage is caused by the excretion of metabolites of the agents known as acrolein (Cox 1979; Talar-Williams *et al.* 1996). The mainstay of management of the condition is prevention by using Sodium 2-mercaptoethane sulphonate (Mesna), which detoxifies acrolein and other urotoxic metabolites.

While the syndromes of radiation and chemotherapy-induced cystitis are well recognized it is also important not to miss a genuine UTI. For this reason, urine should be tested for culture and sensitivity whenever a patient presents with suspicious symptoms.

Intravesical chemotherapy cystitis

Intravesical therapy with cytotoxic agents or BCG is now commonly used in the treatment of early stage transitional cell carcinoma of the bladder. Both types of therapy can result in a cystitis-like syndrome, which will not respond to antibiotic therapy. Symptoms can be managed by reassurance and by encouraging patients to drink plenty of fluids. Low-grade fever or slight malaise may occur in a large proportion of patients. If fever higher than 38.5 °C persists for longer than 24 hours and does not resolve with antipyretic therapy or if fever higher than 39.5 °C is encountered, treatment with isoniazid (300 mg daily for 3 months) is necessary. Systemic BCGosis is generally manifested as pulmonary or hepatic disease and is a serious condition. This form of disease warrants a combination of isoniazid and rifampin for 6 months with the addition of ethambutol in acutely ill patients. Pyridoxine is added to any long courses of isoniazid treatment. BCG sepsis is a rare (0–4%) yet life-threatening condition that should be treated with standard life support methods as well as triple drug therapy. BCG-induced cystitis has a characteristic appearance on cystoscopy and biopsy. It is essential to exclude persistent carcinoma *in situ* from BCG cystitis, and biopsy is mandatory for this purpose. In any case of local or systemic illness with BCG, it is also important to evaluate common urinary pathogens as a cause and treat appropriately.

Table 6.4 National Institutes of Health (NIH) classification of prostatitis

- Acute bacterial prostatitis
- Chronic bacterial prostatitis
- Non-bacterial prostatitis
- Prostatodynia

Prostatitis (Table 6.4)

Acute bacterial prostatitis is usually caused by Gram negatives such as *E. coli*, *Pseudomonas* spp., or Gram-positive enterococci. It is characterized by low back pain, fever, chills, perineal pain, frequency, urgency, and dysuria. Rectal examination reveals a tender, firm prostate. Prostatic massage is contraindicated because of pain and risk of inducing septicaemia. Any transurethral instrumentation should be avoided, and if acute urinary retention develops this is best relieved by suprapubic catheter insertion. Antibiotics capable of penetrating the prostate such as quinolones or trimethoprim, should be used for 4 weeks.

Chronic bacterial prostatitis is usually caused by Gram negatives, *E. coli*, *Pseudomonas* spp., Gram-positive staphylococcus, streptococcus and diphtheroids. It presents with low back pain, perineal pain, and irritative voiding symptoms. Rectal examination reveals a tender prostate gland. Diagnosis is clinched by segmental urinary culture (Stamey's test). Urine sample is collected as follows: first 10 ml (VB1), midstream (VB2), expressed prostatic secretion (EPS), and 10 ml following the massage (VB3). If EPS shows >15 WBC/high power field or VB3 grows more bacteria than VB2, infection could be localized to the prostate. The treatment includes antibiotics such as trimethoprim, ofloxacin for 4–6 weeks, and anti-inflammatory and antimuscarinic agents.

Non-bacterial prostatitis is the most common prostatitis syndrome. The exact cause is unknown. It is associated with inflammatory cells in EPS and no definite organisms. Clinical feature is similar to chronic bacterial prostatitis. Presumed organisms include ureaplasma and chlamydia. It is treated empirically with minocycline, erythromycin, or ofloxacin. Symptomatic relief is obtained with α-blockers and anti-inflammatory agents.

Prostatodynia

Prostatodynia is related to pelvic floor dysfunction and not associated with UTI or inflammation in the prostate. Some relief is obtained with α-blockers such as tamsulosin hydrochloride.

The other form of prostatitis seen in cancer patients is related to BCG treatment (granulomatous prostatitis). Granulomatous prostatitis can be an asymptomatic finding in 20–30% of patients and may cause elevated serum prostate-specific antigen. This condition is symptomatic in approximately 1% of cases. Very rarely this may need isoniazid therapy.

Urethritis and sexually transmitted infections

Sexually transmitted infections should always be remembered in sexually active cancer patients particularly younger males receiving neutropenogenic chemotherapy regimens. The most common sexually transmitted syndrome is urethritis, which is usually caused by organisms including *Neisseria gonorrhoeae, Chlamydia trachomatis, Ureaplasma urealyticum, Mycoplasma genitalium*, and *Trichomonas vaginalis*. The usual presentation is with dysuria and urethral discharge. However, many infected females are asymptomatic, often identified by contact tracing. A urethral swab in males and swab from endocervix in females should be taken for culture and is often diagnostic. Ceftriaxone 250 mg intramuscularly is the drug of choice. Azithromycin 1 g (oral) or doxycycline 100 mg twice a day is the drug of choice for chlamydial urethritis.

Lymphogranuloma venerum is caused by *C. trachomatis*. It presents as a firm, painless penile papule (may ulcerate) associated with painful inguinal lymphadenopathy, fever, headache, and nausea. Serology is diagnostic and doxycycline is effective. Primary syphilis presents with a painless, 'punched out' penile ulcer; diagnosis is made by serological assay for antibodies to *Treponema pallidum* and penicillin G is the drug of choice. Chancroid is caused by *Haemophilus ducreyi* and presents as a painful genital ulcer, often associated with lymphadenopathy; it responds to erythromycin.

Epididymo-orchitis

Acute epididymitis is a clinical syndrome consisting of pain, swelling, and inflammation of the epididymis of less than 6 weeks. It has to be differentiated from torsion and testicular tumours. Ultrasound examination does not exclude torsion and is important in differentiating from tumour. Descending infections from urethra usually are the cause. The causative organisms include Gram-negative bacteria in younger men and sexually transmitted infection (chlamydia) in sexually active men. Ciprofloxacin 500 mg twice a day for 4 weeks or ofloxacin 200 mg twice daily for 2 weeks is the drug of choice. Azithromycin 1 g single dose is recommended for sexually active men. They should also be counselled regarding contact tracing.

References

Cox PJ. (1979). Cyclophosphamide cystitis—identification of acrolein as the causative agent. *Biochemical Pharmacology*, 28, 2045–2049.

Elshaikh MA, Ulchaker JC, Reddy CA, *et al.* (2005). Prophylactic tamsulosin (flomax) in patients undergoing prostate 125I brachytherapy for prostate carcinoma: final report of a double-blind placebo-controlled randomized study. *International Journal of Radiation Oncology, Biology, Physics*, 62, 164–169.

Hirsch HH and Steiger J. (2003). Polyomavirus BK. *Lancet Infectious Diseases*, 3, 611–623.

Kauffman CA, Vazquez JA, Sobel JD, *et al.* (2000). Prospective multicenter surveillance study of funguria in hospitalized patients. the national institute for allergy and infectious diseases (NIAID) mycoses study group. *Clinical Infectious Diseases*, 30, 14–18.

Korzeniowski OM. (1991). Urinary tract infection in the impaired host. *Medical Clinics of North America*, 75, 391–404.

Parsons CL, Greenspan C, Moore SW, and Mulholland SG. (1977). Role of surface mucin in primary antibacterial defense of bladder. *Urology*, 9, 48–52.

Pedersen-Bjergaard J, Ersboll J, Hansen VL, *et al.* (1988). Carcinoma of the urinary bladder after treatment with cyclophosphamide for non-Hodgkin's lymphoma. *New England Journal of Medicine*, 318, 1028–1032.

Prasad KN, Pradhan S, and Datta NR. (1995). Urinary tract infection in patients of gynecological malignances undergoing external pelvic radiotherapy. *Gynecologic Oncology*, 57, 380–382.

Reid G, Hsiehl J, Potter P, *et al.* (2001). Cranberry juice consumption may reduce biofilms on uroepithelial cells: Pilot study in spinal cord injured patients. *Spinal Cord*, 39, 26–30.

Roberts FJ, Murphy J, and Ludgate C. (1990). The value and significance of routine urine cultures in patients referred for radiation therapy of prostatic malignancy. *Clinical Oncology (Royal College of Radiologists)*, 2, 18–21.

Talar-Williams C, Hijazi YM, Walther MM, *et al.* (1996). Cyclophosphamide-induced cystitis and bladder cancer in patients with Wegener's granulomatosis. *Annals of Internal Medicine*, 124, 477–484.

Chapter 7

Bone and joint infections

Michael Laverick

Introduction

Bone is a common site for metastatic cancer and the majority of malignant bone tumours are secondary. Primary bone tumours, though uncommon, do present a formidable challenge as they occur most frequently in a relatively young age group.

Progress in chemotherapy allowing better disease control, progress in imaging allowing better pre-operative planning, progress in bioengineering improving prosthesis design, and increased understanding of distraction histogenesis have radically altered the approach to the treatment of primary malignant bone tumours. Disease for which only amputation surgery was offered in the past, often with poor outcomes, can now be approached by a combination of chemotherapy and surgery and, while amputation remains an option in many cases there are a wide variety of limb sparing surgical options available. Bone defects created by radical surgical excisions can be treated by metal endopros theses, a variety of allografts (including osteoarticular allograft, intercalary allograft, and allograft–prosthesis composites), arthrodesis, rotationplasty, free vascularized fibular transfer, and distraction osteogenesis techniques.

Infection in the reconstructed limb remains a feared complication common to all these techniques and is the commonest cause of failed reconstruction. Avoidance of infection continues to drive the choice of reconstruction technique and also developments in technique and prosthesis design.

Bone and joint infection is more common in the immune-compromised host. Although the literature relating specifically to the cancer patient is sparse it seems that they will be at increased risk of infection after injury or orthopaedic procedures.

Infection and orthopaedic surgery

Acute osteomyelitis and septic arthritis may result from blood-borne organisms or by inoculation in traumatic or surgical wounds. Acute haematogenous infection is more common in children than in adults and like the bone malignancies of childhood has a predilection for the metaphyses of the long bones, where it may present similarly with pain, swelling, and localized redness and tenderness. Chronic osteomyelitis may arise as the result of failure to eradicate the infecting organism or organisms.

In order to establish treatment protocols for this disease Cierney and colleagues developed the concept of the physiological class of the host (Cierney *et al.* 1985). Patients were described as A, B, or C hosts. A-hosts have a normal physiology, B-hosts will have local (B^L), systemic (B^S), or combined (B^{LS}) deficiency of wound healing. Local factors include extensive scarring, radiation fibrosis, and venous stasis or lymphoedema. Systemic factors include malnutrition, immune deficiency, and malignancy as well as smoking, diabetes, and steroid therapy. C-hosts were those for whom the treatment was likely to be worse than the disease. This classification has been modified so that B-hosts would have local or mild systemic disorder and C-hosts major nutritional or systemic disorder (McPherson *et al.* 2002). B and to a greater extent C-hosts are at increased risk of developing chronic infection, and have a worse outcome. In a study of 174 patients with open long bone fractures the incidence of infection was 4% for type A hosts, 15% for type B, and 30% for type C. Four of the C-hosts had malignancy and were 5.7 times as likely as the A-host group to develop infection when other factors were excluded (Bowen and Widmaier 2005).

Persistent discharging sinuses from chronic osteomyelitis may occasionally result in the development of squamous cell carcinoma (Marjolin's ulcer).

Infection following joint arthroplasty causes the failure of between 1 and 5% of primary arthroplasties. It is more common after revision surgery and in immunocompromised patients (McPherson *et al.* 2002). While *Staphylococcus aureus* remains the commonest pathogen in musculoskeletal infections, *Staphylococcus epidermidis* is the predominant pathogen in the presence of orthopaedic implants and methicillin resistance appears to be even more prevalent in coagulase negative staphylococci than coagulase-positive species (Mohanty and Kay 2004).

Routine precautions to try and prevent contamination of wounds at the time of implantation should include the use of ultra clean air operating theatres, prophylactic antibiotics, antibiotic-impregnated polymethylmethacrylate cement when used, and the avoidance of wound drainage. Simple measures such as reducing the number of people in operating theatre and reducing their movement have also been shown to be effective (Ritter 1999). Nonetheless contamination of the prosthesis, emanating from either the patient or the operating environment may occur in as many as 63% of cases (Davis *et al.* 1999). *Staphylococcus epidermidis* is the predominant contaminating organism.

Bacteria bind readily to most of the materials used in orthopaedic implants, including titanium, cobalt chromium, and stainless steel as well as polymethylmethacrylate bone cement. *Staphylococcus epidermidis* has a particular ability to bind to prosthetic materials and this is further enhanced by the production of an exopolysaccharide polymeric matrix or glycocalyx. This matrix and the colonies of bacteria within it are collectively called a biofilm. Biofilms are not unique to orthopaedic implants, and occur in association with many other implanted medical devices but are very important in the pathogenesis of prosthetic infections (Gristina *et al.* 1984). The ability to form biofilms is not unique to staphylococci, and once formed the matrix can attract other bacterial species to form mixed colonies. The slower growing forms of bacteria such as *Escherichia coli* and *Pseudomonas* spp. appear to promote biofilm production.

Bacteria within biofilms are resistant to several hundred times the normal bactericidal concentrations of standard antibiotics. A number of hypotheses exist for this protective effect, including the protective effects of the enveloping polysaccharide and phenotypic variation of bacteria. Antibiotic perfusion through the biofilm is limited by the molecular structure and charge distribution in the glycocalyx as well as pH gradients. Slow growing bacteria are less susceptible to antimicrobials and multidrug-resistant genes may be upgraded (Byers *et al.* 2000). Infecting bacteria, introduced at the time of implantation or by haematogenous spread, can remain dormant on the surface of an implant for many years until an alteration in host immunity or a change in local conditions such as loosening of the implant or periprosthetic fracture permits the proliferation of bacteria shed by the biofilm and the development of overt infection.

Attempts at prevention of the formation of biofilms are concentrated on promoting integration of the implant with the host bone. A stable integrated interface is resistant to bacterial colonization (Gristina 1987). Integration may be promoted by use of different materials such as titanium alloys (Sovak *et al.* 2000), by altering the texture of implant surfaces, by coating with hydroxyapatite (Furlong and Osborn 1991; Dumbleton and Manley 2004) and possibly by the incorporation of bone morphogenetic proteins (Wikesjo *et al.* 2001).

Attempts to eradicate biofilms include the application of pulsed electromagnetic fields, which are used to promote fracture healing and also appear to promote penetration of biofilms by some antibiotics in experimental models (Pickering *et al.* 2003). Ultrasound can dislodge bacteria from biofilms on the surface of explanted prostheses and thereby improve the rate of culture of pathogenic bacteria (Trampuz *et al.* 2003).

Although organisms are frequently inoculated at the primary surgical procedure, infection of prosthetic joints and other implants can occur by haematogenous spread from other infected sites but also as the result of transient bacteraemia. Prosthetic joint infection is second only to cardiac valve replacement as the site of serious infective complications following endoscopy. The risk of infection associated with non-cardiac predisposing conditions has been evaluated in the literature by Zuckerman *et al.* (1994) who reported on 486 consecutive patients undergoing gastrointestinal endoscopic procedures who were prospectively evaluated for the development of infectious complications. The most common non-cardiac risk factor for the development of infectious complications, noted in nine (1.9%) of the 486 patients, was the presence of a prosthetic joint (Zuckerman *et al.* 1994). In a different study of 16 cases of bacteraemia associated with endoscopy, septic arthritis developed in the one patient who had a prosthetic joint (Schlaeffer *et al.* 1996).

While routine antibiotic prophylaxis is not recommended for procedures such as dental extraction there are other procedures that do justify their use particularly in the immune-compromised patient. These procedures include upper gastrointestinal tract endoscopy, when a procedure such as biopsy, dilatation of stricture, or cholangiography. The American Academy of Orthopaedic Surgeons has added that antibiotics should be given to any patient undergoing a procedure that is associated with a substantial risk of mucosal injury or to any patient who has a potentially increased risk of haematogenous prosthetic joint infection. Patients at increased risk include: (1) those who are immunocompromised (whether because of an inflammatory arthropathy, underlying disease, medication, or radiation therapy); (2) those with type 1 diabetes; (3) those who have had a joint replacement within the previous 2 years; (4) those who have had a previous prosthetic joint infection; (5) those who are malnourished; and (6) those with haemophilia. Patients undergoing colonoscopy are at risk of prosthetic infection and should be given prophylactic antibiotics (Cornelius, *et al.* 2003). Clearly many patients, especially where the bone cancer is secondary will be at risk during this type of procedure. Many of these risks clearly apply to the cancer patient.

Infected total joint replacement is treated by one- or two-stage revision. Two-stage revision involves the removal of infected components and other foreign or necrotic materials and temporary insertion of antibiotic impregnated bone cement followed by staged definitive reimplantation of components, typically about 6 weeks later. There is considerable morbidity in the phase between stages as the patient is frequently confined to bed with an unstable limb. One stage revision is becoming more popular, but is possible only when components are well anchored and when the causative organism is known and sensitive to antibiotics. Implant survival in revision hip surgery for infection is much lower when the causative organism is a resistant strain

(Huo and Muller 2004). If the patient is unfit or refuses revision surgery long-term antibiotic suppression is an alternative but side-effects and the emergence of resistant strains remain concerns.

The orthopaedic management of bone cancer

Metastatic disease

Osseous involvement is the presenting feature of 23% of metastatic adenocarcinoma and operative treatment is indicated for most impending or actual fractures through metastatic lesions of the long bones. Pathological fractures have been reported to occur in 9–29% of patients who have bone metastases, depending on the location of the lesion. The most common sites of pathological fractures are the proximal ends of the long bones. Harrington reported that 258 (65%) of 399 fractures occurred in the femur, whereas only 68 (17%) were in the humerus (Harrington 1977). In deciding whether to select internal fixation or prosthetic reconstruction for the treatment of a pathological fracture in a patient who has metastatic bone disease, the surgeon must consider several factors. First, as these patients often have a limited life expectancy, rapid recovery is imperative both for maintaining the quality of life and for adjuvant treatment. Second, successful fracture-healing often is unpredictable for reasons such as continued local tumour growth, poor bone quality, poor nutritional status, and the effects of chemotherapy and radiotherapy.

The results of a retrospective study of the operative treatment of 166 metastatic lesions of the humerus and the femur in 147 patients indicate that mechanical failure is the major problem for the orthopaedic surgeon dealing with metastases (Yazawa et al. 1991). Femoral lesions were treated with a variety of implants including endoprostheses (28 patients), total joint prostheses (13 patients), screws and side-plates (nine patients), and intramedullary devices (18 patients). Failure of fixation or prosthetic replacement was reported in 11 (9%) of 119 patients who had a femoral lesion as compared with only two (4%) of 46 who had a fracture of an upper extremity. The rate of failure was high (three of nine patients) for fractures of the proximal part of the femur that were treated with a compression screw. Intramedullary fixation and prosthetic replacement augmented with methylmethacrylate were the most successful methods.

Primary bone tumours

Primary osteosarcoma is the third most common malignant tumour in adolescence after leukaemia and lymphoma and 75% of all cases occur between age

10 and 25 years. The tumour typically arises in the metaphyses of long bones, particularly the distal femur, proximal tibia, and proximal humerus—all areas of rapid bone growth (Mirra 1989). Lesions may also occur primarily in the diaphysis and can extend into the epiphysis.

Secondary osteosarcomas are associated with Paget's disease of bone or arise in a bone that has had previous irradiation. Both types are aggressive, destructive lesions of bone and have a dismal prognosis, usually with a rapid progression to distant metastasis. The use of chemotherapy may be beneficial, but the patients with these secondary osteosarcomas are usually more than 50 years and do not tolerate the chemotherapy as well as younger patients do (Gibbs 2001).

Ewing's sarcoma is the second most common primary malignant bone tumour. Although Ewing originally believed that the tumour was of vascular origin, recent cytogenetic and immunohistochemical studies have supported a neural cell origin (Dellatre *et al.* 1994; Scotlandi *et al.* 1996; West 2000). Eighty per cent of cases affect patients who are less than 20 years. The tumour presents most frequently in the femur, tibia, and pelvic girdle but can occur in any bone. Classic teaching is that Ewing's sarcoma is confused with bone infection because of fever and raised inflammatory markers at presentation (Durbin *et al.* 1998), but this is only present in 30% and other presentations such as limp or palpable swelling are at least as common. In a Swedish study of the presentation of malignant bone tumours (Widhe and Widhe 2000) Ewing's sarcoma was misdiagnosed as osteomyelitis in three of 47 cases as was one of 102 osteosarcomas. This and other misdiagnoses contributes to a significant delay in diagnosis of Ewing's sarcoma with 28% of patients being diagnosed 6 months after initial presentation to a doctor and 10% of osteosarcomas similarly delayed.

Traditional treatment consisted of surgery or radiotherapy, and the rate of survival was between 5% and 10%. When adjuvant chemotherapy was added in the 1970s, survival improved and the treatment of the primary site became more controversial. Currently, surgical resection has become the treatment of choice in the multidisciplinary management of Ewing sarcoma.

Current management protocols provide long-term survival rates of between 60% and 80% for patients without clinically apparent metastatic disease at presentation. Patients who have clinically apparent metastases at presentation fare considerably worse, with 5-year survival rates of between 10% and 20%. When pulmonary metastases develop after completion of therapy and the metastases can be resected, a 5-year survival rate of 20–40% can be expected.

Adamantinomas are rare, slow growing tumours occurring predominantly in the diaphysis. Adamantinoma is highly radio-resistant, and chemotherapy has not been shown to be effective. This, and their limited propensity for metastasis and local recurrence, has meant that they are often selected for limb-sparing reconstructive surgery. This type of surgery has been associated with a good outcome with 84% final limb salvage rates (Qureshi *et al.* 2000). The authors noted a high incidence of complications but did not specifically comment on infection.

In many ways, the presentation of a patient with a *chondrosarcoma* is similar to that of a patient with a metastatic carcinoma. Unfortunately, the diagnosis of chondrosarcoma may not be considered, and as a result, the patient's care may be compromised. Metastatic carcinoma occurs more frequently than does chondrosarcoma, and most older patients presenting with a destructive bone lesion will have a metastatic lesion, but in the patient presenting with a destructive radiolucent lesion of bone where there is no history of a carcinoma or myeloma a primary chondrosarcoma should be considered.

Treatment of chondrosarcomas is primarily surgical and it is important to ensure wide surgical margins, though this may be difficult in some tumours of the axial skeleton (Fiorenza *et al.* 2001). It has not been proved that limb-salvage surgery, with the risk of an inadequate margin, is justified when an alternative procedure, such as amputation, with a wide margin is possible. Patients who do undergo limb preserving surgery are at similar risk of infection in their reconstruction whether prosthetic or biological.

Limb salvage in the treatment of primary bone tumours

The success of surgical management of any primary bone tumour is dependent on the ability to attain wide surgical margins. This can be accomplished either by limb-sparing resection or by amputation. There does not appear to be any significant difference in long-term survival between patients who undergo amputation and those who have a limb-sparing procedure provided that wide margins are obtained (Rougraff *et al.* 1994). Since the introduction of neoadjuvant chemotherapy in 1975 an increasing number of limb salvage procedures have been performed. Limb-sparing surgery is indicated for patients in whom wide margins can be obtained without sacrificing so much tissue that the remaining limb is non-functional or non-reconstructible. The determining factor is the ability to spare or repair major nerves and blood vessels. There must also be adequate soft-tissue coverage obtained either locally or by tissue transfer techniques to ensure survival of the reconstruction. The overall reconstruction should function as well as, or better than, an appropriate prosthesis after an amputation. The options for reconstructing the skeletal defect include osteoarticular allograft, intercalary allograft, a metal endoprosthesis, an allograft–prosthesis composite, arthrodesis, rotationplasty, free vascularized fibular transfer, and distraction osteogenesis techniques. Interestingly limb salvage has been shown to be cost-effective in comparison with amputation and patients generally prefer limb salvage (Grimer et al. 1997).

Endoprosthetic replacement

Endoprosthetic replacement of resected bone offers the most rapid return to function after treatment of primary bone tumours. Given the predilection of both primary and secondary tumours to the metaphysic of the long bones this frequently means a prosthetic joint. Standard implants are frequently not suitable for reconstruction and a variety of modular and customized implants have been developed (Kotz et al. 1986). Extensive soft tissue resection as well as pre- and postoperative chemotherapy increase the rate of infection with initial reported rates of 2.9–9.7% (McDonald et al. 1990).

Endoprostheses have been carried out most commonly for lesions of the distal and proximal femur and the results in these locations are the most favourable. Grimer and colleagues reported the development of endoprostheses for the replacement of the proximal tibia after resection in 151 patients (Grimer et al. 1999). They recognized that their high early incidence of infection (36%) was related to inadequate soft tissue cover and abrasive materials. By modifying the surgical technique to include a medial gastrocnemius flap to cover the prosthesis they were able to reduce the rate to 12%. Of 28 patients developing infection 17 came to amputation, seven had two staged revision (six successfully) and four had persistent infection controlled by antibiotics. Aseptic loosening and breakage of components were other causes of failure.

The problem of endoprosthetic replacement in the growing child has been addressed by a number of methods. In the older child it is common practice to insert a prosthesis longer than the segment of bone removed in anticipation of future growth. Other solutions involve the insertion of extensible implants. Implants may be extended by mechanisms that include worm drives or implantable collars around the prosthesis. Spring-loaded devices have also been used. The more invasive the technique of lengthening the more likely the lengthening procedure is to introduce infection. The anatomical site of treatment appears to influence the outcome in this regard with fewer infections reported in upper limb prosthetic replacements. The proximal humerus is the fourth most common site for primary malignancy and surgical treatment may involve removal of the physis that is responsible for more than 80% of humeral growth. It is not acceptable to leave the limb short by more than a few centimetres. Ayoub and colleagues reported the result of lengthening proximal humeral prostheses. Eleven patients had a total of 44 lengthenings without deep infection (Ayoub *et al.* 1999). Interestingly it appears that diaphyseal endoprosthesis in the femur and tibia may also be inserted without deep infection (Abudu *et al.* 1996).

Allograft

The use of massive allografts to treat bone defects has been limited in the United Kingdom but used extensively in the United States. Allografts may be intercalary (inserted between two segments of the same long bone) or may include a joint or be incorporated with a prosthetic joint replacement. Typically allografts are fixed to the host bone by metal implants such as plates and screws or intramedullary nails and are thus susceptible to implant-related infection. Ortiz-Cruz and colleagues reported on the long term results of 104 intercalary allografts in 100 patients over an 18-year period (Ortiz-Cruz *et al.* 1997). Eighty-four per cent of the grafts were considered successful with the main causes of failure being infection and fracture. Failure was more likely with more advanced lesions and when adjuvant chemotherapy or radiotherapy were used. In contrast with prosthetic replacements the majority of failures occurred early (within the first 3–4 years). Of the 15 limbs in which the procedure failed, four were salvaged with use of a second allograft and three, with some other technique. For eight of the 100 patients, amputation was performed. Two amputations were for recurrent tumour and the remaining six because of unresolved infection.

In Asian countries, including Japan, allograft can be difficult to obtain for socio-religious reasons and similar techniques are performed by recycling the resected tumour-bearing bone after irradiation, autoclaving, or pasteurization. Theses treatments may cause weakness and loss of osseoinductivity in the replanted bone. More recently reimplantation after cryotherapy with liquid nitrogen has been described (Tsuchiya *et al.* 2005). Seven complications occurred in 28 patients including three deep infections (11%) and two local recurrences. In conventional hip revision surgery vancomycin impregnated allografts have been used to try and reduce infection rates (Buttaro *et al.* 2005).

Free fibular transfer

Free vascularized transfer for the treatment of skeletal defects was first described by Taylor in 1975 (Taylor *et al.* 1975) and use of the technique for defects left after excision of bone tumours by Weiland *et al.* (1977). The transferred fibula hypertrophies under load. Complication rates are as high as 50% although most resolve and do not influence the final outcome. Infection, however, occurs in 10% and may necessitate further extensive plastic surgical treatment or amputation. Development of infection is recognized to be associated with poorly vascularized recipient beds after reoperations due to tumour recurrence, fibrous scarring or previous non-union (Hsu *et al.* 1997).

Distraction osteogenesis

Distraction osteogenesis refers to the production of new bone between vascular bone surfaces created by an osteotomy and separated by gradual distraction. Although the first successful lengthening was reported by Codivilla a century ago (Codivilla 1905) techniques were unreliable and complications frequent until the method was refined by Ilizarov. He emphasized the importance of soft tissue preservation and a gentle corticotomy to divide the bone (Ilizarov 1989). Slow rhythmic distraction, typically 1 mm a day in four increments, using a circular external fixator attached to the bone with tensioned wires produces not only reliable bone regeneration but also stimulates the growth of other tissues including muscle, skin, and nerve (Ilizarov 1989).

Ilizarov coined the term bone transport for the application of distraction osteogenesis to fill intercalary defects of the long bones. He described a wide variety of strategies, primarily for the replacement of diaphyseal defects including acute shortening and relengthening of the tibia, transport of a bone segment across the intercalary defect, and transport of all or part of the fibula to replace massive tibial defects. Variations of the technique specifically for reconstruction after excision of malignant bone tumours have been refined by the group from Kanazawa (Tsuchiya *et al.* 1997). The same group have also described reconstruction of metaphyseal and epiphyseal defects after excision of osteosarcomas around the knee (Tsuchiya *et al.* 2002). A drawback of distraction osteogenesis techniques is the necessity of wearing the external fixation device for a prolonged period. Reconstruction of a 10 cm tibial defect could not infrequently take a year of treatment. To attempt to shorten treatment times, fixator treatment has been combined with the use of an intramedullary rod, and indeed fully implantable lengthening devices are now available. Other modalities used to accelerate bone healing include the use of recombinant human bone morphogenetic proteins and low intensity ultrasound. Concern remains that the activation of osteogenesis by these techniques may itself be potentially carcinogenic but to date there is only one report of malignancy at the site of distraction osteogenesis and this was where the primary pathology was known to have malignant potential (Ohmori *et al.* 1996).

Callus distraction techniques can also be applied using monolateral fixators and these may be better tolerated in the femur and humerus. The use of biological reconstruction techniques normally avoids the need to leave implanted metal or other materials and therefore should reduce the problems of chronic infection. Superficial infections are frequent at the sites of pin and wire insertion, however, and published results of biological reconstruction in the cancer patient are too few to draw definite conclusions at present.

Rotationplasty

Rotationplasty can be used as an alternative to amputation in patients with malignant bone tumours of the proximal, distal, or entire femur, and proximal tibia. A further indication is malignant bone tumours in children under 10 years of age as an alternative to an extendible endoprosthesis. It can also be performed as a second-line surgical procedure after failure, e.g. because of infection, of a limb-salvage procedure.

Rotationplasty was first performed by Borggreve in 1927 on a patient with a fused knee and consequent limb-length inequality secondary to tuberculosis. In 1950, Van Nes used rotationplasty in patients with a congenital defect of the femur. Its application in the treatment of malignant bone tumours, however, was first described by Kristen, Knahr and Salzer in 1975 and Salzer *et al.* in 1981 who used it as an alternative to above-knee amputation in a patient with osteosarcoma of the distal femur. In 1986 a modification of the procedure by Winkelmann allowed it to be used in patients with malignant tumours of the proximal femur with or without involvement of the hip as well as of the lower pelvis. Although infection rates are low other major complications such as arterial and venous thrombosis, loosening of the prosthesis and psychological sequelae restrict its use (Hardes *et al.* 2005).

Conclusions

Although bone cancer may initially be diagnosed as infection, leading to delays in treatment, the main effects of infection are felt in the results of reconstructive treatment of bone cancer. The introduction and refinement of chemotherapy regimens for bone cancer have enabled surgeons to obtain adequate resection limits for limb-sparing surgery. Resection and reconstruction techniques have been increasingly used to the extent that they now are the standard treatment in the majority of situations. Whatever method of limb reconstruction is chosen, infection remains a challenging problem and is likely to contribute to the failure of reconstruction. Amputation remains the ultimate surgical solution for failed reconstruction as well as remaining a primary treatment option in some circumstances. Improvements in prosthetic design and utilization and in biological reconstruction techniques offer hope of further improvements in the outcome of limb salvage for patients with malignant bone tumours.

References

Abudu A, Carter SR, and Grimer RJ. (1996). The outcome and functional results of diaphyseal endoprostheses after tumour excision. *Journal of Bone and Joint Surgery, British Volume*, **78B**, 652–657.

Ainscow DA and Denham RA. (1984). The risk of haematogenous infection in total joint replacements. *Journal of Bone and Joint Surgery, British Volume*, **66**, 580–582.

Ayoub KS, Fiorenza F, Grimer RJ, Tillman RM, and Carter SR. (1999). Extensible endoprosthesis of the humerus after resection of bone tumours. *Journal of Bone and Joint Surgery, British Volume*, **81B**, 495–500.

Bowen TR and Widmaier JC. (2005). Host classification predicts infection after open fracture. *Clinical Orthopaedics and Related Research*, **433**, 205–211.

Buttaro MA, Pusso R, and Piccaluga F. (2005). Vancomycin supplemented impacted bone allograft in infected hip arthroplasty. *Journal of Bone and Joint Surgery, British Volume*, **87B**, 314–319.

Byers RJ, Cox AJ, and Freemont AJ. (2000). The pathology of infected joint replacement. *Current Orthopaedics*, **14**, 243–249.

Cara JA, Forriol F, and Cañadell, J. (1993). Bone lengthening after conservative oncologic surgery. *Journal of Paediatric Orthopaedics Part B*, **2**, 57–61.

Cierney G, Mader JT, and Penninck JJ. (1985). A clinical staging system for adult osteomyelitis. *Contemporary Orthopaedics*, **10**, 17–37.

Codivilla, A. (1905). On the means of lengthening, in the lower limbs, the muscles and tissues which are shortened through deformity. *American Journal of Orthopaedic Surgery*, **2**, 353–363.

Cornelius LK, Reddix RN, and Carpenter JL. (2003). Periprosthetic knee joint infection following colonoscopy—a case report. *Journal of Bone and Joint Surgery, American Volume*, **85A**, 2434–2436.

Davies N, Kay PR, Panigrahi H, et al. (1999). Intraoperative bacterial contamination in operations for joint replacement. *Journal of Bone and Joint Surgery, British Volume*, **81B**, 886–889.

Delattre O, Zucman J, Melot T, et al. (1994). The Ewing family of tumors—a subgroup of small-round-cell tumors defined by specific chimeric transcripts. *New England Journal of Medicine*, **331**, 294–299.

Dumbleton J and Manley MT. (2004). Current concepts review—hydroxyapatite-coated prostheses in total hip and knee arthroplasty. *Journal of Bone and Joint Surgery, American Volume*, **86A**, 2526–2540.

Durbin M, Randall RL, James M, et al. (1998). Ewing's sarcoma masquerading as osteomyelitis. *Clinical Orthopaedics and Related Research*, **357**, 176–185.

Fiorenza F, Abudu A, Grimer RJ, *et al.* (2002). Risk factors for survival and local control in chondrosarcoma of bone. *Journal of Bone and Joint Surgery, British Volume*, **84B**, 93–99.

Furlong RJ and Osborn JF. (1991). Fixation of hip prostheses by hydroxyapatite ceramic coatings. *Journal of Bone and Joint Surgery, British Volume*, **73B**, 741–745.

Gibbs CP. (2001). Instructional Course Lectures The American Academy of Orthopedic Surgeons Malignant Bone Tumors. *Journal of Bone and Joint Surgery, American Volume*, **83A**, 1728–1745.

Grimer RJ, Carter SR, and Pynsent PB. (1997). The cost-effectiveness of limb salvage for bone tumours. *Journal of Bone and Joint Surgery, British Volume*, **79B**, 558–561.

Grimer RJ, Carter SR, Tillman, RM, *et al.* (1999). Endoprosthetic replacement of the proximal tibia. *Journal of Bone and Joint Surgery, British Volume*, **81B**, 488–494.

Gristina AG. (1987). Biomaterial centered infection: microbial adhesion versus tissue integration. *Science*, **237**, 1588–1595.

Gristina AG, Costerton JW, and McGanity PLJ. (1984). Bacteria-laden biofilms: a hazard to orthopaedic prostheses. *Infections in Surgery*, 655–662.

Hardes J, Gosheger G, Hoffmann C, Ahrens H, Winkelmann W, and Vachtsevanos L. (2005). Rotationplasty Type B1 versus Type B111a in children under the age of ten years. *Journal of Bone and Joint Surgery, British Volume*, **87B**, 395–400.

Harrington KD. (1977). The management of malignant pathological fracture. In: Instructional Course Lectures. The American Academy of Orthopaedic Surgeons, Vol. 26, pp. 147–162. St Louis, MO: CV Mosby.

Hsu RW-W, Wood MB, Sim FH, and Chao EYS. (1997). Free vascularised fibular transfer for reconstruction after tumour resection. *Journal of Bone and Joint Surgery*, **79B**, 36–42.

Huo MH and Muller MS. (2004). What's new in hip arthroplasty? *Journal of Bone and Joint Surgery, American Volume*, **86A**, 2341–2553.

Ilizarov GA. (1989a). The tension-stress effect on the genesis and growth of tissues: Part 1. The influence of stability of fixation and soft tissue preservation. *Clinical Orthopaedics and Related Research*, **238**, 249–262.

Ilizarov GA. (1989b). The tension-stress effect on the genesis and growth of tissues: Part 2. The influence of the rate and frequency of distraction. *Clinical Orthopaedics and Related Research*, **238**, 263–281.

Kotz R, Ritschl P, and Trachtenbrodt J. (1986). A modular femur tibia reconstruction system. *Orthopaedics*, **9**, 1639–1652.

McDonald DJ, Capanna R, and Gherlinzoni F. (1990). Influence of chemotherapy on perioperative complications in limb salvage surgery for bone tumors. *Cancer*, **65**, 1509–1516.

McPherson EJ, Woodson C, and Holtom P. (2002). Periprosthetic total hip infection. Outcomes using a staging system. *Clinical Orthopaedics and Related Research*, **403**, 8–15.

Meyer GW and Artis AL. (1997). Antibiotic prophylaxis for orthopedic prostheses and GI procedures: report of a survey. *American Journal of Gastroenterology*, **92**, 989–991.

Mirra JM. (1989). *Bone Tumors: clinical, radiologic, and pathologic correlations*. Philadelphia, PA: Lea and Febiger.

Mohanty SS and Kay PR. (2004). Infection in joint replacements. Why we screen MRSA when MRSE is the problem? *Journal of Bone and Joint Surgery, British Volume*, **86B**, 266–268.

Ohmori K, Matsui H, Kanamori M, Yudoh K, Yasuda T, and Terahata S. (1996). Malignant fibrous histiocytoma secondary to fibrous dysplasia. A case report. *International Orthopaedics*, **20**, 385–388.

Ortiz-Cruz E, Gebhardt MC, Jennings LC, Springfield DS, and Mankin HJ. (1997). *Journal of Bone and Joint Surgery, American Volume*, **79A**, 97–106.

Pickering SA, Bayston R, and Scammell BE. (2003). Electromagnetic augmentation of antibiotic efficacy in infection in orthopaedic implants. *Journal of Bone and Joint Surgery, British Volume*, **85B**, 588–593.

Qureshi AA, Schott S, Mallin B, and Gitelis S. (2000). Current trends in the management of adamantinoma of the long bones. *Journal of Bone and Joint Surgery, American Volume*, **82A**, 1122–1131.

Ritter M. (1999). The operating room environment. *Clinical Orthopaedics and Related Research*, **369**, 103–109.

Rougraff BT, Simon MA, Kneisl JS, Greenberg DB, and Mankin HJ. (1994). Limb salvage compared with amputation for osteosarcoma of the distal end of the femur. A long-term oncological, functional, and quality-of-life study. *Journal of Bone and Joint Surgery, American Volume*, **A76**, 649–656.

Schlaeffer F, Riesenberg K, Mikolich D, Sikuler E, and Niv Y. (1996). Serious bacterial infections after endoscopic procedures. *Archives of Internal Medicine*, **156**, 572–574.

Scotlandi K, Serra M, Manara MC, *et al.* (1996). Immunostaining of the p30/32MIC2 antigen and molecular detection of EWS rearrangements for the diagnosis of Ewing's sarcoma and peripheral neuroectodermal tumor. *Human Pathology*, **27**, 408–416.

Sovak G, Weiss A, and Gotman I. (2000). Osseointegration of Ti6A14V alloy implants coated with titanium nitride by a new method. *Journal of Bone and Joint Surgery, British Volume*, **82B**; 290–296.

Taylor GI, Miller GD, and Ham FJ. (1975). The free vascularised bone graft: a clinical extension of microvascular techniques. *Plastic and Reconstructive Surgery*, **55**, 533–544.

Trampuz A, Osmon DR, Hanssen AD, Steckelberg JM, and Patel R. (2003). Molecular and antibiofilm approaches to prosthetic joint infection. *Clinical Orthopaedics and Related Research*, **414**, 69–88.

Tsuchiya H, Tomita K, Minematsu K, *et al.* (1997). Limb salvage using distraction osteogenesis. a classification of the technique. *Journal of Bone and Joint Surgery, British Volume*, **79B**, 403–411.

Tsuchiya H, Abdel-Wanis ME, Sakurakichi K, Yamashiro T, and Tomita K. (2002). Osteosarcoma around the knee. Intraepiphyseal excision and biological reconstruction. *Journal of Bone and Joint Surgery, British Volume*, **84B**, 1162–1166.

Tsuchiya H, Yamamoto N, Nishida H, Tomita K, Wan SL, and Sakayama K. (2005). Reconstruction using an autograft containing tumour treated by liquid nitrogen. *Journal of Bone and Joint Surgery, British Volume*, **87B**, 218–225.

Weiland AJ, Daniel RK, and Riley LH Jr. (1977). Application of the free vascularised bone graft in the treatment of malignant or aggressive bone tumours. *Johns Hopkins Medical Journal*, **140**, 85–96.

West DC. (2000). Ewing sarcoma family of tumors. *Current Opinions in Oncology*, **12**, 3–9.

Widhe B and Widhe T. (2000). Initial symptoms and clinical features in osteosarcoma and Ewing sarcoma. *Journal of Bone and Joint Surgery, American Volume*, **A82**, 667–674.

Wikesjo UME, Sorensen RG, and Wozney JM. (2001). Augmentation of alveolar bone and dental implant osseointegration: clinical implications of studies with rhBMP-2. *Journal of Bone and Joint Surgery, American Volume*, **83A**, 136–145.

Yazawa Y, Frassica FJ, Chao EYS, Pritchard DJ, Sim FH, and Shives TC. (1990). Metastatic bone disease. A study of the surgical treatment of 166 pathologic humeral and femoral fractures. *Clinical Orthopaedics and Related Research*, **251**, 213–219.

Zuckerman GR, O'Brien J, and Halsted R. (1994). Antibiotic prophylaxis in patients with infectious risk factors undergoing gastrointestinal endoscopic procedures. *Gastrointestinal Endoscopy*, **40**, 538–543.

Chapter 8

Virus infections

Eithne MacMahon and Dakshika Jeyaratnam

Introduction

This chapter addresses viral infections including human immunodeficiency virus (HIV) in patients with solid and haematological malignancies, including those treated with haematopoietic stem cell transplantation (HSCT). The greater frequency and severity, atypical presentation and the challenges of diagnosis, management, and prevention of virus infections in cancer patients are discussed, with separate sections highlighting the specific issues in HSCT and HIV infection. The differential diagnosis of clinical syndromes is tabulated, supplemented by specific discussion of the most important viruses. Herpes simplex virus (HSV) and varicella zoster virus (VZV) are covered under skin and soft tissue infections (Chapter 9). The role of viruses in the pathogenesis of malignancy is discussed elsewhere, eg. Chapter 2.

Many factors contribute to the risk of virus infection in cancer patients. The underlying malignancy and the therapy administered diminish host defences, an effect greatly exacerbated by HSCT, graft versus host disease (GVHD) and consequent immunosuppressive therapy. The patient's age, sex, prior and persistent infections, immunization history, underlying illnesses, travel history, hobbies, animal contact, and risk behaviours, together with geographical location, season and nosocomial or community exposure to circulating viruses all contribute to each patient's ever-changing susceptibility to virus infection and disease. The usual principles of infectious diseases may no longer apply. Cardinal diagnostic features that reflect host response, rather than the infection *per se*, may be absent, e.g. parvovirus or measles infection without fever or rash. Patients are prone, not only to more severe manifestations of locally circulating viruses, but also to life-threatening consequences of usually benign opportunistic pathogens, e.g. cytomegalovirus (CMV). Expectations of finding a single unifying diagnosis to account for signs and symptoms are less, especially in the severely immunocompromised, where several different infectious agents may simultaneously be contributing to the clinical picture.

Table 8.1 lists the viruses of concern in cancer patients, and the additional opportunistic pathogens to consider in HIV-infected patients or following HSCT. Table 8.2 lists the wide range of viruses to consider according to clinical presentation. Of note, fever may be absent despite active infection. A careful history should be taken, seeking clues to possible infectious and non-infectious causes.

Serological responses may be delayed or absent, and difficulties in interpretation of results are compounded by passive acquisition of antibodies in blood and blood products, including platelets and immunoglobulin. Acute or reactivated virus infections should therefore be diagnosed by direct methods, using rapid diagnostic tests to detect viral antigens or nucleic acid where possible.

The various viral pathogens vary in their mode and ease of transmission. At one end of the spectrum, the influenza viruses, transmitted by aerosol, warrant respiratory isolation of cases. For others, spread primarily by droplet or intimate contact, prevention of transmission focuses on strict hand washing and contact precautions.

Table 8.1 Viruses of major concern in different clinical settings

	Solid organ tumour, leukaemia, lymphoma	Haematopoietic stem cell transplantation	HIV
HSV 1&2	●	●	●
VZV	●	●	●
CMV		●	●
EBV		●	●
HHV6		●	
HHV8			●
Adenoviruses		●	
Community respiratory viruses (CRVs)	●	●	
Parvovirus B19		●	●
HBV	●	●	●
HCV		●	●
JC virus			●
BK virus		●	
Molluscum contagiosum virus			●
HPV			●

CRVs: respiratory syncytial viruses; parainfluenza virus 1, 2, 3, 4; influenza A, B, C; rhinoviruses; coronaviruses.

Table 8.2. The main viruses to consider in the differential of clinical syndromes in the immunocompromised host

Clinical syndrome	Virus	Additional notes
Skin		
Maculopapular skin rash	Parvovirus-B19 ETV EBV CMV ADV HHV6 HHV7 Measles Rubella HIV-seroconversion illness (HBV)	Rash may be transient or atypical in the immunocompromised host. In cases of measles and parvovirus the rash may be absent. Measles is severe, frequently complicated and potentially fatal. Parvovirus is typically a biphasic illness, the virus infects nucleated red cells causing anaemia, and fever in the first phase followed by a rash and arthropathy. In the immunocompromised host disease can be monophasic with pancytopenia and no rash. Treatment is with intravenous immunoglobulin (IVIG). Prolonged infectivityhas been described. Rubella has been reported as a benign illness in immunocompromised children.
Vesiculopustular skin rash	VZV HSV ETV (vaccinia (Small Pox vaccine) Cowpox Monkeypox)	Shingles (VZV) can be multi-dermatomal or disseminate cutaneously and/or viscerally, with substantial morbidity and mortality. Cowpox has been associated with fatality in the immunocompromised host. In June 2003 there was an outbreak of monkeypox in the USA resulting from contact with infected prairie dogs.
Skin ulceration	HSV VZV CMV	
Papular skin rash	MCV HPV HSV VZV (HBV HCV EBV)	Widespread MCV is uncommon in HIV negative immunocompromised individuals. The extent of the lesions is inversely correlated with the CD4 count in HIV-positive patients. Cervical intraepithelial neoplasia caused by HPV is an AIDS defining illness. HBV, HCV, HSV, and EBV are associated with erythema nodosum.
Kaposi sarcoma	HHV8	May also be mucosal, visceral
Infectious mononucleosis-like illness	EBV CMV HIV-seroconversion illness (HHV6 HHV7)	Usually diagnosed serologically but maybe unreliable in the immunocompro-mised host. For transplant patients a negative pre-transplant serology, and virus detection by PCR makes the diagnosis.
Myelosuppression	CMV HHV6 Parvovirus-B19	

Table 8.2 *Continued*

Clinical syndrome	Virus	Additional notes
Respiratory		
Upper RTI	CRV ADV (EBV)	
Lower RTI	CRV CMV ADV (VZV ETV Measles HSV HHV6)	Measles giant cell pneumonia can occur without a rash.
Otitis media	CRV	
Sinusitis	CRV	
Gastrointestinal		
Oral ulceration	HSV VZV CMV	HSV gingivo-stomatitis has been associated with mucositis. CMV may cause mouth ulcers in HIV infection.
Oral hairy leucoplakia	EBV	Responds during antiviral therapy.
Warts	HPV	Effective treatment now available: Imiquimod.
Herpangina	Coxsackie-A	
GI ulceration	CMV HSV VZV (EBV)	HSV may cause proctitis. VZV may cause upper GI ulceration.
Acute diarrhoeal illness ± vomiting	GIV ADV CMV HIV	GIV and ADV: Detection by electron microscopy if $> 10^6$/ml of stool, or other rapid detection method. Norovirus causes projectile vomiting, which may be prominent (winter vomiting disease, WVD), and nosocomial and community outbreaks. WVD is characterized by a 12–60-hour illness. Nausea and abdominal cramps are common, fever may occur and diarrhoea is variable. CMV colitis causes diarrhoea, which may be bloody and is usually associated with fever. HIV causes diarrhoea only. HSV has been associated with diarrhoea in HIV.
Hepatitis	CMV ADV EBV HBV HCV HAV (HSV VZV HHV6 ETV HEV)	
Genitourinary		
Haemorrhagic cystitis	BK ADV (CMV HSV HHV6)	

Table 8.2 *Continued*

Clinical syndrome	Virus	Additional notes
Nervous system		
Meningitis	ETV HSV (HIV seroconversion illness CMV EBV LCM HHV6 ADV WNV, VZV WEE EEE Mumps)	Meningitis may occur in association with new or recurrent genital herpes infection. Meningitis is the most common extra-salivary gland manifestation of mumps, often occurring in the absence of parotid gland swelling.
Peripheral nervous system illness	CMV ETV HIV VZV	VZV may cause transverse myelitis. CMV in HIV infection (CD4 < 50 cells/ml) can cause polyradiculopathy. ETV including polioviruses may cause paralysis. OPV virus rapidly reverts to virulence and accounted for most recent cases of polio in developed countries. HIV can cause vacuolar myelopathy.
Encephalomyelitis/ encephalopathy	ETV HSV CMV JC (VZV, Mumps, Measles, ADV EBV WNV HHV6, Rubella, WEV EEV)	Mumps encephalitis may be due to CNS infection or to post-infectious encephalomyelitis. Measles encephalitis is well described in the immunosuppressed. Measles inclusion body encephalitis may occur following measles exposure in leukaemics and other immunocompromised patients, presenting up to 1 year later. EBV-driven lymphoproliferative disease/lymphoma is associated with both primary and persistent infection. Encephalitis maybe a feature of primary EBV infection. JC causes progressive multifocal leucoencephalopathy (PML) in severely immunocompromised hosts. (WNV is also seen in North America and Europe).

[1] Uncommon causes are in brackets. Geographical variation may apply.

[2] Abbreviations (in alphabetical order): acquired immunodeficiency syndrome (AIDS). Adenovirus (ADV). BK virus (BK). Community respiratory viruses (CRV), *see below*. Eastern equine encephalitis virus (EEE). Enterovirus (ETV). Epstein–Barr virus (EBV). Gastrointestinal (GI). GI viruses (GIV), *see below*. Hepatitis A virus (HAV). Hepatitis B virus (HBV). Hepatitis C virus (HCV). Herpes simplex virus (HSV). Human herpesvirus (HHV). Human immunodeficiency virus (HIV). Human papillomavirus (HPV). JC virus (JC). Lymphocytic choriomeningitis virus (LCM). Molluscum contagiosum virus (MCV). Oral polio vaccine (OPV). Respiratory tract illness (RTI). Varicella zoster virus (VZV). West Nile virus (WNV). Western equine encephalitis virus (WEE).

[3] Collective groups of viruses. CRV: respiratory syncytial virus, influenza virus A–C, parainfluenza virus 1–4, metapneumovirus, rhinovirus, coronavirus (including SARS). GIV: noroviruses, rotaviruses, calicivirus, astroviruses.

Haematopoietic stem cell transplantation (HSCT)

Among cancer patients, HSCT recipients bear the brunt of viral complications.

Following the transplant conditioning, three consecutive phases have been recognized, with the risk of different infections paralleling the depression and recovery of different leucocyte lineages. During pre-engraftment (phase I, <30 days after transplantation), when neutropenia and breaches of mucocutaneous barriers predominate, HSV reactivation is the only common viral manifestation. During the early post-engraftment phase (phase II, 30–100 days) when cellular immunity is impaired and acute GVHD may warrant immunosuppression, reactivation of latent virus infections in the graft and/or host may present clinically (CMV, Epstein–Barr virus (EBV), human herpesvirus type 6 (HHV6), BK virus). This timetable of viral infection hails from the early era of HSCT, predating strategic developments in the nature and manipulation of HSC, conditioning regimens, use of haematological growth factors, management of GVHD, and the prevention of viral disease.

While all HSCT recipients are at risk of virus-induced morbidity and mortality, in general the risk is lowest for autologous and syngeneic HSCT, higher for matched related allogeneic transplants and greatest for 'alternate' donor HSCT. 'Alternate' includes matched unrelated donors (MUD), mismatched related donors, and umbilical cord blood (UCB). Acute and chronic GVHD and their treatment add to the risk of infection. The varying frequency and timing of opportunistic infections according to the type of HSCT has been reviewed (Wingard 1999).

In HSCT, myeloablative conditioning regimens rapidly result in the loss of T-cells, B-cells, and the accumulated immune memory of the recipient. More recently, the non-myeloablative reduced-intensity conditioning HSCTs (RIC-HSCT) or 'mini-allos' have facilitated treatment of a broader spectrum of patients. Acquiring donor leucocytes, while retaining their own clones, recipients become immunological chimeras. These patients are spared the high-risk initial pre-engraftment phase but the requirement for immunosuppressive therapy to control GVHD predisposes to infection.

Pre-transplant screening of donors and recipients is mandatory (Department of Health 2000; US Department of Health & Human Services 2000). After careful history, examination, and serological/nucleic acid screening, potential allogeneic donors with evidence of, or at risk of, HIV1, HIV2, hepatitis B virus (HBV), hepatitis C virus (HCV), and human T-cell lymphotropic virus (HTLV) 1 or 2 are generally excluded. However, HBV- and HCV-positive donors may warrant consideration on an individual case basis following careful risk assessment and specialist advice. Testing of prospective allogeneic and autologous recipients for these infections is likewise routine, identifying patients who warrant careful reconsideration of the risks/benefit and require careful monitoring and management if HSCT is undertaken.

Recipient and donor are also routinely screened for CMV and in many centres the recipient's EBV, HSV, and varicella zoster virus (VZV) immunoglobulin G (IgG) status is also determined. Unless there is evidence of recent primary infection in the donor, evidence of herpesvirus infections do not exclude donors but serve to indicate the recipient risk and to some extent determine management. Following primary infection with viruses of the herpes family, infection persists lifelong, together with virus-specific IgG, and can reactivate causing clinical symptoms. Both CMV and EBV can be transmitted in the HSCT, together with virus-specific immune cells. But passive transfer of donor immune memory is unpredictable.

HSCT recipients should commence an individually tailored programme of vaccination. Live vaccines are contraindicated until 24 months post-transplant and in all patients with chronic GVHD and/or receiving immunosuppressive therapy (US Department of Health & Human Services 2000; Ljungman *et al.* 2005).

Human immunodeficiency virus

While a full discussion is beyond the scope of this chapter, here we outline the salient features of infection and current approaches to management. Following infection HIV infects CD4-positive cells resulting in cytolysis and high-level plasma viraemia. Subsequently the viral load falls, with recovery of the CD4 count and HIV-specific seroconversion within 3 months. Primary infection may be asymptomatic or manifest clinically as a mononuclear-like syndrome, termed seroconversion illness. For a median of 10 years, HIV infection is clinically quiescent, despite the continued massive turnover of virus and CD4-positive cells. Ultimately, however, increasing lymphopenia is manifest by progression to AIDS and opportunistic infections/tumours. HIV1 accounts for the vast majority of cases world-wide. HIV2, predominant in West Africa, is associated with a slower progression of disease.

As shown in Table 8.1, the spectrum of opportunistic virus infections seen in HSCT, and in AIDS, are somewhat different and nor do they share the same predominant clinical manifestation. For example, CMV pneumonitis, a major threat in HSCT recipients, is rarely a feature of end-stage HIV infection, where CMV instead typically causes potentially sight-threatening retinitis. With the advent of highly active anti-retroviral therapy (HAART), opportunistic infections are now much less common in developed countries, with cases largely confined to late presentations and therapeutic failures.

Management of HIV patients on HAART has become increasingly complex, with individualized therapy necessitating both the input of a specialist HIV physician and sophisticated laboratory services. The optimal timing for initiation of HAART remains controversial. Therapy comprises at least two drugs selected from 20 or more antiretroviral agents of several different classes including nucleoside and non-nucleoside reverse transcriptase inhibitors, protease inhibitors, and fusion inhibitors. The therapeutic benefit is monitored by serial measurements of plasma viral load and CD4+ counts. The detection of drug resistance mutations (by genotypic analysis and/or virtual phenotyping) in the patient's viral RNA permits the substitution of more effective therapy. Successful HAART restores immune function, prevents opportunistic infections and may allow the discontinuation of prophylaxis (USPHS/IDSA 2000; The EACS Euroguidelines Group 2003). Unfortunately the reconstitution of the immune system that results from HAART may exacerbate opportunistic infections, e.g. CMV retinitis.

While the risk of HIV-associated Kaposi's sarcoma and non-Hodgkin's lymphoma has declined in the HAART era, the risk of other malignancies, e.g. lung cancer has increased (Clifford *et al.* 2005; Engels and Goedert 2005). Whether immunodeficiency is a contributory factor is unknown but disproportionately high rates of smoking and other risk factors (HBV, HCV, human papillomavirus infections) among individuals living with HIV/AIDS in developed countries have been implicated in the higher risk of associated malignancies (Engels and Goedert 2005).

Unless all HAART options have already been exhausted, immune restoration, if possible, facilitates chemotherapy and allows closer approximation to the usual dosage regimens. However, HAART does not restore the patient to an even playing field, with CMV detection in blood continuing to identify patients with a poor prognosis (Deayton *et al.* 2004). Extra vigilance is also required as newer immunosuppressive agents, e.g. Rituximab, add to the risk of toxicity (Spina *et al.* 2005). Management of malignancy in these HIV patients warrants multidisciplinary input including expertise in infectious diseases and the management of HIV.

Cytomegalovirus

CMV infection is common among adults in developed nations of whom approximately 60% are seropositive. Primary infection is usually subclinical but CMV then persists lifelong, with asymptomatic reactivation in body tissues facilitating transmission via saliva, blood, body fluids, organs, and tissues. Serological detection of CMV IgG thus identifies infected individuals.

This typically benign course of infection in the immunocompetent stands in stark contrast to that in immunodeficient patients, for whom CMV poses a major threat. Although CMV can cause disease in patients with haematological malignancies and solid organ tumours, cases are uncommon (Torres et al. 2005). Most morbidity and mortality attributable to CMV occurs in those with deficient T-cell immunity (HSCT and solid organ transplant recipients or HIV-infected individuals), with manifestations including fever, hepatitis, and upper or lower gastrointestinal ulceration. However, CMV preferentially targets certain organs in the different patient groups: causing pneumonitis and myelosuppression in HSCT recipients, and encephalopathy and polyradiculopathy in end-stage HIV infection.

CMV manifests a broad cellular and tissue tropism *in vivo*, persisting in CMV-seropositive recipients after destruction of immune defences following myeloablative HSCT, or transmitted to seronegative recipients with the stem cells. With the loss of host/virus *status quo*, CMV reactivation and replication, i.e. 'CMV infection' is the rule, frequently culminating in end-organ disease. CMV infection is defined as the isolation of virus or detection of viral components (proteins or nucleic acid) in body fluids or tissue. The term 'CMV syndrome' has been used where CMV infection is accompanied by fever and bone marrow suppression, but the use of this terminology has been discouraged in HSCT, as other viruses, e.g. HHV6 or HHV7, or adenovirus might be responsible (Ljungman et al. 2002b). In the internationally agreed definitions of CMV end-organ diseases, CMV pneumonia is defined as the presence of signs or symptoms of pulmonary disease together with the detection of CMV in the bronchoalveolar lavage fluid or lung tissue by a non-polymerase chain reaction (PCR) based method (Ljungman et al. 2002b). CMV pneumonia may be immunopathologically mediated and although not subjected to rigorous evaluation, the use of high-dose intravenous immune globulin (IVIG) in addition to ganciclovir is the accepted standard of care (Grundy et al.1987; Emanuel et al. 1988; Reed et al. 1988). Even with treatment, CMV pneumonitis carries a high mortality with only a 50% survival rate. There is no evidence to support the use of IVIG to treat other manifestations of CMV disease.

The risk of disease is greatest in CMV-seropositive recipients (R+) but whether the use of a CMV-seropositive donor (D+) rather than a seronegative donor (D−) improves survival is controversial (Kollman et al. 2001; Ljungman et al. 2003a). CMV-seronegative HSCT recipients (R−) with CMV D+ are also at risk (albeit much less) therefore, where possible, a CMV D− should be used (Ljungman et al. 2004). Prospective CMV D− R− should only receive blood products which are either leucodepleted or from CMV-seronegative blood donors, and all R− advised how to avoid CMV acquisition (US Department of Health & Human Services 2000; Ljungman *et al*. 2004). Immunosuppressive therapy to prevent or treat GVHD increases the risk of CMV disease and while recent years have seen improved survival rates among recipients of matched related transplants, these benefits have not been extended to the recipients of 'alternate' grafts. Although uncommon, CMV disease in seropositive autologous recipients has a morbidity and mortality comparable with that in allogeneic recipients (Reusser *et al*. 1990; Ljungman *et al*. 1994).

The burden of illness and death from CMV disease in allogeneic recipients, despite the use of antiviral therapy, emphasized the need for preventative strategies and two main themes have emerged.

In routine prophylaxis, all at-risk patients receive antiviral therapy for a predetermined period, usually until 100 days post-transplant. Several different drugs are available. Aciclovir and valaciclovir are not sufficiently active to treat CMV infection but as prophylactic agents have been shown to reduce the incidence of infection but not CMV disease (Prentice *et al*. 1994; Ljungman *et al*. 2002a). Possible beneficial effects on survival are controversial (Prentice *et al*. 1994). Owing to limited efficacy, surveillance and pre-emptive therapy is still required (US Department of Health & Human Services 2000; Ljungman *et al*. 2004). Intravenous ganciclovir prophylaxis does reduce CMV disease but is associated with late-onset CMV disease and a significant risk of neutropenia, and does not increase survival (Li *et al*. 1994; Winston *et al*. 2003). Valganciclovir, the oral prodrug of ganciclovir with improved oral bioavailability, has yet to be evaluated for prophylaxis.

The pre-emptive approach is based on routine weekly surveillance testing to detect CMV infection in blood, peripheral blood leucocytes or plasma, using a sensitive test (pp65 antigenaemia or nucleic acid testing) with a high positive predictive value for CMV disease (Meyers *et al*. 1990; Einsele *et al*. 1995; Boeckh *et al*. 1996). Positive test results trigger the administration of pre-emptive antiviral therapy until 100 days post-transplant, or for a minimum of 3 weeks, or until CMV is undetectable, followed by resumption of weekly surveillance. Nucleic acid testing is useful when neutropenia precludes the detection of antigenaemia. Quantitative PRC viral load measurements are more predictive of disease than qualitative tests and also have a role in monitoring therapeutic response and in determining the duration of CMV therapy (Emery *et al*. 2000; Mattes *et al*. 2004). Pre-emptive therapy has been shown to reduce the risk of CMV disease and mortality (Einsele *et al*. 1995). Intravenous ganciclovir and foscarnet are both effective (Reusser *et al*. 2002). Unlike ganciclovir, foscarnet does not cause neutropenia but requires close monitoring for electrolyte imbalance. The use of oral formulations place of intravenous ganciclovir is currently under investigation. Cidofovir requires only weekly administration but, due to the high risk of nephrotoxicity, remains a second-line agent.

Clearly the pre-emptive approach requires sophisticated laboratory support but avoids the expense and toxicity associated with the routine administration of antivirals over long periods to patients who might never have developed symptoms. Routine ganciclovir prophylaxis is associated with delayed CMV-specific immune reconstitution and the development of late CMV disease (Li *et al.* 1994). It may also increase the risk of developing antiviral drug-resistant CMV.

Guidelines have recommended that all at-risk patients (D− R+, D+ R+, and D+ R−) be placed on a CMV disease prevention programme from engraftment until 100 days post-transplant. Either approach may be used but, where possible, the pre-emptive strategy is preferred over routine prophylaxis for the relatively low risk D+ R− patients (US Department of Health & Human Services 2000). According to the more recently published European recommendations, all allogeneic HSCT recipients should be under CMV surveillance whether or not CMV prophylaxis has been administered, to continue for at least 100 days (Ljungman *et al.* 2004). Patients at risk of late disease, i.e. those with acute or chronic GVHD, alternate transplants, or prior CMV reactivation, require longer surveillance (Ljungman *et al.* 2004).

In the future, the prevention of CMV disease may not depend solely on antiviral agents: the massive *in vivo* expansion of allogeneic donor-derived CMV-specific T-cells following short-term culture *in vitro*, raises the prospect of adoptive transfer as a realistic possibility (Peggs *et al.* 2003).

Adenoviruses

Long since known to be a threat to immunocompromised children, adenoviruses are now increasingly recognized as an important cause of morbidity and mortality in adults with HSCT (Jalal *et al.* 2005). There are at least 50 adenovirus serotypes causing outbreaks of symptomatic infection mainly in childhood, manifest as upper respiratory tract symptoms, gastroenteritis, and keratoconjunctivitis (Walls *et al.* 2003). After primary infection, adenovirus persists in lymphoid tissues. Following HSCT, reactivated infection may result in asymptomatic shedding or localized or disseminated disease. Reactivation has been detected in surveillance cultures in about 10% of adults within 3 months of HSCT. Localized disease manifests primarily in the respiratory, gastrointestinal, or urinary tracts. Recently, adenovirus has been implicated as a cause of nephritis in HSCT patients of all ages (Bruno *et al.* 2004). Disseminated disease involves at least two organ systems, often causing pneumonia and/or hepatitis, but encephalitis is rare. As is the case with CMV, adenovirus pneumonia is not preceded by upper respiratory symptoms. Adenovirus infection is significantly associated with poor outcome and an increased risk of mortality post-HSCT (Bruno *et al.* 2003).

Risk factors for reactivation include young age, allogeneic transplant, second allogeneic transplant, alternate graft, and moderate to severe GVHD. Recipients of T-cell-depleted and T-cell-repleted grafts are at risk. Ganciclovir seems to be protective. In a large retrospective study, the patients who received neither pre-emptive nor prophylactic ganciclovir were at significantly higher risk of infection (Bruno *et al.* 2003).

The most important predictor for clinical adenovirus disease is the number of sites from which adenovirus is isolated. One site is associated with disease in 11%, two sites in 40% and three or more sites with disease in 100% reflecting disseminated infection and a low chance of survival (Flomenberg *et al.* 1994).

Treatment of adenovirus infections post-HSCT has not as yet been subject controlled trials. Available evidence casts doubt on the benefit of ribavirin therapy. Although effective *in vitro*, cidofovir has been associated with dose-limiting nephrotoxicity. Paralleling CMV, prevention of adenovirus disease is now focusing on surveillance and administration of early or pre-emptive therapy (Hoffman *et al.* 2001; Ljungman *et al.* 2003b).

Community respiratory viruses

The community respiratory viruses (CRV), including the influenza, parainfluenza (PIV), respiratory syncytial (RSV), rhinoviruses, and metapneumoviruses, do not invade beyond the respiratory tract. They are transmitted by the respiratory route causing upper respiratory tract symptoms after a short incubation period. In myelosuppressed patients with leukaemia, or recent HSCT however, infection frequently descends to the lower respiratory tract, causing pneumonia (Whimbey *et al.* 1997). These viral pneumonias carry a high mortality, but in contrast to systemic viral infections (CMV, adenovirus), which start abruptly, the preceding upper respiratory infection provides an opportunity for potentially life-saving pre-emptive therapy.

The epidemiology of CRV infections mirrors that in the community, with influenza and RSV cases largely confined to the winter season, while PIV occurs year round with summertime peaks (Nichols *et al.* 2001b). Infections are highly contagious, spreading readily between patients, visitors and staff.

CRV are transmitted by droplet particles, and spread primarily by contact with contaminated surfaces. Influenza, the most infectious of the CRVs, is also transmitted by aerosol. Control of infection is hampered by the capacity of asymptomatic individuals to transmit infection and the prolonged virus shedding in immunocompromised patients. Prevention of nosocomial acquisition and outbreaks in both inpatient and outpatient facilities requires strict infection control precautions (Harrington *et al.* 1992).

In HSCT patients with respiratory symptoms, CRV infections were detected in over 30% in prospective winter surveillance but in just 2% in a non-seasonal European multicentre study. Notably, RSV accounted for approximately 50% of cases in both studies (Whimbey *et al.* 1996; Ljungman 2001). This section addresses the more readily diagnosed CRVs commencing with RSV and PIV, followed by influenza.

In virus-specific studies in adult patients with leukaemia, RSV was detected in 10%, and PIV in 6.2% of those with acute respiratory illnesses (Whimbey *et al.* 1995; Marcolini *et al.* 2003). Retrospective analysis of 10 year's data from Seattle, showed attack rates of 4.5% for RSV and 7.1% PIV (90% PIV-3) in HSCT recipients (Nichols *et al.* 2001b). RSV is associated with a high risk of pneumonia with 32% HSCT cases progressing from upper respiratory infection and a further 8% presenting directly. Of the HSCT recipients with PIV infection, 13% of the 87% presenting with only upper respiratory symptoms later developed pneumonia. Risk factors that have been associated with progression of CRV to pneumonia include lymphopenia, neutropenia, infection in the pre-engraftment phase, alternate donor, acute or chronic GVHD, steroids and other immunosuppressive therapy, and underlying lung disease (Harrington *et al.* 1992; Champlin and Whimbey 2001; Nichols *et al.* 2001b).

The mortality rate of established RSV or PIV pneumonia is high in leukaemic and HSCT patients (Whimbey *et al.* 1995; Marcolini *et al.* 2003). In HSCT recipients with RSV pneumonia, mortality is 60–80% despite treatment, and between 35% and 75% in PIV pneumonia (Harrington *et al.* 1992; Lewis *et al.* 1996; Whimbey *et al.* 1996; Ghosh *et al.* 2000; Nichols *et al.* 2001b). Allogeneic recipients with PIV early post-HSCT and those with co-pathogens are at greatest risk (Lewis *et al.* 1996; Nichols *et al.* 2001a), as are lymphopenic leukaemia patients (Marcolini *et al.* 2003).

The main approaches to treatment of RSV or PIV pneumonia have entailed the use of the antiviral agent ribavirin and various immunoglobulin preparations. Ribavirin can be given intravenously, orally, or as an aerosol using a small particle aerosol generator but is associated with significant toxicity. The aerosol may induce bronchospasm and is often poorly tolerated, and is not suitable for use in mechanically ventilated patients. Teratogenicity in rodents warrants caution regarding inhalation exposure of pregnant staff (Rodriguez *et al.* 1987). Both oral and intravenous preparations may cause dose-related haemolytic anaemia.

As yet there are no data from controlled clinical trials, but uncontrolled case series indicate the futility of any treatment strategy in patients requiring mechanical ventilation. Given promptly however, aerosolized ribavirin with or without IVIG or RSV-specific monoclonal antibody, has been associated with resolution of RSV pneumonitis in a few non-ventilated patients (Whimbey *et al.* 1995; Whimbey *et al.* 1996; McColl *et al.* 1998). Used pre-emptively, aerosolized ribavirin has been associated with cessation of upper respiratory symptoms and reduced progression to RSV pneumonitis, but clearance of viral shedding is unreliable (Sparrelid *et al.* 1997; McColl *et al.* 1998; Adams *et al.* 1999; Ghosh *et al.* 2000; Chakrabarti *et al.* 2001). Trials of early therapeutic intervention to pre-empt RSV pneumonia are currently underway.

Early therapy of PIV pneumonia with ribavirin, with or without immunoglobulin, has not reliably reduced either mortality or viral shedding, prompting suggestions that immunosuppressive therapy should be reduced or stopped early in PIV infection (Wendt *et al.* 1992; Lewis *et al.* 1996; Chakrabarti *et al.* 2001; Nichols *et al.* 2001a,b).

Vigilance is required to help minimize the threat of CRV in HSCT units. The results of controlled trials of pre-emptive therapy are not yet available but active daily clinical surveillance of HSCT patients for symptoms of CRV has nevertheless been recommended to facilitate early diagnosis and to prevent nosocomial transmission (US Department of Health & Human Services 2000; Dykewicz 2001). Nasopharyngeal aspirate, throat washings, bronchoalveolar lavage, or lung biopsy samples are suitable for rapid detection and should be tested promptly. Nasopharyngeal aspirates are often poorly tolerated and thrombocytopenia should be corrected before sampling. If suspicion remains high despite a negative result, fresh samples should be tested. Despite the current lack of a recommended strategy, consideration of pre-emptive therapy of RSV with aerosolized ribavirin and/or an immunoglobulin preparation should be considered, taking account of potential drug toxicities (US Department of Health & Human Services 2000; Dykewicz 2001).

The influenza viruses are subject to constant change, with different strains circulating giving rise to epidemic years, and genetic shift to new pandemic subtypes of influenza A. Immunocompromised patients, including HSCT recipients, are at risk of fatal pneumonia. Asplenic/hyposplenic patients may be at special risk of secondary bacterial pneumonia. In contrast to the other CRVs, HSCT recipients can be afforded some protection during influenza season through pre- and post-transplant vaccination together with annual vaccination of household contacts (US Department of Health & Human Services 2000; Dykewicz 2001). Post-transplant vaccination is not recommended until 6 months after HSCT. The protection afforded by vaccination depends on how closely the vaccine components resemble the viruses circulating in that season. Specific anti-influenza agents provide an important additional line of defence. The older M2 blockers, amantadine and rimantadine, are only effective against influenza A. Furthermore, the rapid and predictable generation of resistant virus, undiminished in virulence, has precluded the use of these agents for both prophylaxis and treatment in an outbreak. Fortunately, resistance does not appear to be rapidly induced by the recently developed neuraminidase inhibitors, oseltamivir and zanamivir. These drugs are effective against influenza A and B and avian strains, and are licensed for both prophylaxis and treatment of influenza (Moscona 2005).

Epstein–Barr virus

Most adults have had prior asymptomatic or symptomatic primary EBV infection. Infection is not cleared but persists for life in latently infected B-lymphocytes. These cells can be grown *in vitro* as immortalized lymphoblastoid cell lines but in the normal host are controlled by vigorous EBV-specific immune responses mediated mainly by cytotoxic T-lymphocytes (CTLs) (Cohen 2000).

In the absence of effective T-cell immunity, EBV-driven proliferation of latently-infected B-cells may present clinically as post-transplant lymphoproliferative disease (PTLD). The majority present in the first 6 months post-HSCT with diverse clinical features ranging from infectious mononucleosis-like illness to an occult mass lesion in any organ or tissue. The tumours may be polyclonal or monoclonal and are histologically diverse. Detection of EBV-encoded RNAs (EBERs) by *in situ* hybridization is required to confirm EBV association (MacMahon and Ambinder 1994).

While all HSCT recipients are at risk, this varies considerably (0.5–22%) depending on the presence of major risk factors, including primary EBV infection post-HSCT, alternate donor, *in vivo* or *in vitro* T-cell depletion, GVHD, and CMV infection (Curtis *et al.* 1999). As EBV infection is cleared by myeloablative conditioning, EBV is usually acquired from a seropositive donor or intimate contact (Gratama *et al.* 1988).

Treatment of established PTLD is of limited success. Reduction of immunosuppression remains paramount. While surgery may be life-saving in localized disease, chemotherapy and radiotherapy are of limited efficacy. The benefits of antiviral therapy and of α-interferon with IVIG are unclear. More recently, both anti-CD20 antibody (rituximab) therapy and adoptive therapy with donor-derived EBV-specific CTLs have met with some success.

Given the high morbidity and mortality even with treatment, the major focus is on prevention of PTLD. This includes preventing exposure through careful hygiene and intimate contact (US Department of Health & Human Services 2000). Consideration should be given to avoiding T-cell depletion, or to using an agent, which depletes both B- and T-cell fractions (alentuzumab or MacCampath) as this manipulation is associated with a lower risk for PTLD. These measures are of particular importance in the more vulnerable, EBV-seronegative recipients.

EBV viral load monitoring with the early institution of pre-emptive therapy, paralleling the approach to CMV, has been proposed. Possible approaches include antiviral agents, rituximab and adoptive transfer of CTLs. High EBV viral loads, however, are seen in many patients who do not develop PTLD. The positive predictive value may be improved by considering viral load measurements together with the presence of risk factors (Gartner *et al.* 2002). In a recent study of HSCT patients with alternate donors, the predictive value of a high EBV DNA level on more than two occasions was only 50%. As all eight patients in this study were successfully treated with rituximab and/or CTLs, the authors suggest that EBV viral load testing instead be used to facilitate early diagnosis with prompt treatment in patients with clinical and radiological features consistent with PTLD (Wagner *et al.* 2004).

Hepatitis B and C

Individuals with prior HBV are at risk of reactivation as a result of immunosuppressive or cytostatic therapy. Up to 50% of hepatitis B surface antigen (HBsAg)-positive patients may develop disease ranging from mild to fulminant hepatitis.

The reverse transcriptase inhibitors, lamivudine and now adefovir, are licensed for treatment of hepatitis B. Used in patients with hepatitis flare after fludarabine-based treatment for non-Hodgkin's lymphoma, lamivudine treatment failed in three of five patients and was associated with the generation of lamivudine-resistant mutant strains (Picardi *et al.* 2003). The results of small studies have shown that primary prophylaxis with lamivudine may be a better approach to preventing disease in HBsAg-positive patients undergoing treatment for solid and haematological malignancies (Rossi *et al.* 2001; Idilman *et al.* 2004; Dai *et al.* 2004).

Prospective HSCT recipients testing HBsAg positive require evaluation of hepatitis markers, measurement of plasma viral load and specialist advice. Surface antigen negative, core antibody positive individuals have an approximate 1 in 10 risk of reactivation and should be regularly monitored for appearance of surface antigen post-HSCT.

HBsAg-positive patients are at high risk of morbidity and mortality after HSCT. Autologous and allogeneic recipients have a 36% and 81% respective risk of abnormal liver function tests. The clinical manifestations are widely variable but allogeneic recipients have a 16% risk of fulminant hepatitis. Patients with high viral loads are at greatest risk of disease, including HBV 'e' antigen negative individuals who may have pre-core mutant virus. The timing of hepatic impairment is variable, but often coincides with withdrawal of immunosuppression. Prior infection with HBV may increase the mortality in patients with liver failure due to hepatic GVHD or veno-occlusive disease (VOD) (El-Sayed et al. 2004).

Optimal management of HBsAg-positive patients to prevent hepatitis B disease post-HSCT has yet to be defined. Minimizing steroid therapy is an important component of prevention. Steroids directly increase HBV replication due to the presence of a glucocorticoid-responsive element in the HBV genome. Use of an HBV-seropositive donor may result in clearance of HBsAg in the recipient, particularly if the donor is core antibody as well as surface antibody positive. Donor vaccination may prove to have a role in prevention. Hepatitis B specific immunoglobulin and antiviral agents have been used but the use of α-interferon is limited due to the increased risk of GVHD. For optimal management, specialist supervision is required to take account of the risk of drug toxicity, induction of resistance, and of flare-ups on withdrawal of treatment.

HCV IgG indicates either current or resolved hepatitis C infection. Detection of HCV RNA identifies those with chronic hepatitis. HCV genotype and load are routinely used to determine the dose and duration of anti-HCV therapy (pegylated α-interferon 2B and ribavirin) in immunocompetent individuals. As 85% of infected individuals become chronic carriers, at least two negative RNA tests are required to rule out ongoing infection. Prospective donors with hepatitis C infection are excluded following pre-transplant screening.

After allogeneic HSCT, acute flares of hepatitis occur in about one-third of HCV-positive patients, usually after withdrawal of immunosuppression. Hepatitis is mild or moderate and the risk of fulminant disease is low but HCV is also a significant risk factor for VOD (El-Sayed et al. 2004). Long-term HSCT survivors are at risk of cirrhosis and hepatocellular carcinoma.

Ribavirin has been used for prophylaxis of severe HCV disease but use of pegylated α-interferon is limited by concerns about the increased risk of GVHD.

Gastrointestinal viruses

This group comprises the rotaviruses, noroviruses, caliciviruses, and astroviruses, which cause gastroenteritis in immunocompetent and immunocompromised hosts. All have short incubation periods and are spread via the faeco-oral route, contaminated food, water and surfaces, and by aerosol (from projectile vomit). Illness is usually self-limiting and there are no therapeutic agents available.

Noroviruses are the most common cause of gastroenteritis outbreaks in hospitals, sometimes requiring ward closure. Cases among staff are a key feature in nosocomial outbreaks. Early collection of samples (faeces and/or vomitus) is important as only 50% cases yield positive results with the more widely available tests. Given that outbreaks may cause major disruption of clinical services, prompt control measures must be instituted once viral gastroenteritis is suspected, for which guidelines exist incorporating nursing strategies and cleaning (Chadwick et al. 2000).

BK virus

BK virus (BKV) is a polyoma virus that is ubiquitous in humans. More than 80% adults have BKV infection. After childhood acquisition, BKV remains latent in the kidney, lymphoid tissue, and leucocytes (Leung et al. 2005). Reactivation can occur and is probably responsible for the BKV viruria, which is seen in approximately 50% of HSCT recipients (Arthur et al. 1986). This has been associated with post-engraftment haemorrhagic cystitis (HC) in HSCT (Erard et al. 2005) and less frequently in non-transplant cancer patients (Fogazzi et al. 2002). Consequently, BKV has been implicated in HC pathogenesis in such patients. Supporting this hypothesis, in HSCT a high BKV viral load in urine has been associated with a higher risk of HC and an increase in the viral load precedes the onset of haematuria (Leung et al. 2005). In addition, BK viraemia detected before or during HC has been independently associated with HC, and higher peak plasma levels and bladder biopsies containing BKV nucleic acid have been described during HC (Erard et al. 2004, 2005). However, a direct causative role has not been established as BKV viruria is also commonly asymptomatic (Erard et al. 2005) often coupled with the presence of more than one potential cause of HC during one episode (Leung et al. 2005).

HC is graded 1–4 progressing from microscopic haematuria to macroscopic haematuria with clot retention and urinary tract obstruction (Erard *et al.* 2005; Leung *et al.* 2005). BKV HC is clinically indistinguishable from chemical-induced, adenovirus, CMV, and GVHD-associated HC, which are all well described in HSCT recipients.

The diagnosis of BKV HC rests upon clinical symptoms and signs, the detection of BKV and the exclusion of other aetiologies. A urine specimen should be sent for cytological and if possible, electron microscopy examination, as well as viral culture. Cytology allows the identification of human polyomavirus-induced cytopathological changes of the urinary epithelial cells. Electron microscopy, which can also be performed on urinary sediment or tissue, may identify human polyomaviruses. However, neither specifically identifies BKV. Viral culture is slow and may take up to 4 weeks. Enzyme-linked immunosorbent assays for the detection of viral antigens and BKV nucleic acid detection are faster, but the latter requires sophisticated laboratory expertise. Owing to the frequency of asymptomatic shedding, the detection of BKV viruria has a low positive predictive value for HC (Erard *et al.* 2004). Though not yet routinely available, nucleic acid detection methods for the quantification of viraemia and viruria, and for use on tissue, are employed by some HSCT centres and these are likely to supersede the currently available diagnostic tests.

Spontaneous resolution of both BKV-associated HC and asymptomatic shedding is well described. Analgesia and supportive therapy is paramount, and patients with severe or persistent (>7 days) symptoms should be referred to a urologist, who may perform bladder irrigation (Leung *et al.* 2005). There are case reports of successful treatment of BKV HC in HSCT patients with intravenous vidarabine and with cidofovir, and vidarabine may prevent progression from asymptomatic viruria to cystitis (Kawakami *et al.* 1997; Held *et al.* 2000; González-Fraile *et al.* 2001). However, as the urine viral load has been reported to be in decline/at baseline at the point of haematuria, some have debated the role of antivirals (Leung *et al.* 2005). Quinolone antibiotics have an inhibitory effect upon BKV and it has been suggested that their indication is extended beyond prophylaxis against Gram-negative sepsis, to include the prevention of BKV HC (Leung *et al.* 2005).

Acknowledgement

The authors would like to thank Alice Gem for secretarial assistance with this chapter.

References

Adams RH, Christenson JC, Petersen FB, and Beatty PG. (1999). Pre-emptive use of aerosolized ribavirin in the treatment of asymptomatic pediatric marrow transplant patients testing positive for RSV. *Bone Marrow Transplantation*, **24**, 661–664.

Arthur RR, Shah KV, Baust SJ, Santos GW, and Saral R. (1986). Association of BK viruria with hemorrhagic cystitis in recipients of bone marrow transplants. *New England Journal of Medicine*, **315**, 230–234.

Boeckh M, Gooley TA, Myerson D, Cunningham T, Schoch G, and Bowden RA. (1996). Cytomegalovirus pp65 antigenaemia-guided early treatment with ganciclovir at engraftment after allogeneic bone marrow transplantation: a randomized double-blind study. *Blood*, **88**, 4063–4071.

Bruno B, Gooley T, Hackman RC, Davis C, Corey L, and Boeckh M. (2003). Adenovirus infection in hematopoietic stem cell transplantation: effect of ganciclovir and impact on survival. *Biology of Blood and Bone Marrow Transplantation*, **9**, 341–352.

Bruno B, Zager RA, Boeckh MJ, *et al.* (2004). Adenovirus nephritis in hematopoietic stem-cell transplantation. *Transplantation*, **77**, 1049–1057.

Chadwick PR, Beards G, Brown D, *et al.* (2000). Management of hospital outbreaks of gastro-enteritis due to small round structured viruses. *Journal of Hospital Infection*, **45**, 1–10.

Chakrabarti S, Collingham KE, Holder K, Fegan CD, Osman H, and Milligan DW. (2001). Pre-emptive oral ribavirin therapy of paramyxovirus infections after haematopoietic stem cell transplantation: a pilot study. *Bone Marrow Transplantation*, **28**, 759–763.

Champlin RE and Whimbey E. (2001). Community respiratory virus infections in bone marrow transplant recipients: the M.D. Anderson Cancer Center experience. *Biology of Blood and Marrow Transplantation*, **7**, 8S–10S.

Clifford GM, Polesel J, Rickenbach M on behalf of the Swiss HIV Cohort Study, *et al.* (2005). Cancer risk in the Swiss HIV Cohort Study: associations with immunodeficiency, smoking, and highly active antiretroviral therapy. *Journal of the National Cancer Institute*, **97**, 425–432.

Cohen JI. (2000). Epstein–Barr virus infection. *New England Journal of Medicine*, **343**, 481–492.

Curtis RE, Travis LB, Rowlings PA, *et al.* (1999). Risk of lymphoproliferative disorders after bone marrow transplantation: a multi-institutional study. *Blood*, **94**, 2208–2216.

Dai MS, Wu PF, Lu JJ, Shyu RY, and Chao TY. (2004). Preemptive use of lamivudine in breast cancer patients carrying hepatitis B virus undergoing cytotoxic chemotherapy: a longitudinal study. *Supportive Care in Cancer*, **12**, 191–196.

Deayton JR, Sabin CA, Johnson MA, Emery VC, Wilson P, and Griffiths PD. (2004). Importance of cytomegalovirus viraemia in risk of disease progression and death in HIV-infected patients receiving highly active antiretroviral therapy. *Lancet*, **363**, 2116–2121.

Department of Health Advisory Committee on the Microbiological Safety of Blood and Tissues for Transplantation. *Guidance on the microbiological safety of human organs, tissues and cells used in transplantation [Online].* 2000 [cited 07 October 2005]; [55 screens]. Available from URL: http://www.dh.gov.uk/assetRoot/04/07/90/53/04079053.pdf

Dykewicz CA. (2001). Guidelines for preventing opportunistic infections among hemapoietic stem cell transplant recipients: focus on community respiratory virus infections. *Biology of Blood and Marrow Transplantation*, 7, 195–225.

Einsele H, Ehninger G, Hebart H, *et al.* (1995). Polymerase chain reaction monitoring reduces the incidence of cytomegalovirus disease and the duration and side effects of antiviral therapy after bone marrow transplantation. *Blood*, 86, 2815–2820.

El-Sayed MH, El-Haddad A, Fahmy OA, Salama II, and Mahmoud HK. (2004). Liver disease is a major cause of mortality following allogeneic bone-marrow transplantation. *European Journal of Gastroenterology, and Hepatology*, 16, 1347–1354.

Emanuel D, Cunningham I, Jules EK, *et al.* (1988). Cytomegalovirus pneumonia after bone marrow transplantation successfully treated with the combination of ganciclovir and high-dose intravenous immune globulin. *Annals of Internal Medicine*, 109, 777–82.

Emery VC, Sabin CA, Cope AV, Gor D, Hassan-Walker AF, and Griffiths PD. (2000). Application of viral load kinetics to identify patients who develop cytomegalovirus disease after transplantation. *Lancet*, 355, 2032–2036.

Engels EA and Goedert JJ. (2005). Human immunodeficiency virus/acquired immunodeficiency syndrome and cancer: past, present and future. *Journal of the National Cancer Institute*, 97, 407–409.

Erard V, Storer B, Corey L, *et al.* (2004). BK virus infection in hematopoietic stem cell transplant recipients: frequency, risk factors, and association with postengraftment hemorrhagic cystitis. *Clinical Infectious Diseases*, 39, 1861–1865.

Erard V, Kim HW, Corey L, *et al.* (2005). BK DNA viral load in plasma: evidence for an association with hemorrhagic cystitis in allogeneic hematopoietic cell transplant recipients. *Blood*, 106, 1130–1132.

Flomenberg P, Babbitt J, Drobyski WR, *et al.* (1994). Increasing incidence of adenovirus disease in bone marrow transplant recipients. *Journal of Infectious Diseases*, 169, 775–781.

Fogazzi GB, Furione M, Saglimbeni L, Gattiù M, Cant M, and Tarantino A. (2002). BK and JC polyomavirus infection in a patient with chronic lymphocytic leukaemia and renal failure. *Nephrology Dialysis Transplantation*, 17, 1534–1536.

Gartner BC, Schafer H, Marggraff K, *et al.* (2002). Evaluation of use of Epstein–Barr viral load in patients after allogeneic stem cell transplantation to diagnose and monitor posttransplant lymphoproliferative disease. *Journal of Clinical Microbiology*, 40, 351–358. [Erratum in: *Journal of Clinical Microbiology*, 40, 2316.]

Ghosh S, Champlin RE, Englund J, *et al.* (2000). Respiratory syncytial virus upper respiratory tract illnesses in adult blood and marrow transplant recipients: combination therapy with aerosolized ribavirin and intravenous immunoglobulin. *Bone Marrow Transplantation*, 25, 751–755.

González-Fraile MI, Cañizo C, Caballero D, *et al.* (2001). Cidofovir treatment of human polyomavirus-associated acute haemorrhagic cystitis. *Transplant Infectious Disease*, 3, 44–46.

Gratama JW, Oosterveer MA, Zwaan FE, Lepoutre J, Klein G, and Ernberg I. (1988). Eradication of Epstein–Barr virus by allogeneic bone marrow transplantation: implications for sites of viral latency. *Proceedings of the National Academy of Sciences of the United States of America*, 85, 8693–8696.

Grundy JE, Shanley JD, and Griffiths PD. (1987). Is cytomegalovirus interstitial pneumonitis in transplant recipients an immunopathological condition? *Lancet*, **ii**, 996–999.

Harrington RD, Hooton TM, Hackman RC, *et al.* (1992). An outbreak of respiratory syncytial virus in a bone marrow transplant center. *Journal of Infectious Diseases*, **192**, 987–993.

Held TK, Biel SS, Nitsche A, *et al.* (2000). Treatment of BK virus-associated hemorrhagic cystitis and simultaneous CMV reactivation with cidofovir. *Bone Marrow Transplantation*, **26**, 347–350.

Hoffman JA, Shah AJ, Ross LA, and Kapoor N. (2001). Adenoviral infections and a prospective trial of cidofovir in pediatric hematopoietic stem cell transplantation. *Biology of Blood and Marrow Transplantation*, **7**, 388–394.

Idilman R, Arat M, Soydan E, *et al.* (2004). Lamivudine prophylaxis for prevention of chemotherapy-induced hepatitis B virus reactivation in hepatitis B carriers with malignancies. *Journal of Viral Hepatitis*, **11**, 141–147.

Jalal H, Bibby DF, Tang JW, *et al.* (2005). First reported outbreak of diarrhea due to adenovirus infection in a haematology unit for adults. *Journal of Clinical Microbiology*, **43**, 2575–2580.

Kawakami M, Ueda S, Maeda T, *et al.* (1997). Vidarabine therapy for virus-associated cystitis after allogeneic bone marrow transplantation. *Bone Marrow Transplantation*, **20**, 485–490.

Kollman C, Howe CW, Anasetti C, *et al.* (2001). Donor characteristics as risk factors in recipients after transplantation of bone marrow from unrelated donors: the effect of donor age. *Blood*, **98**, 2043–2051.

Leung AYH, Yuen K-Y, and Kwong Y-L. Polyoma BK virus and haemorrhagic cystitis in haematopoietic stem cell transplantation: a changing paradigm. *Bone Marrow Transplantation*, advance online publication, 26 September 2005, doi:10.1038/sj.bmt.1905139.

Lewis VA, Champlin R, Englund J, *et al.* (1996). Respiratory disease due to parainfluenza virus in adult bone marrow transplant recipients. *Clinical Infectious Diseases*, **23**, 1033–1037.

Li CR, Greenberg PD, Gilbert MJ, Goodrich JM, and Riddell SR. (1994). Recovery of HLA-restricted cytomegalovirus (CMV)-specific T-cell responses after allogeneic bone marrow transplant: correlation with CMV disease and effect of ganciclovir prophylaxis. *Blood*, **83**, 1971–1979.

Ljungman P. (2001). Respiratory virus infections in stem cell transplant patients: the European experience. *Biology of Blood and Marrow Transplantation*, **7**, 5S–7S.

Ljungman P, Biron P, Bosi A, *et al.* (1994). Cytomegalovirus interstitial pneumonia in autologous bone marrow transplant recipients. *Bone Marrow Transplantation*, **13**, 209–212.

Ljungman P, de La Camara R, Milpied N, Volin L, Russell CA, Crisp A, and Webster A; Valacyclovir International Bone Marrow Transplant Study Group. (2002a). Randomized study of valacyclovir as prophylaxis against Cytomegalovirus reactivation in recipients of allogeneic bone marrow transplants. *Blood*, **99**, 3050–3056.

Ljungman P, Griffiths P, and Paya C. (2002b). Definitions of cytomegalovirus infection and disease in transplant recipients. *Clinical Infectious Diseases*, **34**, 1094–1097.

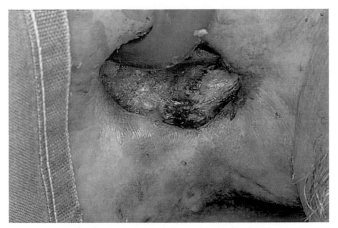

Plate. 1 Wound breakdown around tracheostomy site following laryngectomy.

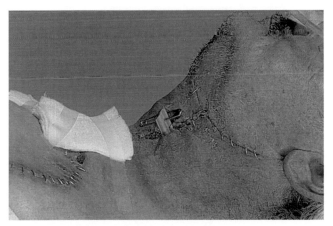

Plate. 2 Salivary fistula following pharyngolaryngectomy.

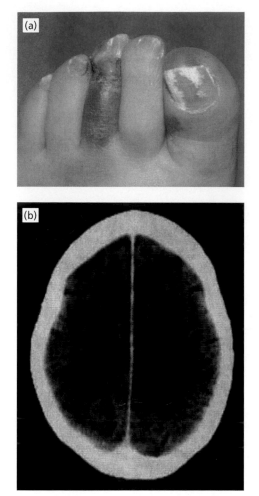

Plate. 3 Male 60y AML neutropenic after chemotherapy for 21 days. Generalised skin rash (haemorrhagic 1–2cm papules). Right parietal lesion. Cause: *Acremonium* I sp.. Origin: chronic toe nail infection.

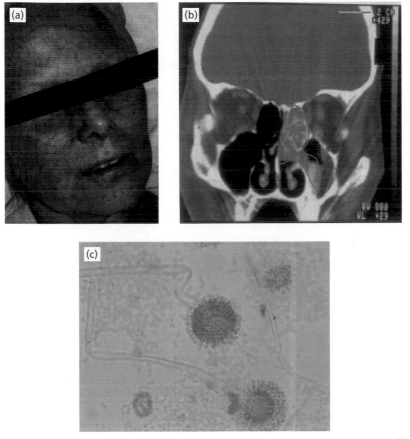

Plate. 4 Female 45 AML neutropenic after chemotherapy for 14 days. Sinusitis and brain lesion due to *Aspergillus flavus*.

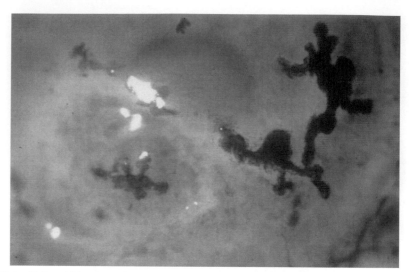

Plate. 5 Dendritic ulcers due to HSV, stained with Rose Bengal.

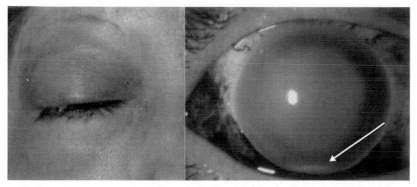

Plate. 6 Hypopyon (arrow) due to endophthalmitis in an elderly lady with metastatic disease. The cornea is hazy and the contents of the eye look yellow due to severe inflammation caused by the infection.

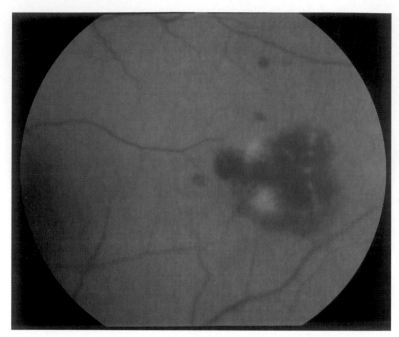

Plate. 7 Roth Spots seen in a case of endophthalmitis in an elderly man with cerebral glioma.

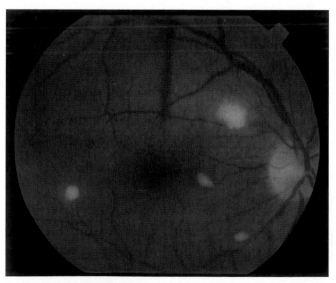

Plate. 8 Candida lesions of the retina in a 56 year old woman recovering from major bowel surgery for malignancy.

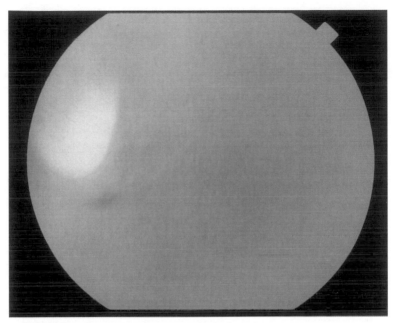

Plate. 9 Fusarium retinitis in a teenager with leukaemia.

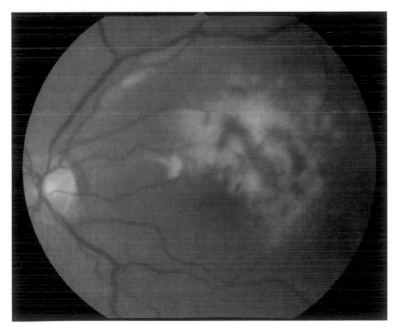

Plate. 10 CMV Retinitis in a 60 year old man on systemic immunosuppression.

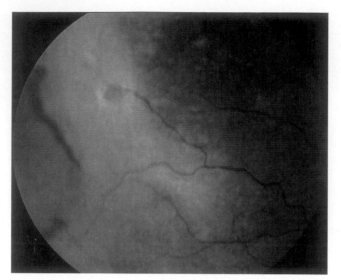

Plate. 11 PORN complicated by a retinal tear in a leukamic patient with leukopenia.

Ljungman P, Einsele H, Frassoni F, *et al.* (2003a). Donor CMV serological status influences the outcome of CMV seropositive recipients after unrelated donor stem cell transplantation: an EBMT Megafile analysis. *Blood*, **102**, 4255–4260.

Ljungman P, Ribaud P, Eyrich M, *et al.* (2003b). Cidofovir for adenovirus infections after allogeneic hematopoietic stem cell transplantation: a survey by the Infectious Diseases Working Party of the European Group for Blood and Marrow Transplantation. *Bone Marrow Transplantation*, **31**, 481–486.

Ljungman P, Reusser P, de la Camara R, *et al.* (2004). Management of CMV infections: recommendations from the Infectious Diseases Working Party of the EBMT. *Bone Marrow Transplantation*, **33**, 1075–1081.

Ljungman P, Engelhard D, de la Camara R, *et al.* (2005). Vaccination of stem cell transplant recipients: recommendations of the Infectious Diseases Working Party of the EBMT. *Bone Marrow Transplantation*, **35**, 737–746.

MacMahon EME and Ambinder RF. (1994). In situ hybridization to detect latent Epstein–Barr virus in routinely fixed specimens. *Reviews in Medical Virology*, **4**, 251–260.

Marcolini JA, Malik S, Suki D, Whimbey E, and Body GP. (2003). Respiratory disease due to parainfluenza virus in adult leukaemia patients. *European Journal of Clinical Microbiology and Infectious Diseases*, **22**, 79–84.

Mattes FM, Hainsworth EG, Geretti AM, *et al.* (2004). A randomized, controlled trial comparing ganciclovir to ganciclovir plus foscarnet (each at half dose) for preemptive therapy of cytomegalovirus infection in transplant recipients. *Journal of Infectious Diseases*, **189**, 1355–1361.

McColl MD, Corser RB, Bremner J, and Chopra R. (1998). Respiratory syncytial virus infection in adult BMT recipients: effective therapy with short duration nebulised ribavirin. *Bone Marrow Transplantation*, **21**, 423–425.

Meyers JD, Ljungman P, and Fisher LD. (1990). Cytomegalovirus excretion as a predictor of cytomegalovirus disease after marrow transplantation: importance of cytomegalovirus viremia. *Journal of Infectious Diseases*, **162**, 373–380.

Moscona A. (2005). Neuraminidase inhibitors for influenza. *New England Journal of Medicine*, **353**, 1363–1373.

Nichols WG, Corey L, Gooley T, Davis C, and Boeckh M. (2001a). Parainfluenza virus infections after hematopoietic stem cell transplantation: risk factors, response to antiviral therapy, and effect on transplant outcome. *Blood*, **98**, 573–578.

Nichols WG, Gooley T, and Boeckh M. (2001b). Community-acquired respiratory syncytial virus and parainfluenza virus infections after hematopoietic stem cell transplantation: the Fred Hutchinson Cancer Research Center experience. *Biology of Blood and Marrow Transplantation*, **7**, 11S–15S.

Peggs KS, Verfuerth S, Pizzey A, *et al.* (2003). Adoptive cellular therapy for early cytomegalovirus infection after allogeneic stem-cell transplantation with virus-specific T-cell lines. *Lancet*, **362**, 1375–1377.

Picardi M, Pane F, Quintarelli C, *et al.* (2003). Hepatitis B virus reactivation after fluderabine-based regimens for indolent non-Hodgkin's lymphomas: high prevalence of acquired viral genomic mutations. *Haematologica*, **88**, 1296–1303.

Prentice HG, Gluckman E, Powles RL, *et al.* (1994). Impact of long-term acyclovir on cytomegalovirus infection and survival after allogeneic bone marrow transplantation. *Lancet*, **343**, 749–753.

Reed EC, Bowden RA, Dandliker PS, et al. (1988). Treatment of cytomegalovirus pneumonia with ganciclovir and intravenous cytomegalovirus immunoglobulin in patients with bone marrow transplants. Annals of Internal Medicine, 109, 783–788.

Reusser P, Fisher LD, Buckner CD, Thomas ED, and Meyers JD. (1990). Cytomegalovirus infection after autologous bone marrow transplantation: occurrence of cytomegalovirus disease and effect on engraftment. Blood, 75, 1888–1894.

Reusser P, Einsele H, Lee J, et al. (2002). Randomized multicenter trial of foscarnet versus ganciclovir for preemptive therapy of cytomegalovirus infection after allogeneic stem cell transplantation. Blood, 99, 1159–1164.

Rodriguez WJ, Bui RH, Connor JD, et al. (1987). Environmental exposure of primary care personnel to ribavirin aerosol when supervising treatment of infants with respiratory syncytial virus infection. Antimicrobial Agents and Chemotherapy, 31, 1143–1146.

Rossi G, Pelizzari A, Motta M, and Puoti M. (2001). Primary prophylaxis with lamivudine of hepatitis B virus reactivation in chronic HBsAg carriers with lymphoid malignancies treated with chemotherapy. British Journal of Haematology, 115, 58–62.

Sparrelid E, Ljungman P, Ekelöf-Andström E, et al. (1997). Ribavirin therapy in bone marrow transplant recipients with viral respiratory tract infections. Bone Marrow Transplantation, 19, 905–908.

Spina M, Jaeger U, Sparano, et al. (2005). Rituximab plus infusional cyclophosphamide, doxorubicin, and etoposide in HIV-associated non-Hodgkin lymphoma: pooled results from 3 phase 2 trials. Blood, 105, 1891–1897.

The EACS Euroguidelines Group. (2003). European guidelines for the clinical management and treatment of HIV-infected adults in Europe. AIDS, 17 (Suppl. 2), S3–S26.

Torres HA, Kontoyiannis DP, Bodey GP, et al. (2005). Gastrointestinal cytomegalovirus disease in patients with cancer: a two decade experience in a tertiary care cancer center. European Journal of Cancer, 41, 2268–2279.

US Department of Health, and Human Services Centers for Disease Control and Prevention (CDC). (2000). Guidelines for preventing opportunistic infections among hemopoietic stem cell transplant recipients. Recommendations of CDC, the Infectious Disease Society of America, and the American Society of Blood and Marrow Transplantation. Morbidity and Mortality Weekly Report. Recommendations and Reports, 49 (RR-10), 1–128.

USPHS/IDSA Prevention of Opportunistic Infections Working Group. (2000). 1999 USPHS/IDSA guidelines for the prevention of opportunistic infections in persons infected with human immunodeficiency virus. Clinical Infectious Diseases, 30 (Suppl. 1), S29–S65.

Wagner HJ, Cheng YC, Huls MH, et al. (2004). Prompt versus preemptive intervention for EBV lymphoproliferative disease. Blood, 103, 3979–3981.

Walls T, Shankar AG, and Shingadia D. (2003). Adenovirus: an increasingly important pathogen in paediatric bone marrow transplant patients. Lancet Infectious Diseases, 3, 79–86.

Wendt CH, Weisdorf DJ, Jordan MC, Balfour HH Jr, and Hertz MI. (1992). Parainfluenza virus respiratory infection after bone marrow transplantation. New England Journal of Medicine, 326, 921–926.

Whimbey E, Couch RB, Englund JA, et al. (1995). Respiratory syncytial virus pneumonia in hospitalized adult patients with leukemia. Clinical Infectious Diseases, 21, 376–379.

Whimbey E, Champlin RE, Couch RB, *et al.* (1996). Community respiratory virus infections among hospitalized adult bone marrow transplant recipients. *Clinical Infectious Diseases*, **22**, 778–782.

Whimbey E, Englund JA, and Couch RB. (1997). Community respiratory virus infections in immunocompromised patients with cancer. *American Journal of Medicine*, **102**(3A), 10–18.

Wingard JR. (1999). Opportunistic infections after blood and marrow transplantation. *Transplant Infectious Disease*, **1**, 3–20.

Winston DJ, Yeager AM, Chandrasekar PH, Snydman DR, Petersen FB, and Territo MC; Valacyclovir Cytomegalovirus Study Group. (2003). Randomized comparison of oral valacyclovir and intravenous ganciclovir for prevention of cytomegalovirus disease after allogeneic bone marrow transplantation. *Clinical Infectious Diseases*, **36**, 749–758.

Chapter 9

Skin infections in the cancer patient

Roderick J. Hay

Introduction

In many parts of the world infections of the skin are the commonest manifestations of skin disease. This is because the major factors determining the risk of infection are the ease of transmission of the organisms and their intrinsic pathogenicity rather than the underlying condition of the host. Many skin pathogens cause disease in a variety of different human hosts irrespective of the host's underlying immune status. Infections such as bacterial pyoderma (impetigo), dermatophytosis or ringworm, scabies and viral warts (human papillomavirus or HPV infections) are all examples of these common infections (Table 9.1). Their transmission is generally determined by simple risk factors for exposure, such as communal activities including use of public swimming pools, overcrowding, and sometimes, lack of hygiene. Opportunities for spread between individuals under these circumstances are frequent.

These infections are also seen in the immunosuppressed patient. Generally in such individuals their prevalence is no commoner, and sometimes less frequent, than that seen in the healthy population. The reasons for reduced prevalence may reflect a lower opportunity for spread due, for example, to reduction of communal activities. However, in immunologically predisposed patients skin infections may present with clinical manifestations that are either similar to those seen in normal individuals or more widespread, atypical in presentation or recalcitrant to therapy. For instance the lesions of furunculosis (staphylococcal boils) in the neutropenic patient may be widely distributed rather than clustered in one region or there may be an abnormal evolution of infection such as occurs in disseminated *Fusarium* infections originating from an infected toenail in the severely neutropenic patient. In short the presence of immunosuppression does not affect the prevalence of the infection but may alter its clinical expression (Chren *et al* 1995).

Table 9.1 Infections in the cancer patient

Organism	Infection in healthy host	Infection in cancer patient
Bacteria		
Staph. aureus	Impetigo, furunculosis, carbuncles, toxic shock	Similar. But wide spread furunculosis is more common
Group A Streptococci	Impetigo, cellulitis, necrotizing fasciitis	Similar
Rare:		
Gram-negative bacteria	Folliculitis	Similar
Bartonella henselae	Bacillary angiomatosis	Rare in lymphoma
Nocardia spp.	Primary cutaneous nocardiosis	Rare but usually a manifestation of disseminated nocardiosis
Mycobacterium tuberculosis	Lupus vulgaris, scrofuloderma, tuberculosis verrucosa cutis	Miliary tuberculosis
Fungi		
Dermatophytes	Tinea corporis, cruris, capitis, etc., onychomycosis	Altered expression, e.g. large lesions
Superficial candidosis	Oral, vaginal, cutaneous	Oral candidosis follows chemotherapy, radiation to head and neck and extensive antibiotics
Malassezia infection	Pityriasis versciolor, seborrhoeic dermatitis, *Malassezia* folliculitis	Similar. *Malassezia* folliculitis in patients in ITU
Viruses		
Herpes simplex virus	Cold sores, eczema herpeticum	Same but also risk of disseminated cutaneous herpes simplex
Varicella zoster virus	Herpes zoster	Same but extensive zoster seen in immunosuppressed patients
Human papilloma virus	Viral warts	Same but can be very extensive and chronic in immunosuppressed
Herpes type 8	Kaposi's sarcoma	Mainly associated with HIV/AIDS
Molluscum contagiosum	Molluscum contagiosum	More extensive in immune suppressed
Ectoparasites		
Sarcoptes scabei	Scabies	Similar but risk of crusted scabies in immunosuppressed patient

However, in addition, there are certain infections due to a variety of opportunistic pathogens, which only cause disease in the presence of some underlying change in host resistance. Examples include bacterial angiomatosis due to *Bartonella henselae*. Systemic fungal infections presenting with skin lesions provide a further example.

Microbiology of the normal skin

The normal human skin is host to a diverse population of bacteria, fungi, and ectoparasites whose numbers are generally held in balance by the normal immune system. The normal bacteria that can be isolated are a variety of different coryneforms, *Staphylococcus epidermidis, Staph. saprophyticus, Propionibacterium acnes*, and micrococci. Their distribution is variable, some favouring sebaceous follicles while others are most often found in intertriginous areas. Other bacteria such as *Brevibacterium* spp. may also colonize specific sites such as the soles or web spaces of the feet. Even in the severely immunosuppressed patient these organisms seldom if ever cause skin disease, although they may enter the circulation, if there is an appropriate entry site, such as a subcutaneous cannula or intravenous line. There have been no studies that show that this normal spectrum of commensal organisms changes in severely immunosuppressed patients with cancer. Although intuitively this is likely as antibiotic therapy and stay in hospital, among other factors, are all known to predispose to changes in colonization rates by the resident microbes.

The fungi that form part of this normal flora are lipophilic yeasts of the genus *Malassezia*, organisms that frequently cluster within the openings of hair follicles. Again they rarely cause skin infections, although in some diseases associated with T-cell-mediated immunosuppression, such as Cushing's syndrome or in solid organ transplant patients, they can cause pityriasis versicolor (*M. globosa*) or folliculitis (a variety of *Malassezia* species). Haematogenous dissemination of *Malassezia* infections is also possible, although generally where this has been reported it is mainly seen in newborn infants rather than those with underlying disease. *Candida* (see below) is a part of the normal oral, gastrointestinal tract, and vaginal flora. It is seldom isolated from healthy skin.

The only ectoparasite present on normal human skin is the mite, *Demodex folliculorum*. It is usually found in sebaceous follicles on the face. Despite many attempts to link this with human disease in either the otherwise healthy or those with underlying disease there is no evidence that it is a pathogen under any circumstances in humans.

Transient carriage of pathogenic microbes

In addition to the normal residents there are some organisms that are transiently carried on the human skin or mucosal surfaces. The term transient in this context implies that carriage is not continuous but fluctuates with time. Many of these organisms potentially cause superficial or internal infections. An estimated 44% of the normal population carries *Staphylococcus aureus* in the anterior nares and a lower proportion Group A streptococci in the throat. *Staph. aureus* can also be carried on the hands and fingers. Carriage rates of staphylococci increase in patients with an atopic background or on diseased skin such as eczema. The carriage rates of *Staph. aureus* rise in patients in hospital.

Gram-negative bacteria such as *Pseudomonas* can also be transiently carried on the hands or on broken skin surfaces. These organisms are not long-term residents but can cause disease under appropriate circumstances.

Among the fungi *Candida* species, including *Candida albicans*, are normal residents of the oral cavity and vaginal mucosa in some 25% of the population, the prevalence rising in hospitalized patients. The pathogenic status of *Candida* spp. is affected by changes in the local environment and local infections such as oral or oesophageal candidosis may result from a variety of changes, ranging from chemotherapy to radiotherapy, which can affect the balance between commensal status and invasive disease. Defects affecting numbers and function of T lymphocytes or neutrophils predispose to increased carriage of *Candida* as well as increased risk of infection. This does not affect all forms of *Candida* infection and vaginal candidosis is uncommonly associated with immunosuppression.

Host immunity and carriage of micro-organisms

The interaction between the different factors affecting regulation of the growth of commensals on the skin is poorly understood but there is sufficient evidence to show that the ecological balance between normal and overgrowth is a delicate one. Factors that remove or alter the prevailing situation in favour of one or more organism such as occurs with antibiotic therapy may affect this balance but infection is not necessarily the outcome. Such factors include: immunosuppression particularly changes that affect T-lymphocyte numbers or function, reduction of surface lipids, increased skin humidity and carbon dioxide content (after occlusion) and the presence of prostheses, which facilitate formation of biofilms on the skin or mucosal surfaces. Other factors include ultraviolet radiation.

The skin's defence system is equally complex as it relies on a combination of intrinsic mechanisms which are:

- *Physical*: a layer of dead but heavily keratinized cells acts as a highly effective physical barrier to entry of organisms. The cells of the lower levels of the epidermis are bound by a system of complex intercellular bridges and disruption of cell binding, leading to penetration of organisms is rare under normal circumstances
- *Mechanical*: epidermal proliferation, which leads to outward growth of cells from the epidermal basal layer, is mediated by direct stimulation but is also amplified by locally produced cytokines. It is a partial barrier to penetration by the larger invasive organisms from the outer epidermis, which are invading against the direction of cell growth.
- *Intrinsic inhibitors*: inhibitory molecules include medium chain length fatty acids in sebum or epidermal peptides with antimicrobial activity.
- *Acquired immune responses*: T-lymphocyte-mediated immunological responses are known to be important in controlling certain infections particularly those due to the pathogenic fungi. The antigen-presenting cells of the skin are the Langerhans' cells usually found in the basal and suprabasal layers of the epidermis. Keratinocytes, the principal cells of the epidermis, are immunologically active as immature cells in the basal and immediate suprabasal layers and can produce different chemokines as well as interacting with lymphocytes.
- *Innate immune responses*: neutrophils can be activated directly by microbial products. Phagocytic cells such as neutrophils can migrate through the dermis and into the epidermis. While there is no evidence that they play a part in controlling the intrinsic skin flora they are mobilized in response to many infections. Equally some bacteria, including *Staph. aureus* produce superantigens, which directly stimulate T lymphocytes.

Bacterial infections

The commonest cutaneous bacterial pathogens *Staph. aureus* and Group A streptococci cause a variety of different infections of the skin. They are not normal commensals on the skin surface and infections are usually associated with increased carriage rates on the skin or adjacent structures. *Staph. aureus* is most often carried in the anterior nares, the axillae or the perineum or on skin lesions such as plaques of psoriasis or eczema. Group A streptococci are carried in the throat.

The common infections due to Staph. aureus are:

+ impetigo (and ecthyma)
+ folliculitis
+ furunculosis

whereas the main infections due to pathogenic streptococci are impetigo or cellulitis (Davies *et al* 1996).

These infections are well described in the dermatological literature and are generally no commoner in the cancer patient than in the rest of the population.

Impetigo

Impetigo an infection caused by *Staph. aureus* or Group A streptococci, is chiefly seen in children and is no longer very common in most industrialized societies. The main clinical forms of infection are non-bullous or bullous intertrigo, the former accounting for the majority of cases of infection. In non-bullous impetigo areas of the skin are covered by clusters of crusted and weeping erythematous lesions. In bullous impetigo lesions initially form into blisters although these rupture rapidly leaving open and denuded patches. Both forms are itchy. The bullous form, which is most often seen in infants, is always caused by *Staph. aureus*, whereas either staphylococci or streptococci can cause the non-bullous variety.

There is no specific connection with cancer and most cases of impetigo are seen in perfectly healthy children.

Ecthyma

Likewise there is no relationship between deeper ulcerative infections of the epidermis caused by staphylococci or streptococci in the skin, ecthyma, and cancer. Lesions present as deep crusted and punched out scabs and ulcers. This is accentuated by climate; it is more common in humid tropical environments or where the infected site is covered.

Generalized skin lesions due to staphylococcal infections

The most extensive infections are staphylococcal scalded skin syndrome due to the presence of *Staph. aureus* strains which are producing exfoliatoxin A or B (ET-A or ET-B) and streptococcal or staphylococcal toxic shock syndrome, but neither of these is specifically associated with cancer. In scalded skin there is widespread erythema followed by exfoliation of the skin at mid-epidermal level. The lesions are tender and skin shows a tendency to slough away on fingertip pressure. The condition is most often seen in infants. Whereas in toxic shock syndrome the skin becomes red and oedematous and the patients develops hypotension and signs of shock.

Staphylococcal follicular infections

The commonest of these, staphylococcal folliculitis, is seen commonly in hair bearing sites such as the scalp, the beard area, and the lower legs. It is often precipitated by trauma or by shaving, e.g. leg shaving in young women. Furuncles or boils are sporadic infections caused by *Staph. aureus* and, although often said to be associated with immunodeficiency states, it is not common for these to be found on investigation of patients with recurrent furunculosis. They generally present as a single or localized cluster of tender fluctuant erythematous nodules that contain pus. In the later stages of the formation of a boil the lesion develops a clear pustular centre (pointing). Treatment involves drainage and the appropriate antibiotic such as flucloxacillin. However, in the cancer patient other causes of cutaneous abscesses should be considered; in those with any defect in immunity affecting T-lymphocyte function these would include nocardiosis or systemic fungal infections such as cryptococcosis and such abscesses should always be cultured.

A larger cluster of infected follicles which leads to a large skin abscess is called a carbuncle.

However there are some conditions where there is a connection between the common staphylococcal infections and cancer. These include the following.

Secondary wound infection

There is a relationship between anticancer chemotherapy and secondary wound infection. Here there is an increased risk of secondary bacterial infection of wounds such as tracheotomies or skin ulcers due to *Staph. aureus* if the patient had received chemotherapy within the preceding 2 weeks (Penel *et al* 2004).

Cellulitis

Cellulitis is a subdermal infection that presents with erythema and tenderness over the affected area. The patient may have systemic symptoms such as fever and chills as well as nausea and vomiting. When the infection is confined strictly to the upper dermis it is called erysipelas, although this may be difficult to distinguish from other forms of cellulitis. Commonly cellulitis is caused by streptococci, classically members of Group A (Davies *et al* 1996).

Cellulitis may develop in the presence of primary or secondary lymphoedema. Obstruction of the lymphatics appears to predispose to recurrent episodes of bacterial infection of varying degrees of severity. In patients with lymphatic obstruction secondary to cancer or surgery it is not unusual to encounter episodes of recurrent swelling and erythema. The risk factors for the development of cellulitis have been mainly investigated in relation to carcinoma of the breast. It is clear here that removal of axillary lymph glands is an important predisposing cause but aspiration of a serous collection and excision of a large amount of breast tissue are also risk factors (Brewer *et al* 2000). The same is true of surgery involving removal of local lymph glands elsewhere, e.g. inguinal glands following surgery for vulval carcinoma (Gould *et al* 2001). Cellulitis following irradiation has also been reported in breast cancer (Hughes *et al* 1997) and maxillary squamous cell carcinoma (Penel *et al* 2004). Cellulitis may occur within 30 days of operations that result in removal of lymphatic tissue or may develop as a late complication.

Generally there are two clinical forms of inflammatory reaction, which are referred to as cellulitis.

- The first is limited in extent with erythema and pain within an area of lymphoedema. The patient may feel slightly unwell but does not experience severe symptoms such as chills.

- The second form is of acute onset and is more symptomatic with fever, erythema and swelling and severe pyrexia and rigors.

In neither case is it usually possible to isolate an organism but in the latter there is often objective evidence of Group A streptococcal infection such as a raised ASO or anti-DNAase titre. It is assumed that Group A streptococci are responsible for the first form as well and that this is simply part of the spectrum of virulence exhibited by different strains of Group A streptococci, but it is possible that other streptococci, e.g. Group G may be involved.

Management of acute cellulitis depends on the use of oral antibiotics, which cover streptococci, e.g. penicillin, or, in the severe cases, intravenous antibiotics are necessary.

It is more difficult to prevent recurrent episodes as there are few published studies that have shown effective measures. Recent work has shown that key risk factors for cellulitis include the presence of potential entry sites. On the feet, for instance, cracking between the two webs such as that caused by tinea pedis would be an example. The treatment of skin infections including dermatophyte infections of the feet is a logical approach to management. However, there are no studies that have firmly established this as a means of prevention. In lymphatic filariasis where lymphoedema is a major chronic complication there is evidence that regular skin surface hygiene through washing and local disinfection with agents such as povidone, or chlorhexidine reduce the frequency of acute inflammatory episodes. While these have not been extended to cancer patients with lymphoedema it would be a simple measure to take. However, in many of the more severe cases and where it is not possible to suppress recurrent episodes of cellulitis it will be necessary to use long-term suppressive therapy with oral penicillin V continued indefinitely if necessary.

It is also important to recognize that in some cancer patients other organisms can cause cellulitis (Vartivarian *et al* 1994). In neutropenic patients cellulitis spreading from the orbit on to the face or internally through the hard palate can be caused by fungi invading surrounding tissue from the paranasal sinuses. The causes are either zygomycete fungi (Mucormycosis or Aspergilli (*A. fumigatus* but often *A. flavus* causes infections in this site in this site)). Facial cellulitis should be investigated thoroughly with cultures and histopathology if necessary and imaging procedures to understand the extent of infection. This may include a biopsy of the affected tissue as this is often the best way of revealing the organisms. Fungal cellulitis may carry a poor prognosis particularly if it is caused by a zygomycete fungus, but the organisms can be seen in biopsies and have a characteristic appearance of large strap-like hyphae in tissue section. Frozen sections will provide a rapid diagnosis. Magnetic resonance imaging or CT scan of the head and neck focusing on the paranasal sinuses shows the extent of infection and bone involvement in cases of fungal cellulitis. This is important as medical treatment is supplemented by surgical removal of non-viable tissue. Extensive clearance of the infected paranasal sinuses is normally essential for effective treatment. The value of other antifungals such as lipid associated amphotericin B (AmBisome—liposomal; Abelcet—colloidal dispersion; or Amphocil—suspension of lipid microdiscs) is inferred from case reports but not established through formal clinical trials. Likewise there is some evidence to support the use of hyperbaric oxygen but again it has not been the subject of a comparative study.

Necrotizing fasciitis

Necrotizing fasciitis is the name given to an infection, which may start as a cellulitis but proceeds to invade deeper subcutaneous tissue often leading to considerable local necrosis and toxaemia leading in some cases to death (Childers *et al* 2002). This may develop as an acute or hyperacute reaction leading to rapid deterioration or it may be subtle, developing with little warning and little or no pyrexia, or occur following surgery where there are postoperative complication such as leakage of gastrointestinal anastomoses. At the late stages there may be gas in the tissue and it has been suggested that the description of these conditions should be broader, necrotizing subcutaneous infections, which would include all disease where, in addition to subcutaneous infection, there is extensive necrosis. This would include gas gangrene, some forms of mucormycosis and the most frequent forms of necrotizing fasciitis.

The latter is generally caused by one of two infections either Group A streptococcal infection or a polymicrobial infection, which may include both aerobic and anaerobic bacteria. Cancer may be an underlying disease in patients with this infection, particularly where previous gastrointestinal surgery is involved (Hang *et al* 2003).

The presenting signs are localized and subsequently spreading erythema and tenderness together with pyrexia. The evolution of the infection may be accompanied by the onset of high fever and shock. In some patients blisters develop in the overlying skin and the skin may be indurated. A characteristic late feature is the finding that in the overlying skin there is reduction of sensory detection, reported by patients to be dulled sensation, indicating severe underlying oedema and necrosis. If this condition is suspected magnetic resonance imaging scan can show the presence of considerable subcutaneous infection with fascial thickening with fluid and gas and surgical exploration is necessary. A rapid frozen section though may identify the true cause. The necrotic area should be removed with an extensive fasciotomy and the patient put on appropriate antibiotics. A Gram smear of the excised tissue may rapidly reveal chains of streptococci, or other bacteria, and appropriate antibiotic therapy should be given. Generally treatment is started with a broad-spectrum therapy, e.g. piperacillin plus in some cases metronidazole. However, antibiotics alone are not sufficient and surgery plus supportive care will be needed. In some cases it has been possible to replace the skin flap back on the excised tissue bed.

The prognosis has improved in recent years but the mortality remains at 15–20%. Early detection is the key to preventing morbidity and death.

Gram-negative bacteria

Pseudomonas causes a variety of different skin conditions ranging from green nails to folliculitis associated with contaminated hot tubs or whirlpools (Korten *et al* 1992).

Pseudomonas infections of the nails causes a characteristic greenish discoloration beneath the nail plate. It can also case a painful form of interdigital infection on the feet, which is often mistaken for tinea pedis but is usually tender. Again greenish discoloration on the edge of the area of eroded skin provides a clue to the real nature of the infection. Gram-negative bacteria have also been associated with a painful form of folliculitis on the trunk associated with use of whirlpools, Jacuzzis or hot tubs. It follows contamination of the drainage outlet with bacteria.

However, there are two infections which may occur in superficial or subcutaneous tissues in cancer patients.

1 Bacteraemia due to Gram-negative bacteria is one of the complications of the management of patients with cancer. While it may be due to a number of different organisms, *Pseudomonas* species are commonly isolated. With most bacteraemias the signs of infection are non-specific and confined to pyrexia and hypotension. With *Pseudomonas* species a characteristic skin lesion may accompany the infection, ecthyma gangrenosum. This is a large and necrotic skin lesion 2–3 cm in diameter and usually covered by a black eschar. It starts as a tender purplish indurated circular patch in the skin becoming necrotic as it develops into a haemorrhagic bullous lesion, which then ruptures leaving the dry eschar. The lesion seldom progresses further and will shrink slowly with specific treatment.

Gram-negative rods can usually be seen in biopsy material or smears, along with necrotizing vasculitis in the dermal blood vessels. Lesions should always be cultured as other organisms such as *Aeromonas hydrophila*, *Aspergillus* spp., and *Fusarium* spp. can cause similar necrotic areas. The use of an aminoglycoside and piperacillin or methicillin would be appropriate.

2 *Pseudomonas* can also cause a destructive form of otitis externa known as malignant otitis externa in neutropenic patients. Here the patient has pain and haemorrhagic exudation from the external auditory canal along with hearing loss. Invasion of adjacent structure such as bones and the internal ear is a risk and debris taken from exudative otitis must be cultured as other organisms, notably *Aspergillus* spp., can cause a similar pattern on infection. Extensive debridement of the area together with antibiotics are the best approaches to therapy.

Bartonella infections—bacillary angiomatosis

These infections due to *Bartonella quintana* or *B. henselae* are rare in most patient groups but previously they would have been considered under the eponym of cat scratch fever. Bacillary angiomatosis is the form of infection seen mainly in immunosuppressed individuals and a history of cat scratch or bite is rare. It has become clear over recent years that the condition bacillary angiomatosis is seen predominantly in patients with HIV/AIDS. The condition has also been recorded in those with acute leukaemia.

Epidemiologically the risk factors for the two infections are distinct as *B. henselae* is mainly associated with exposure to cats or fleas, whereas *B. quintana* is associated with low socio-economic status. Cat exposure ranges from owning a cat to being scratched or bitten, whereas socio-economic status mainly relates to homelessness.

The lesions are small red nodules or papules very similar in appearance to pyogenic granulomas. They may be protruberant and surrounded by a small collarette of scales. Deeper cutaneous lesions are erythematous nodules. Disseminated lesions in the liver and other sites may occur.

The diagnosis is made by biopsy with histopathology or polymerase chain reaction for *Bartonella* species playing the key role in diagnosis. The histology shows proliferation of capillaries and endothelial cells. Clumps of bacilli can be seen with Warthin–Starry-stained sections.

The condition responds to treatment with erythromycin or an alternative macrolide such as clarithromycin or a rifamycin (rifampicin).

Nocardia infections

Members of the actinomycete genus, *Nocardia*, cause a number of different patterns of infection, which may present in the skin or subcutaneous tissue ranging from mycetoma caused by *Nocardia brasiliensis* to disseminated cutaneous infection due to *N. asteroides* or *N. otidiscaviarum*. Rarer species are *N. nova* and *N. farcinica*. More commonly in cancer patients *Nocardia* infections present as disseminated internal infections that affect the lung or brain. However, two patterns of cutaneous nocardiosis can be seen in cancer patients. The first is primary cutaneous nocardiosis, which usually presents with either a localized abscess or lymphocutaneous spread where there is an ascending chain of nodules along a lymphatic (Ye *et al* 1996). These nodules may discharge pus or heal spontaneously. More commonly in immunosuppressed individuals skin lesions of nocardiosis are due to haematogenous spread and these present as multiple, skin abscesses; all such patients presenting with skin lesions due to *Nocardia* species should be investigated for internal spread. The organisms are not difficult to isolate from the lesions and can be seen as weakly acid fast filaments in histological sections or smears. Treatment with cotrimoxazole, macrolide antibiotics, e.g. erythromycin, aminoglycosides such as amikacin or imipenem are all used.

Cutaneous mycobacterial infections

Infections of the skin due to tuberculous or non-tuberculous mycobacteria are uncommon. The skin infections due to *Mycobacterium tuberculosis* have been divided into three main entities whose clinical evolution depends on a number of factors, key among which are the route of infection and the state of host immunity.

Cutaneous inoculation with *M. tuberculosis* or *M. bovis* that produces a wart-like clinical form of disease is an infection, where there are few organisms (paucibacillary), called tuberculosis verrucosa cutis. It occurs in the presence of a high level of host immunity in contrast to direct cutaneous inoculation without immunity, tuberculous chancre, which generally presents as a solitary ulcer.

The second clinical type reflects direct spread to the skin from a contiguous structure. It is most commonly represented by scrofuloderma, a paucibacillary form, which arises typically secondary to lymph gland disease in the neck. Here there is a purplish and infiltrated plaque over the lymph nodes with ulceration and it also occurs when the level of immunity is high. Neither of these forms is specifically associated with the cancer patient. The final form reflects dissemination to the skin following spread through the bloodstream. In the presence of poor host immunity this is represented by miliary tuberculosis, which is multibacillary—papules and pustules are widely distributed around the skin—but when there is a higher level of immunity, the clinical form most often seen is lupus vulgaris. This is a solitary plaque often on the face and neck which atrophies but causes considerable scarring and sometimes severe facial destruction.

None of these forms is particularly associated with cancer, although in patients with HIV infection the manifestations of cutaneous tuberculosis are often different with miliary cutaneous tuberculosis, tuberculous ulcers.

Likewise, a severe reaction to BCG inoculation can be expected in anyone with severely compromised T-cell immunity where extensive local infection and ulceration due to the BCG bacillus can occur.

Rarely a variety of non-tuberculous mycobacteria such as *M. fortuitum* or *M. haemophilum* cause skin infections, which usually present as either local abscesses and disseminated nodular dermatitis. *M. avium intracellulare* infections are particularly associated with HIV but although present in the skin there are often no clinical signs of infection apart from papules, nodules, or abscesses on rare occasions.

Leprosy

There is no evidence that leprosy may develop as a complication of cancer. However, there are a numbers of studies that have indicated that leprosy patients appear to have a higher incidence of squamous cell carcinomas—often associated with poorly healing neurotropic ulcers and that the rate of progression of malignant neoplasms is more rapid in patients with lepromatous leprosy, in other words those with compromised T-lymphocyte-mediated responses to leprosy.

Fungi

The only fungi that are commensals of the surface of the epidermis or within the openings of the sebaceous follicles are the lipophilic yeasts belonging to the genera *Malassezia*. The commonest of these species on human skin are *M. globosa* and *M. sympodialis*. There are another six species of this genus and it is likely that as molecular classification is applied more widely there will be more. These fungi are normal skin residents, having the highest density on the scalp, face, and upper chest and back. They are known to cause disease in certain circumstances notably after exposure to sunlight and in warm and tropical environment when they cause the infection pityriasis versicolor. In addition they can cause a form of folliculitis sometimes in patients in the intensive care unit. They also contribute to the pathogenesis of seborrhoeic dermatitis. However, although *M. globosa*, for instance causes the vast majority of cases of pityriasis versicolor differentiation between species does not aid the management of these conditions; the diagnosis relies on direct microscopy of skin scrapings. Rarely in low birthweight neonates these yeasts cause fungaemia.

Candida species are not normally resident on the skin. However, they can be found in the oral cavity and the vagina as commensal organisms. The figures for carriage by healthy populations vary from study to study, but overall some 25% of individuals have oral colonization by *Candida* species. The commonest organism isolated is *Candida albicans*. This can be found temporarily on the skin itself on the hands but is more usually carried in moist areas such as the toe web spaces or in the groins where it can also cause a localized infection, intertrigo.

For other fungi presenting with skin disease all infections are exogenous and therefore exposure to them is the rate-limiting step in determining the prevalence of infection The common superficial infections due to fungi are the dermatophyte infections (dermatophytosis or ringworm), superficial candidosis or *Malassezia* infections. Dermatophyte infections are common in all patients and cause conditions such as tinea pedis, corporis, or capitis as well as infections of the fingernails, onychomyocosis. *Candida* is the cause of thrush, a common superficial infection of the oral or vaginal mucosal surfaces presenting with white plaques on an erythematous background. The main *Malassezia* infection is pityriasis versicolor where the skin is covered small or confluent hyper- or hypopigmented scaling patches. With the exception of oral candidosis (see below) none is particularly associated with cancer patients.

Systemic infections due to fungi are also seen in rare circumstances and infection of the skin can arise from this process, usually after haematogenous dissemination.

Disseminated candidosis for instance may affect the skin leading to nodules and papules scattered over the trunk and limbs. These are generally non-specific in clinical appearance and the diagnosis is only made after biopsy. Likewise the rare endemic fungal pathogens seen in parts of the USA or tropics can cause skin lesions after haematogenous dissemination. Generally, these are unusual in cancer patients, although they are important in those with HIV infection. Cryptococcosis, which may occur in patients with AIDS but also T-cell lymphoma, may lead to the appearance of small nodules or ulcers with raised edges on the skin. Histoplasmosis may produce similar lesions. In South-east Asia the organism *Penicillium marneffei* produces an infection that can produce similar changes.

Cancer and fungal infections of the skin

Superficial fungal infections

Dermatophytosis or tinea is common in all populations and there is no evidence to support the view that it is more common in patients with cancer. Onychomycosis though has been shown to have a higher incidence in cancer patients (Sigurgeirsson and Steingrimsson 2004) and, although the study was based on a community sample defined using photographs of potential lesions, the risk of developing onychomycosis in patients with cancer was about three times greater that a normal population. However, there are no known abnormal clinical features of these infections in cancer patients. The exception is certain systemic *Fusarium* infections that are seen in the neutropenic cancer patient. Here often the earliest sign of infection is swelling around a proximal nail fold on the feet. Often the patient has pre-existing discoloration on the nail usually affecting the superficial aspect of the nail plate, which shows a white discoloration and sometimes subungual discoloration. Swelling of the nail fold is followed by generalized swelling of the toe or affected digit and the patient is ill and febrile. Distal skin signs of haematogenous dissemination of *Fusarium* are circular plaques like lesions with central purplish discoloration. The organisms can be seen in biopsy material or cultures from the skin. Treatment with high doses of lipid-associated amphotericin can be used but success rates remain low.

For other nail infections treatment is similar to that used in otherwise healthy patients, although in some immunosuppressed patients it is necessary to use a longer course, i.e. more than 3 months at higher doses.

There is also an indirect relationship between cancer and prior irradiation treatment of scalp ringworm where there is a clear increased risk of non-melanoma skin cancer, mainly basal cell carcinomas developing years later in the irradiated area (Shore *et al* 2003). There is also evidence that there is an increased risk of brain and thyroid cancers forming in response to mean doses of irradiation of 1.4 Gy up to 39 years after the initial exposure to radiation.

Candidosis

Candida infections are caused by *Candida albicans* and a variety of other species such as *C. glabrata, C. tropicalis*, and *C. krusei*. As stated previously *Candida* is usually a commensal that can be isolated from the mouth but it can cause superficial infection in patients with underlying disease. Predisposing factors include lesion leading to a break in the skin or mucosal surface such as ulcers, antibiotic therapy, neutropenia, and T-lymphocyte abnormalities. Oropharyngeal candidosis is one of the commonest complications seen in immunosuppressed cancer patients or those receiving head and neck irradiation.

The usually presenting signs are the appearance of white plaques on a friable mucosal base on the hard or soft palate or buccal mucosa, less commonly the tongue (plaque-type candidosis). However, it may also present with more insidious lesions that are sore particularly when eating or drinking and difficult to distinguish from mucositis, (erythematous candidosis). There are no white plaques. In such cases extension of the infection to the oesophagus is common. The infection in either case may extend to the angles of the lips, cheilitis, and this may be a presenting sign indicating that there is more extensive oral *Candida* infection.

The infection can be diagnosed by taking a swab and examining a potassium hydroxide treated or Gram-stained smear by direct microscopy.

Treatment with an antifungal agent such as oral fluconazole or itraconazole is usually successful. Oral nystatin is a less satisfactory alternative. In neutropenic patients with severe mucositis tolerance of anti-*Candida* treatments may present problems as fluconazole syrup or itraconazole often taste sickly to patients with inflamed mucosae. It is important to treat oral candidosis in the immunocompromised patient symptomatically rather than persist with treatment to suppress recurrent infection if possible. Continuous treatment of oral *Candida* infection in the face of continuing immunosuppression is a potent risk factor for the development of azole resistance.

Systemic mycosis and the skin

Systemic fungal infections may present with skin lesions in the cancer patient. These are not common but the main types seen are:

- Invasive candidiasis. This occasionally presents with scattered skin nodules in a febrile patient with diffuse myalgia. The lesions are tender and non-specific and unless the organism is also isolated from blood cultures the only way of diagnosing the condition is by skin biopsy.

- Aspergillosis. Rarely, *Aspergillus* infections present as either cold abscesses or ecthyma gangrenosum-like lesions.

- Zygomycosis (mucormycosis). Infections due to zygomycete fungi such as *Absidia, Rhizomucor*, or *Rhizopus* may present with necrotic lesions adjacent to the paranasal sinuses or skin (McCarty *et al* 2004).

- In lymphoma patients and those with HIV/AIDS patients with infections due to *Histoplasma capsulatum, Cryptococcus neoformans*, and *Penicillium marneffei* may present with multiple skin papules and small ulcers often with a central area of softening like the lesions seen in molluscum contagiosum. These are accompanied by generalized haematogenous dissemination of infection.

While presentation of systemic mycoses with skin lesions is not common their importance serves to underline the need to biopsy unexplained skin lesions occurring in the cancer patient.

Viral infections of the skin

There are no viruses that are naturally resident on the normal human skin. Therefore, the presence of virus indicates the presence of the disease. The main pathogens seen in the human skin are the viruses of the HPV family, the herpes viruses, notably human herpes viruses (HHV)1 and 2, varicella zoster virus (VZV, now HHV3), HHV6 (slapped cheek syndrome), and HHV8 (Kaposi's sarcoma, molluscum contagiosum). Other infections such as measles that present as exanthems or manifestations of deep infection are covered elsewhere.

Human papillomaviruses

These are DNA viruses that belong to a large family of papilloma, viruses some of which infect animals and are often host specific in their choice, e.g. bovine papillomaviruses. The HPVs are a very large group of genetically typable viruses of which there are now over 70 recognized varieties. However, the main diseases are associated with specific HPV types seen below.

The commonest of these infections the warts are seen in all groups and are no more common in cancer patients (Table 9.2). However, the management of the common warts and plantar warts may be more complex in that as a result of immunosuppression they may be recalcitrant and very large. The treatment of HPV infections depends on the use of local destructive therapies such as cryotherapy, podophyllin, tricholacetic acid, surgery, electrodissection, laser ablation (Lauchli *et al* 2003), or bleomycin. Immunomodifiers such as imiquimod has hardly been more successful, although there appear to be some better cure rates for mucosal lesions—yet these have not been subject to direct comparative studies.

There are no assured cures for wart infections (Table 9.3) and in an extensive systematic review of the results of treatment Gibbs (Gibbs *et al* 2002) showed that there were very few comparative studies of sufficient weight on which

Table 9.2 HPV Associations with skin disease

Skin or mucosal infection	HPV type (only common associated forms are shown)
Common, plantar, mosaic warts	1, 2, 4
Plane warts	3, 10
Butcher's warts	7
Bowen's disease (some)	16
Epidermodysplasia verruciformis	3, 5, 8, 12, 36–38
Condyloma acuminata	6, 11
Intra-epithelial neoplasia, e.g. cervical dysplasia, bowenoid papulosis	16
Buschke Lowenstein tumour (giant condyloma)	6, 11
Florid oral papillomatosis	6, 11

Table 9.3 Treatments used for viral warts

Cytotoxic	Salicylic acid, Lactic acid, hydrochloric acid, trichloracetic acid podophyllin 10–25% (anogenital). Podophyllotoxin Bleomycin, 5 fluorouracil
Surgical/ablative	Cryotherapy Electrosurgery, laser, photodynamic therapy
Immunotherapy	Diphencyprone, Dintirocholobenzene (DNCB), Squaric acid, Imiquimod Interferon α
Occlusion	Duct tape
Other	Acupuncture Herbal Hypnosis

therapeutic advice could be based. It was also clear that recovery rates after treatment with over-the-counter products such as salicylic acid preparations versus cryotherapy are no different. It is possible to destroy individual wart lesions with ablative therapy; however, the recurrence rates are high. Sensitization of warts using diphencyprone is a more valuable approach to treatment, although patients are subjected to severe discomfort. However, there are no studies reporting the merits of this treatment in cancer patients.

Surgical or laser excision is the main treatment for intraepithelial neoplasms such as cervical dysplasia or Bowenoid papulosis.

The main interest in the relation between HPV infections and cancer is a causative one as a number of cancers, ranging from cervical carcinoma to some forms of squamous cancer of the skin associated with epidermodysplasia verruciformis, are derived from HPV lesions (Zur Hausen 1999, Iftner *et al* 2003). The mechanisms for deregulation of normal cell growth leading to cancer are incompletely understood. However, some of the early expressed products of the HPV genomes such as E6 and E7 have an effect on the cell cycle (O'Connor *et al* 2001). E6 for instance promotes degradation of P53, which in turn leads to loss of cell cycle arrest where there is damage to cellular DNA. It appears that the HPV types that are more likely to be associated with intraepithelial or frank carcinomas are more efficient at P53 degradation. E7 gene products promote DNA replication again leading to uncontrolled growth.

Vaccine studies using both mono- and multivalent HPV products based on HPV16 or HPV18 are currently in clinical trial for the prevention of cervical carcinoma.

Molluscum contagiosum

Molluscum contagiosum is a member of the pox viruses and is caused by one of two molecular subtypes (MCV1 and -2). It is a benign and self-limiting infection seen in infants and young adults usually, affecting the face of trunk in children and the genitalia in adults where it is sexually transmitted. The lesions are small 0.2-cm papules and they usually have a central plug of soft keratinous material. These vary in size and can be surrounded by a ring of eczema. Lesions are generally scattered on the trunk, face, or thighs. In HIV-positive patients it gives rise to large numbers of lesions often on the face, which are pleomorphic and atypical. This infection has not been reported as a particular problem in cancer patients. Other pox viruses that cause disease of the human skin such as cow pox, monkey pox, or orf are uncommon infections, which are also not specifically associated with cancer.

Human herpes infections

Herpes simplex

Herpes simplex infections or HSV infections type 1 and 2 are common in all areas. They cause disease such as cold sores and herpetic whitlows as well as disseminated infections. Herpes simplex infections are spread directly and the virus usually gains entry after viral shedding, e.g. with saliva or in the case of type 2 by sexual contact. Figures for prevalence rates for the two infections are not certain but at least 30% of the population are thought to have been infected by type 1 virus. Primary infections are those that occur in patients without prior exposure but in common with other members of this family a hallmark of infection is the ability to cause latent infection, in this case in the dorsal root ganglia of the central nervous system. A number of factors have been implicated in reactivation of infection, which range from sun exposure to a febrile reaction.

The typical lesions of herpes infection are small papules that cluster in area such as at one side to the mouth or lip. These develop over 24–48 hours into vesicles. The infection lasts for 3–6 days, although secondary infection with bacteria, such as *Staph. aureus*, is common. Immunosuppressed patient are more susceptible to recurrent disease and indeed in HIV/AIDS reactivation is often accompanied by deep ulceration and prolonged atypical infection. However, other situations encountered in the management of cancer do not appear to reactivate infection such as head and neck irradiation (Epstein *et al* 2002). Events resulting in very severe immunosuppression such as bone marrow transplantation may also result in a different pattern on infection—generalized dissemination to both the skin and other sites. Here the lesions are not simply confined to one area but may appear on multiple skin sites but infection of the other mucosal surfaces, the gastrointestinal tract and brain are also seen.

The main treatment for recurrent herpes simplex is topical treatment with aciclovir (5%) or penciclovir (1%). For more severe attacks oral aciclovir or valaciclovir may be used. For chronic suppression in those with very frequent and distressing attacks these can be used continuously. This reduces viral shedding resulting in a lower risk of transmission.

Varicella zoster human herpes virus type 3

VZV or HHV type 3 is the principal cause of two common diseases, chicken pox and shingles. The first is the primary manifestation of the infection, whereas the latter follows endogenous reactivation of latent infection. Chicken pox is predominantly a disease of childhood, whereas zoster usually appears later in life. Both can be associated with cancer, once again usually in the presence of very profound immunosuppression.

Typical cases of zoster present with discomfort or neuraesthesia in the area followed by the appearance of small papules in a dermatomal segment of the skin. These develop over 48 hours into small vesicles. They may also follow the distribution of a cranial nerve adding further complications such a severe corneal ulceration following involvement of the ophthalmic branch of the trigeminal nerve. Atypical forms are seen in some cancer patients and reactivation of latent virus infection can be triggered by radiotherapy or chemotherapy. The commonest form seen in these circumstances is best described as disseminated zoster where there are multiple papules and pustules often preceded by pain but the distribution extends outside the normal 1–2 dermatomal distribution. Like herpes simplex infections these may extend to other sites such as the gastrointestinal tract. In HIV/AIDS the skin lesions are often atypical and may appear verrucose, haemorrhagic, or confluent. Even in the more widespread forms there may be residual pain after disappearance of lesions—post-herpetic neuralgia, although this is more often a feature of localized disease. Herpes zoster occurs in a large proportion of patients in the first year after bone marrow engraftment. These may be atypical with haemorrhagic or ulcerative forms being seen, particularly early after transplant.

Treatment of herpes simplex virus infections is usually confined to the symptoms with analgesia and rest. However, in the cancer patient active - antiviral therapy is advisable. Aciclovir, famciclovir, or valciclovir are usually used in such patients. Treatment is started as soon as possible. Intravenous aciclovir should be used to initiate therapy if the patient is immunosuppressed.

Human herpes virus type 6: exanthem subitum

This disease know as roseola infantum is a common and benign condition that presents with fever and rubelliform rash. It has also been reported in association with acute leukaemia and bone marrow graft recipients (Yoshikawa et al 1996).

Human herpes virus type 8: Kaposi's sarcoma

Kaposi's sarcoma is the name given to a specific tumour that is caused by HHV8. The condition was originally described in Europe among elderly Jewish patients who presented with purplish nodules and plaques usually on the lower limbs. The condition slowly spread and was ultimately fatal. A second form was subsequently described where the disease affected patients at a younger age but they were mainly seen in sub-Saharan Africa and then again the limbs were infiltrated by papules and nodules. The emergence of HIV/AIDS produced a third form where the initial lesions are flatter and appear as small ecchymoses, although they may subsequently become infiltrated or ulcerative. Involvement of multiple sites on the trunk, the mouth, and internal organs such as the lungs can occur. Gastrointestinal involvement may also develop. A similar form is occasionally seen in patients who are immunosuppressed for other reasons. Diffuse Kaposi's sarcoma has been associated in AIDS patients with Castleman's disease and primary effusion lymphoma, although the causal relation is not understood.

The biopsy appearances of Kaposi's lesions are typical with atypical endothelial cells lining vascular channels. These are surrounded by spindle cells. There is a variable lymphocytic infiltrate throughout the lesions.

Superficial lesions may respond well to radiotherapy. Doxirubicin or daunorubicin are effective in widely disseminated cases. However, lesions disappear with the institution of highly active antiretroviral therapy in AIDS patients

Scabies

Scabies is an infestation with the human scabies mite, *Sarcoptes scabei*. The infection affects the stratum corneum of the skin and does not extend beneath. It is common in young adults, the elderly and in many developing countries among infants and children as well as in institutionalized individuals, e.g. in prisons. Close contact and overcrowding predispose to infection. The infection follows transfer of a mite from another human and the mature adult burrowing into the epidermis of the new host creating a small tunnel in the keratin layer. The scabies mite causes considerable itching and lesions, which are papules, and linear tunnels are mainly seen on the hands, wrists, shoulders, lumbar and buttock area, external genitalia, and lower legs. Itching can be intense and is worse at night. This damage is caused by a small number of mites, e.g. 11–15 adults per host.

In immunosuppressed patients the scabies mite may behave atypically and very large numbers are seen leading to superficial crusting of the skin often in the areas of predilection. However, other sites such as the head and the nails may be affected in crusted or Norwegian scabies. This form is seen in patients who are severely immunosuppressed such as AIDS patients. It is rare in cancer patients.

Scabies is transmissible to others. While the normal patterns of scabies can only be transmitted after close contact, the crusted forms can be spread by casual contact including on hospital wards among staff and other patients.

The main treatment is the application of topical scabicides such as benzyl benzoate, gamma benzene hexachloride, malathion, or permethrin. The latter are most effective and can be used once. Treatment of crusted scabies is challenging and it may be necessary to use several treatments; the oral agent ivermectin, which is used to treat acarid infestations in farm animals is also effective in severe forms of scabies.

References

General

Chren MM, Lazarus HM, Salata RA, and Landefeld CS. (1995). Cultures of skin biopsy tissue from immunocompromised patients with cancer and rashes. *Archives of Dermatology*, **131**, 552–555.

Bacterial infections

Davies HD, McGeer A, Schwartz B, *et al.* (1996). Invasive group A streptococcal infections in Ontario, Canada. Ontario Group A Streptococcal Study Group. *New England Journal of Medicine*, **335**, 547–554.

Penel N, Fournier C, Lefebvre D, *et al.* (2004). Previous chemotherapy as a predictor of wound infections in non-major head and neck surgery: Results of a prospective study. *Head & Neck*, **26**, 513–517.

Brewer VH, Hahn KA, Rohrbach BW, Bell JL, and Baddour LM. (2000). Risk factor analysis for breast cellulitis complicating breast conservation therapy. *Clinical Infectious Diseases*, **31**, 654–659.

Gould N, Kamelle S, Tillmanns T, *et al.* (2001). Predictors of complications after inguinal lymphadenectomy. *Gynecologic Oncology*, **82**, 329–332.

Hughes LL, Styblo TM, Thoms WW, *et al.* (1997). Cellulitis of the breast as a complication of breast-conserving surgery and irradiation. *American Journal of Clinical Oncology*, **20**, 338–341.

Vartivarian SE, Papadakis KA, Palacios JA, Manning JT Jr, and Anaissie EJ. (1994). Mucocutaneous and soft tissue infections caused by Xanthomonas maltophilia. A new spectrum. *Annals of Internal Medicine*, **121**, 969–973.

Childers BJ, Potyondy LD, Nachreiner R, *et al.* (2002). Necrotizing fasciitis: a fourteen-year retrospective study of 163 consecutive patients. *American Surgeon*, **68**, 109–116.

Lamy A, Tissot B, and Pigot F. (2003). Perineal necrotizing cellulitis disclosing rectal adenocarcinoma. *Annales de Chirurgie*, **128**, 630–632.

Korten V, Gurbuz O, Firatli T, Bayik M, and Akoglu T. (1992). Subcutaneous nodules caused by Pseudomonas aeruginosa: healing without incision and drainage. *Journal of Chemotherapy*, **4**, 225–227.

Ye Z, Shimomura H, Kudo S, Arao T, Sato Y, and Ono T. (1996). A case of lymphocutaneous nocardiosis with a review of lymphocutaneous nocardiosis reported in Japan. *Journal of Dermatology*, **23**, 120–124.

Fungal infections

Sigurgeirsson B and Steingrimsson O. (2004). Risk factors associated with onychomycosis. *Journal of the European Academy of Dermatology and Venereology*, **18**, 48–51.

Shore RE, Moseson M, Harley N, and Pasternack BS. (2003). Tumors and other diseases following childhood x-ray treatment for ringworm of the scalp. *Health Physics*, **85**, 404–408.

McCarty ML, Wilson MW, Fleming JC, *et al.* (2004). Manifestations of fungal cellulitis of the orbit in children with neutropenia and fever. *Ophthalmic Plastic & Reconstructive Surgery*, **20**, 217–223.

Viral infections

Lauchli S, Kempf W, Dragieva G, Burg G, and Hafner J. (2003). CO_2 laser treatment of warts in immunosuppressed patients. *Dermatology*, 2003; **206**, 148–152.

Gibbs S, Harvey I, Sterling J, and Stark R. (2002). Local treatments for cutaneous warts, systematic review. *British Medical Journal*, **325**, 461–464.

zur Hausen H. (1999). Papillomaviruses in human cancers. *Proceedings of the Association of American Physicians*, **111**, 581–587.

Iftner A, Klug SJ, Garbe C, *et al.* (2003). The prevalence of human papillomavirus genotypes in nonmelanoma skin cancers of nonimmunosuppressed individuals identifies high-risk genital types as possible risk factors. *Cancer Research*, **63**, 7515–7519.

O'Connor DP, Kay EW, Leader M, Murphy GM, Atkins GJ, and Mabruk MJ. (2001). Altered p53 expression in benign and malignant skin lesions from renal transplant recipients and immunocompetent patients with skin cancer: correlation with human papillomaviruses? *Diagnostic Molecular Pathology*, **10**, 190–199.

Epstein JB, Gorsky M, Hancock P, Peters N, and Sherlock CH. (2002). The prevalence of herpes simplex virus shedding and infection in the oral cavity of seropositive patients undergoing head and neck radiation therapy. *Oral Surgery, Oral Medicine, Oral Pathology, Oral Radiology and Endodontics*, **94**, 712–716.

Yoshikawa T, Suga S, and Asano Y. (1996). Human herpes virus 6 infection in bone marrow transplantation. *Blood*, **78**, 1381–1384.

Chapter 10

Infections of the central nervous system

Geoff Scott

Introduction

Cancer and its chemotherapy lead to increased susceptibility to infections. Central nervous system (CNS) infections are rare but commonly fatal and a disappointing outcome in patients who may have otherwise been successfully treated for their tumours. The degree of immunosuppression conferred by the neoplastic disease and its treatment determine what sort of infections can be expected. The greater the degree of immunosuppression, the more likely that infection can arise from otherwise harmless saprophytes. Primary CNS infections with traditional virulent organisms such as the meningococcus and *Haemophilus influenzae* are quite rare in otherwise healthy people so that, although they may occur in patients with cancer, the absolute number of individuals with malignancy who develop community-acquired 'virulent' infections is very low. Nevertheless, B-lymphocyte diseases such as myeloma particularly predispose to pneumococcal infections.

CNS infections are most likely to occur in those who are most immunosuppressed by disease aggravated by chemotherapy, allogeneic or autograft transplantation, radiation, corticosteroids, splenectomy, or underlying human immunodeficiency virus infection. They may also follow neurosurgical procedures.

Leukaemia–lymphoma and allogeneic bone marrow transplantation with profound prolonged neutropenia allow invasive infection with almost any bacterium or fungus or reactivation of protozoa such as *Toxoplasma gondii*. Immunosuppression to prevent graft-versus-host disease further extends the risk beyond the phase of acute susceptibility due to chemotherapy. Lymphoma complicating human immunodeficiency virus infection with CD4 lymphopenia adds a further dimension to the range of potentially pathogenic organisms that have to be considered. The risks are much lower with solid tumours and chemotherapy.

Bacteria and fungi delivered *via* the bloodstream may cause meningoen-cephalitis, brain mass lesions, or abscesses. Some blood-borne causes of these conditions in cancer such as *Listeria monocytogenes*, *Nocardia asteroides*, fungi, and *Toxoplasma gondii* are very rare in healthy individuals. In addition in cancer patients more than one infection may occur in the same individual. Surgery for CNS tumours also presents a special risk of post-surgical sepsis. Bacteria may be inoculated directly into the CNS by surgery for primary and secondary tumours and via ventriculo-peritoneal shunts, extraventricular drains, and Ommaya reservoirs used to administer intraventricular chemotherapy. Lumbar punctures to administer chemotherapy may also

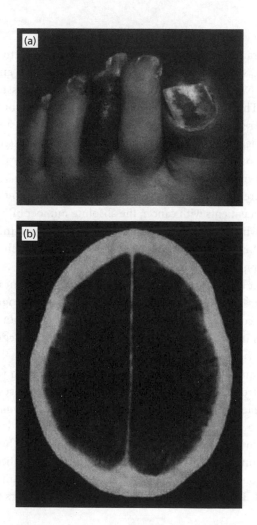

Fig. 10.1 Male 60y AML neutropenic after chemotherapy for 21 days. Generalised skin rash (haemorrhagic 1–2cm papules). Right parietal lesion. Cause: *Acremonium* sp.. Origin: chronic toe nail infection. See colour plate section.

introduce bacteria or fungi, most likely by breaching the blood–brain barrier and causing extravasation of blood containing micro-organisms into the cerebrospinal fluid (CSF).

Viruses tend to cause diffuse or focal encephalitis or myelitis. Infection occurs by reactivation of latent virus in the CNS or by acquisition of new agents usually by the respiratory route.

Making a microbiological diagnosis is the key to selecting optimal therapy. The range of organisms involved, each rare, makes selecting rational empirical therapy extremely difficult. Most patients will already have been exposed to antimicrobials, selecting for resistant organisms, making bacteriological diagnosis difficult and enhancing susceptibility to saprophytes. Imaging has revolutionized the ability to localize infection but also may help to distinguish non-infectious causes. Histological and microbiological examination of CSF and lesional biopsies are crucial to specific diagnosis.

Classification of infections

Infections can be broadly divided into those that cause inflammation of the meninges, diffuse encephalitis, and mass lesions. There may well be an overlap between these conditions but it is convenient to classify them according to the predominant manifestation of the infection. The symptoms, signs, and surrogate markers of CNS infection are usually attenuated by all aspects of immunosuppression. On presentation, the differential diagnosis of any syndrome will include many non-infectious causes, including tumour effects, metabolic abnormalities, or drug toxicity.

Bacteraemia with any organism may occasionally predispose to meningitis. Classically, staphylococci are associated with intravenous line infection or endocarditis and Gram-negative organisms with translocation from the gut. As in non-immunosuppressed individuals, metastatic *Staphylococcus aureus* may settle in bone causing an extradural abscess. Staphylococci are also the most common causes of postoperative sepsis after neurosurgical procedures for primary and secondary intracranial tumours. However, it is in this group of patients that invasive Gram-negative infections with coliforms and pseudomonads, which would hardly ever be seen in immunocompetent individuals, can also occur. Fungi often disseminate in the bloodstream: intracranial embolism and fungal masses commonly occur as part of the syndrome (See fig 10.1). Various virus infections tend to cause encephalitis. Most commonly, these are members of the human herpesviridae, adenovirus, and papovavirus families. Established latent parasites in bradyzoite form, especially *Toxoplasma gondii*, may start to replicate and cause brain cysts and encephalitis.

Clinical approach to diagnosis

Table 10.1 provides a scheme for how to consider and investigate a patient with suspected CNS infection. This cannot be comprehensive but indicates a logical progression of steps to aid investigation and may help to prevent missing an obvious diagnosis.

Table 10.1 Diagnostic approach for investigation of meningoencephalitis or mass central nervous system lesions in cancer

Is this the first presentation of cancer?

If not, what degree of immunosuppression is there? Note stage of disease and treatment.

• Solid tumour

  plus

  chemotherapy

  corticosteroids

  neutropenia

• Haemopoietic malignancy: severity of predicted immunosuppression (e.g. Acute myeloid leukaemia versus Hodgkin's disease)

  plus

  chemotherapy

  corticosteroids

  transplant: allograft or autograft

  graft-versus-host disease

  neutropenia

• Specific malignancy

  —myeloma

  —brain tumour

  plus

  surgery

  chemotherapy: systemic or local

  radiotherapy

  corticosteroids

History

Accurate details of the presenting complaint

• Speed of onset

• Are there any focal symptoms?

Table 10.1 (*Continued*)

Is this part of a wider known syndrome?

* Disseminated
  —tuberculosis
  —bacterial infection
     endocarditis
     line-associated or gut translocation bacteraemia
  —fungal infection
     from lung or sinuses
  —parasitic infection
     toxoplasmosis
* Coincident mumps, chicken pox, measles etc.
* Non-infectious complication of cancer
  —stroke
  —vasculitis
  —drug effects

In the history, check

* Employment and hobbies
* Foreign travel (where exactly, and when, behaviour)
  —arthropod exposure (ticks, mosquitoes, etc.)
   sexual history
* Immunization history

PLUS

* Vaccination history
* Exposure to contacts with infection
* Freshwater swimming/diving
* Drugs: chemotherapy, NSAIDs, penicillin, carbamazepine, Ara-C, sulphas, etc.

Physical examination

* Skin and mouth
  —be prepared to biopsy or aspirate skin lesions
* Sinuses
* Cardiology
* Focal neurology

Rapid assessment to exclude toxic confusional state

* Metabolic
* Drug evaluation and screen

Table 10.1 (*Continued*)

- Sepsis
- Consider paraneoplastic syndromes

Imaging

- Chest X-ray

  —Brain and spinal cord   —masses

  —abscess

  - diffuse change
  - focal change
  - basal or diffuse meningeal enhancement
  - atrophy
  - hydrocephalus

[MRI with gadolinium enhancement is most sensitive but CT may be easier to obtain (e.g. prior to lumbar puncture to prevent herniation/coning). Always ask for 'with contrast' images. High resolution CT with bone windows will show bony defects. Include sinuses and middle ears. Angiography: in special circumstances]

- Other imaging

  —echocardiogram? Transoesophageal preferred to exclude valve lesion

Diagnostic tests

- *Blood culture(s)* preferably before antibiotics (line-associated bacteraemia, endocarditis, etc.)

  —Review blood culture results over the last periods of treatment

- *Review routine blood tests*

  —FBC ESR

  —renal

  —liver

  —albumin, globulin

  —C-reactive protein

  —glucose

  —thyroid

  —Ca^{2+}

  —EDTA (sequestrene) specimen for polymerase chain reaction (PCR), save in virology

- Review: previous serological tests

  —immunity to

     varicella zoster

     Toxoplasma gondii

     measles (in children)

Table 10.1 (*Continued*)

cytomegalovirus

Epstein–Barr virus

Cerebral spinal fluid (CSF): routine

• Cell count

—smear (Giemsa)

neutrophils

mononuclear cells: lymphocytes and monocytes

eosinophils

other

• Bacteria, etc.

—wet prep (counting chamber)

—Gram stain

—motility (*Listeria monocytogenes*)

—acridine orange (stains bacterial DNA and RNA, useful if patient on antibiotics and Gram-stain negative)

—India ink exclusion

—Auramine O or ZN (centrifugation of large volume)

• Culture

—bacterial

—fungal

—viral

—mycobacteria

—special

protozoa

• Antigen tests

—available for meningococci, pneumococci, *Haemophilus influenzae* b, *Cryptococcus neoformans*

Chemistry

• Protein

—CSF/serum albumin ratio

• Glucose

—CSF/blood glucose ratio

• Lactate (high in tuberculosis (TB), bacterial)

• oligoclonal bands (immunoglobulins late >5 days), parallel with serum (IgA brain abscess and TB, IgM Lyme mumps, non-Hodgkin lymphoma) CSF/serum IgG

Save uncentrifuged specimen at −70° C in several aliquots for molecular diagnosis

Table 10.1 (*Continued*)

Brain biopsy

* Histology
  —tumour
  —mass lesions suggesting infection
  > granulomas (mycobacteria, etc.)

  > Splendore–Hoeppli lesion (*Nocardia, Actinomyces*)

  —diffuse changes
  > encephalitis

  > progressive multifocal leucoencephalopathy

  —fungi
  > *Candida* spp.

  > *Aspergillus* spp.

  > mucorales

  (Appropriate travel history)
  > *Histoplasma capsulatum*

  > *Coccidioides immitis*

  > *Penicillium marneffei*
* Culture and DNA probe: appropriate to histological appearance

Specific diagnostic tests

NB *Limitations*: availability (liaison with local laboratory and list of reference laboratories), lack of validation and cost. You can elect not to do a test if the disease is epidemiologically unlikely.

NO TRAVEL

Clotted blood

* dsRNA, autoimmune 'screen'
* Angiotensin-converting enzyme (ACE)
* Save serum
* Serology for
  —toxoplasmosis
  —HIV
  —cytomegalovirus (CMV)
  —Epstein–Barr virus

EDTA blood

  —meningococcus PCR
  —save for further DNA studies (e.g. CMV PCR)

Table 10.1 (*Continued*)

Cerebral spinal fluid

- Herpesvirus PCR
- Enterovirus RNA (reverse transcription–PCR)
- Virus culture
  —herpesviruses
  —enterovirus
  —adenoviruses

Stool and T/S for enterovirus

  Check date of onset

  Convalescent serum 7 days and 14 days

  Mycoplasma

  Legionella

  Chlamydia

  Lyme borreliosis

  mumps

  measles

  influenza

  syphilis

  Leptospira

  Bartonella

  Trophyrema

  REPEAT CSF (insufficient for all tests or evolving disease?)

  large volume TB, etc.

  Oligoclonal bands

  Save CSF and consider further tests

TRAVEL

Many of these will not be relevant, although some patients may have been born abroad. Tests should be selected dependent on details of syndrome and travel history.

World-wide

- Tuberculosis
- Rabies
- Polio

Africa

- Malaria
- Flaviviruses
- Congo-Crimean Haemorrhagic Fever

Table 10.1 (*Continued*)

- West Nile Fever
- If eosinophilia (which does not have to be present)
    - *Taenia solium* (cysticercosis)
    - *Echinococcus* (hydatid)
    - *Trypanosoma* (sleeping sickness)
    - *Strongyloides* (larva migrans)
    - *Schistosoma*
- Other
    - *Rickettsia*
    - *Bartonella*
- Eosinophilic meningitis
    - nematodes
- Any fungus

Europe
    - tick-borne encephalitis
    - *Brucella* spp.
    - Hantavirus
    - *Bartonella*
    - *Rickettsia*

Asia
- Dengue
- Japanese B encephalitis
    - *Schistosoma japonicum*
    - Hantavirus
    - *Rickettsia*
    - *Penicillium marneffei*

America
- West Nile virus
- Western equine encephalitis
- Eastern equine encephalitis
- Venezuelan equine encephalitis
- St Louis virus
- Colorado tick fever
- Fungi
    - *Histoplasma capsulatum*
    - *Coccidioides immitis*

The key to clinical diagnosis is the history. Generally, new symptoms occur in the context of the cancer and its treatment and the stage of cancer and degree of immunosuppression will be well known. Very occasionally, pneumococcal meningitis will be the first sign of, for instance, myeloma. A detailed history of travel and occupational exposure should be taken.

The symptoms rarely come on rapidly even with more virulent organisms. Classical presentation with obtundation, neck stiffness and extension, and photophobia is unusual. This is because the patient is unable to respond to infection by mounting a normal inflammatory response. Patients often have mild changes in cerebral function, headache, fever, and sometimes focal symptoms and signs or convulsions. Insidious onset is a feature of infections with *Mycobacterium tuberculosis*, *Treponema pallidum*, and fungi. Certain specific syndromes such as limbic encephalitis are associated with herpes viruses. Similarly brainstem encephalomyelitis is a feature of *Cryptococcus neoformans* or *Listeria monocytogenes* infections.

The syndrome must be assessed in relation to the degree of immunosuppression by disease and cancer chemotherapy.

The most important first investigation is scanning of the CNS. Both computerized tomographic X-radiographs and magnetic resonance imaging, preferably with, and without, contrast imaging, play a major part in identifying lesions. Generally the latter will show smaller lesions but the former may be more easily obtainable at short notice. A microbiological–pathological diagnosis cannot be made by radiology.

In CNS infection, blood cultures (current or historical) may yield the causative organism. In a new syndrome, however, not too much reliance should be placed on old blood culture results. If the diagnosis is not clear then further invasive procedures are necessary. The simple investigation by lumbar puncture of CSF may be instructive. However, this may be contraindicated if the platelet count is very low. A platelet infusion before the procedure may be necessary but in the worst cases when there is no peripheral increment after platelet infusion, the procedure may simply not be possible. On the other hand, the risk of tentorial herniation following lumbar puncture has been exaggerated.

With profound peripheral neutropenia, there are usually no polymorphonuclear leucocytes in the CSF even in the face of plentiful bacteria. The protein may be elevated and the CSF sugar low in relation to the blood sugar in most pyogenic or tuberculous meningitis, but only if cells are present. If specialist laboratories are available, oligoclonal bands in the CSF compared with bands in the serum may indicate infection or demyelination. None of these tests are precise enough to direct therapy if the microbiology is negative. Known viruses are generally identified by DNA amplification methods. However, it is important to note that many viruses are latent in the CNS, are activated by immunosuppression and it is tempting to ascribe a syndrome to any isolate detected.

Unless a test is 100% sensitive and specific (and no microbiological tests are), the positive-predictive (PVP) and negative-predictive (PVN) values of any test are enormously influenced by the prevalence of the disease in the population, which in this situation, by definition, will tend to be low. This is well illustrated by comparing results in a population with high and low prevalence of a disease. If the sensitivity of a test is 90% (1:10 missed), and specificity 95% (1:20 false positive), for a common disease with expected rate of positivity of 17%, the PVP will be 78%; for an uncommon disease with expected rate of positivity 1%, the PVP will be only 15%. In general, it is tempting for clinicians to fit a syndrome to a positive test result but it is very important to keep an open mind.

Serological tests for antibodies to micro-organisms are generally unhelpful. At best an IgM titre will indicate recent infection, at worst it will be misleading. Polyclonal activation may lead to an anamnestic (memory-derived) response. However, negative antibodies to, for instance, *Toxoplasma* may be very helpful in excluding this disease.

For mass lesions, unless the likely cause can be identified as part of a generalized syndrome by, for example, blood culture or peripheral lesion biopsy, it may be necessary to perform a burr hole and obtain tissue by biopsy for histological and microbiological examination. The biopsies will be small and must not be wasted: the microbiology tests should be dictated by the histological appearance. Therefore, it is important to get rapid histopathology examination performed and the samples for microbiology processing reserved until these are ready.

Meningitis

Patients often present more insidiously than those who are not immunosuppressed. There are often mild symptoms indicating encephalitis. There may be few inflammatory cells in the CSF but many organisms, especially if the patient is neutropenic. This is a poor prognostic feature. If the blood–brain barrier is not disrupted by an inflammatory response, then, theoretically, agents such as penicillin may not penetrate very well. Occasionally an agent circulating in the blood may be introduced by therapeutic lumbar puncture, for example to deliver methotrexate. In patients immunosuppressed but without any neurosurgical procedure, the commonest bacteria causing meningitis include *Streptococcus pneumoniae*, *Streptococcus bovis*, *Staphylococcus aureus*, and *Listeria monocytogenes*. The commonest invasive fungi are *Candida albicans* and *Cryptococcus neoformans*.

CSF protein and glucose (with concurrent blood glucose) will be measured and CSF also examined microscopically for cells and micro-organisms. Cultures will be set up for cultivable organisms and usually enriched in broth for up to 5 days. If there is a mononuclear cell predominance, it may be appropriate to cytospin 100–200 μl of CSF and use appropriate monoclonal antibodies to establish whether the cells are monoclonal thus reflecting malignant disease.

A modest rise in CSF protein ($>0.5 < 1.2$ g/l) and predominant lymphocytosis with normal CSF glucose ($\geq$50% blood glucose) indicate virus infection. Glucose is consumed by cells in pyogenic and mycobacterial or listerial meningitis. Both lead to significant rises in CSF protein but, in general, polymorphonuclear cells predominate with the former and lymphocytes in the latter. These rules are not absolute. It is not unusual in the early phase of viral, tuberculous or listerial meningitis to have a polymorphonuclear cell predominance and virtually normal chemistry.

It is important to try to identify the causative organism and obtain antimicrobial sensitivities in order to direct antimicrobial therapy. There is increasing resistance to commonly used antimicrobials in *S. aureus* and *S. pneumoniae*. Empirical therapy is usually with a broad-spectrum cephalosporin that will penetrate the CSF well (e.g. cefotaxime, ceftriaxone, or ceftazidime) but that will not be active against methicillin-resistant *S. aureus* and some strains of penicillin-resistant pneumococcus. Problems also arise with Gram-negatives, which produce extended spectrum β-lactamase and are resistant to all cephalosporins. Glycopeptides, aminoglycosides, and macrolides do not cross the blood-brain barrier and flucloxacillin, ureidopenicillins, and carbapenems penetrate poorly.

More useful broad-spectrum antimicrobials that do penetrate sufficiently well include chloramphenicol, amoxicillin, sulphonamide, rifampicin, and linezolid. Except for rifampicin, these are bacteriostatic antibiotics that may not work even though adequate concentrations which well exceed the *in vitro* minimal inhibitory concentration are achievable. Although drastic, it may be necessary to place an extraventricular drain to deliver non-absorbable bactericidal antibiotics. Antibiotics should not be delivered into the lumbar cerebrospinal space because they will not be distributed through the whole subarachnoid space. Fungal meningitis requires directed therapy, for example with amphotericin B and 5-fluorocytosine, then fluconazole or voriconazole.

Listeria monocytogenes

L. monocytogenes is found in contaminated unpasteurized dairy products, and other raw food contaminated with animal faeces. Cancer patients are discouraged from eating these products. It may be found as part of the established gut flora in humans and can cause an acute gastrointestinal infection in immunocompetent individuals on acquisition of a large dose. Colonization is encouraged by stomach acid inhibition. Sepsis with acute amnionitis occurs in pregnant women and, although rare, sepsis in neonates and elderly adults carries a mortality of 1:5. Cases have occurred after sigmoidoscopy and colonoscopy. Like *M. tuberculosis*, *Listeria* is an intracellular parasite that can only be controlled by intact cell-mediated immunity.

In cancer patients, treatment with fludarabine and prednisolone seems to be a particular risk and invasive disease is most likely with bone marrow transplantation (Safdar *et al.* 2002). A Gram-positive rod with characteristic motility at room temperature, it can replicate at 4°C, and grows well on simple media. In clinical specimens, the organism may be pleomorphic and Gram-variable but CSF can be examined for motile organisms when *Listeria* is suspected. Although there is much awareness of the risk of listeriosis in cancer patients, the disease is relatively rare. Bacteraemia occurs in our practice ($\approx$220 first febrile neutropenic episodes per annum) less often than once per year and there has not been a case of meningitis in 20 years. An impression that there has been a reduction in cases over the last 10 years suggests that the food industry have now recognized the risk and is testing products for contamination. Translocation and bacteraemic spread leads to infection of the CNS. The organism infects brain tissue as well as causing meningitis so the patient often has decreased consciousness and focal signs. There is particular tropism for the brainstem with asymmetrical cranial nerve palsies, cerebellar, and long tract abnormalities. In much the same way that *M. tuberculosis* infects the brain, there may be multiple brain abscesses with meningitis in about one half of cases.

The recommended treatment is amoxycillin in high dose together with gentamicin. An alternative is to combine the amoxicillin with co-trimoxazole, a regimen that may give a better outcome, perhaps because gentamicin does not cross the blood–brain barrier (Merle-Melet *et al.* 1996). There have been no controlled clinical trials and observations are anecdotal. In patients allergic to penicillin and sulphonamides, perhaps a quinolone with good CSF penetration, such as levofloxacin, is the choice. Relapse is common so patients should be treated for 3 weeks. Patients with abscesses and encephalitis particularly involving the brainstem have a poor prognosis.

Mycobacterium tuberculosis

Tuberculous infections are more common than *Listeria*. Dissemination and CNS involvement may occur in immunocompetent patients.

Immunosuppression allows reactivation of latent infection, which may appear as pulmonary disease and disseminate as though the patient had post-primary miliary spread. The risk of development of true miliary disease is dependent on good cell-mediated immunity.

Meningitis arises from the development and rupture of subependymal microtubercles. About one half of patients have intracranial tuberculomas without meningitis. If meningitis is present, then there should be a lymphocytic infiltration and a relatively low CSF glucose with a high CSF protein level. However, in the early stages and in some who are immunosuppressed, neutrophils may predominate and the sugar is normal. Repeated lumbar puncture is needed to watch the evolution of the CSF changes and a large volume is necessary to increase the chances of seeing mycobacteria. DNA amplification of mycobacterial sequences adds little to good microscopy. The culture will be delayed so treatment must be started empirically. Unfortunately, surrogate markers such as PPD skin test reaction and interferon-γ tests are rarely helpful in deciding whether to treat or not. The treatment is standard, with pyrazinamide penetrating the blood–brain barrier well, and isoniazid and rifampicin penetrating adequately. It is usual to increase the adult dose of isoniazid to 10 mg/kg (usually 600 mg/day). Most patients will already be on corticosteroids for their cancer treatment but it may be necessary to add these or optimize the dose. Rifampicin reduces the bioavailable concentration of corticosteroid by about one half. There is no place for streptomycin or ethambutol in the treatment of tuberculous meningitis, because neither cross the blood–brain barrier.

Cryptococcus neoformans

This asexual haploid capsulate yeast that can undergo sexual recombination under special circumstances was a rare cause of infection before AIDS despite widespread existence in the environment. There are two main variants of this organism. *C. neoformans* var. *neoformans* is cosmopolitan and particularly associated with bird (pigeon, chicken, and turkey) faeces. It contaminates nests and soil. *C. neoformans* var. *gatti* is geographically constrained, mainly to Africa, not associated with guano but more with certain *Eucalyptus* and probably other trees, and is more virulent. Var. *neoformans* is not particularly virulent and infected only five to 10 patients per year before the advent of AIDS in the UK.

The organism is acquired by inhalation and causes a complex of peripheral lesions, with lymph node enlargement analogous to that seen in primary tuberculosis. The organism may then remain dormant. Solitary non-calcified lung nodules may be mistaken for cancer or tuberculoma. Pneumonia and dissemination is then driven by immunosuppression. Cryptococcal meningitis is classically subacute or chronic and presents with headache, fever, and altered mental state and memory. There may be cranial nerve palsies or hydrocephalus. Scanning may reveal nodules in the brain, gyral enhancement, or hydrocephalus. Often in severely immunocompromised patients there are characteristic skin lesions that can be biopsied. Furthermore, blood cultures are often positive and serum cryptococcal antigen (CRAG) is detectable. The changes in the CSF are similar to those of *Listeria* or tuberculosis but capsulate yeasts are easily visualized by India ink exclusion. Noncapsulate forms resemble lymphocytes so further staining is required. The CSF CRAG is positive.

Treatment is with amphotericin B deoxycholate at 0.7 mg/kg or liposomal amphotericin B at 4 mg/kg (Leenders *et al.* 1997). Flucytosine, which crosses the blood–brain barrier well, is added for synergy (Bennett *et al.* 1979). Fluconazole also penetrates well and is used for continuation therapy. Itraconazole (poor penetration) and caspofungin (unreliable activity) are not indicated.

Candida albicans

C. albicans has proved to be the most common cause of cerebral lesions in autopsy studies in cancer patients (Chimelli and Mahler-Araujo 1997). Perhaps this is not surprising given the propensity for candidosis in such patients. Microabscesses, which arise from dissemination into the brain, often rupture into the subarachnoid space causing pachymeningitis. Alternatively, the organism might arise from lumbar puncture, shunts, and extraventricular drains usually after patients have been treated with antibiotics. CSF contains large numbers of lymphocytes, a high protein and a relatively low sugar level. The organism is seen in about half of the cases and grown in most. Non-albicans species may be increasing in frequency as prophylaxis for *C. albicans* is used widely. Hydrocephalus is a complication of fungal growth within the narrow foramina in the brain.

Enterovirus

Enteroviruses are the commonest cause of meningitis in healthy individuals and occur particularly in late summer in temperate climes. Encephalitis and paralytic illness are rare manifestations of infection. There are many serotypes of non-polio Echo and Coxsackie viruses. Chronic excretion of one or more viruses is common especially in poor communities. B-cell-deficient patients are particularly prone to severe infection. Bone marrow transplant recipients have developed very severe illness with chronic encephalitis with fatal outcome (Biggs *et al.* 1990; Acquino *et al.* 1996). Immunoglobulin may be useful though efficacy has not been proved. The antiviral pleconaril may reduce the length of a meningitic illness in healthy children (Rotbart 2002). There is no evidence of benefit yet in severely affected immunocompromised patients.

Meningitis or ventriculitis in patients with cancer receiving neurosurgical procedures

Most infections are secondary to neurosurgical procedures and are usually with *Staphylococcus epidermidis*, *S. aureus*, Gram-negative organisms (coliforms or *Pseudomonas aeruginosa*) or *Propionibacterium* spp. Wound infection classically occurs 10–14 days after surgery. It is presumed that these organisms being normal or abnormal skin flora gain entry directly from the environment to the brain at the time of surgery. However, patients may be transiently bacteraemic at this time and some infections might arise via this route. Patients with a residual extraventricular drain have an inevitable additional risk of secondary infection of the ventricular system.

Pernasal sinus extirpation of a pituitary tumour presents a special risk of inoculation of nasal flora into the pituitary fossa and subsequent meningitis.

It is usually possible to obtain ventricular CSF easily from extraventricular drains or by puncturing the valve of a ventriculoperitoneal shunt system or from an Ommaya reservoir. If these devices are blocked, then they must be removed or changed forthwith. If there is a natural block to CSF flow, lumbar CSF may simply show a high protein but may not reveal a causative organism.

Treatment must be tailored to the organism isolated and sensitivity tests. Often it is necessary to administer antibiotics via an extraventricular drain.

Coagulase-negative staphylococci

Low-grade postoperative wound infection with *S. epidermidis* usually arises from the patient's own skin flora. Similarly, the patient's own bacteria are introduced when extraventricular drains and shunts are inserted and handled. There may be a delay of many months before a shunt infection manifests itself. *S. epidermidis* is extremely adherent to plastic: the development of microcolonies within an extracellular matrix explains persistence and the organisms are in stationary phase and not accessible to antibiotics. Infected shunt systems must be removed. If ventricular drainage is still required, then an extraventricular drain is placed and changed regularly (say, weekly) while antibiotics are given and until there is no evidence of infection. Permanent shunts must not be inserted when there is any suggestion of intraventricular infection (hypercellular CSF, any organism seen or cultured) with the patient *off* antibiotics. Antibiotic sensitivities of coagulase-negative staphylococci are unpredictable and resistance to most antibiotics has been increasing over 20 years. More than 50% of strains are resistant to methicillin and therefore to all β-lactam antimicrobials. Most strains are sensitive to vancomycin, although some are now tolerant and are not killed. Half of strains of *S. haemolyticus* are resistant to teicoplanin.

Staphylococcus aureus

S. aureus excites a greater inflammatory response than most coagulase-negative staphylococci so infections manifest more rapidly after surgery, often with superficial abscess formation. There may be ventriculitis and even para-ventricular abscess formation or the infection may be restricted to the extradural component of the wound. The infection most likely originates from the patient's own flora but may be acquired intraoperatively or postoperatively from external sources. Two important principles of therapy remain: any abscess must be drained and extraventricular drains must be changed regularly. If *S. aureus* is sensitive to methicillin then a wide range of β-lactam antimicrobials would be active including a range of cephalosporins that will cross the blood–brain barrier. Flucloxacillin penetrates rather poorly. If the isolate is methicillin-resistant, then intraventricular vancomycin (with gentamicin if it active) may be the most effective way of curing the ventriculitis. Rifampicin together with trimethroprim or linezolid alone penetrate sufficiently well and offer useful alternatives.

Gram-negative infections

Some patients acquire intraventricular coliform or pseudomonad infection. In hospital practice, these organisms have a high risk of being resistant to many antimicrobials and the sensitivity tests are essential to choose appropriate therapy. If sensitive, cephalosporins are probably the drugs of choice. However, if a strain is shown to be resistant to cefuroxime or cefotaxime and sensitive to ceftazidime, this antibiotic should be regarded as ineffective *in vitro*. Similarly *Klebsiella* spp., *Enterobacter* spp., *Serratia* spp., and *Citrobacter* spp. may have inducible cephalosporinases rendering cephalosporins ineffective. If they are sensitive to fluoroquinolones, then an agent like levofloxacin that penetrates the blood–brain barrier reasonably well would be preferred to ciprofloxacin. Otherwise an extraventricular drain is necessary to administer an aminoglycoside or colistin.

Intraventricular antibiotics must be prepared in a sterile unit in the pharmacy department. Useful drugs include vancomycin 20 mg daily and gentamicin

5 mg daily. Other aminoglycosides are acceptable but clinical experience is not as great as with gentamicin. Amphotericin (0.1–0.5 mg daily) may also be given for yeast infection. Other antibiotics that have been used include colistin (10 mg daily), teicoplanin (5–40 mg daily). Administration of the antimicrobial must be done in such a way that the risk of introducing new nosocomial organisms is kept to a minimum.

Encephalitis

The presentation is often indistinguishable from that of insidious onset meningitis. Alteration in higher cerebral functions and conscious level is common. Patients may have one or more focal neurological sign. Most infections are caused by viruses (herpes viruses, enteroviruses, JC polyomavirus).

JC virus is associated with progressive multifocal leucoencephalopathy

Recognized in 1958, this syndrome classically manifests a variety of rapid onset neurological symptoms and signs, including cognitive impairment (36%), visual field defects, ataxia, and cranial nerve palsy. Hemiparesis occurs in just under half of cases. Later, dementia and signs of global cerebral involvement supervene and progress inexorably to death over a few months though sometimes the disease is fluctuant and persists for several years. JC virus may be detected by DNA amplification in the CSF (Weber *et al.* 1994; De Lucca *et al.* 2000) and the virus is usually excreted in the urine where infection can be detected by cytologists as a basophilic intranuclear inclusion in urothelial cells. The virus can be seen on electron microscopy of the spun deposit and DNA amplification methods used to define the virus. The virus is excreted in a few bone marrow transplant recipients but there is no consistent relationship between viruria and progressive multifocal leucoencephalopathy. The diagnosis is made by cerebral imaging and brain biopsy. Magnetic resonance imaging is more sensitive than computerized tomography. Histology reveals demyelination and nuclear basophilic inclusions in oligodendrocytes. There is no proven effective antiviral therapy, but in AIDS, antiretroviral therapy may lead to a reduction in viral load and some amelioration of the disease process.

Herpes simplex virus

Herpes simplex virus type 1 accounts for about 10–20% of cases of encephalitis (Whitley and Lakeman 1995). Herpes simplex virus type 2 may cause meningitis as part of the primary illness but rarely causes late encephalitis. Most cases of type 1 encephalitis in adults were preceded by clinical or serological evidence of prior established infection but sometimes the virus isolated from brain or CSF is different from that shed in the oropharynx. The patient often has focal encephalitis especially involving the temporal lobe. Diagnosis tends to be made by DNA amplification of herpes simplex virus DNA from the CSF and this has replaced serodiagnosis and brain biopsy as the diagnostic method of choice. The treatment is with high-dose intravenous aciclovir followed by a well-absorbed prodrug such as valciclovir.

Human herpesvirus type 6 and 7

Novel herpes viruses were discovered in the context of AIDS and are now recognized to cause encephalitis in other immunocompromised patients. Human herpes virus (HHV)-6 infects many cells of haematopoietic lineage (T lymphocytes, B lymphocytes, macrophages, megakaryocytes), Epstein–Barr virus (EBV) transformed B lymphocytes and HIV-infected cells. Variant A of the virus is acquired transplacentally, in the neonatal period and through childhood and causes roseola infantum, transient fever alone perhaps with lymphadenopathy, otitis and diarrhoea or febrile convulsions or, more usually, no discernible disease. Variant B sharing 90% nucleic acid homology affects immunocompromised individuals.

Within the context of bone marrow transplantation, HHV6 may reactivate often in association with cytomegalovirus (CMV) and EBV and is implicated in encephalomeningitis in such patients. The virus is intensely neurotropic. However, because the presence of HHV6 DNA is so common, it is tempting to ascribe a syndrome to this virus if the test is positive. Perhaps more important is that HHV6 viraemia may predispose to invasive fungal infection (Dockrell and Paya 2001).

Aciclovir and analogues are not active against HHV6; ganciclovir is poorly active but foscarnet and cidofovir are active *in vitro*. In practice ganciclovir and foscarnet prophylaxis used for the prevention of CMV disease may be effective at preventing HHV6 replication and associated disease.

HHV7, which shares epidemiological properties with HHV6 and may also cause roseola, has not been shown to be associated with syndromes in immunosuppressed patients.

Cytomegalovirus (CSF)

Meningoencephalitis is rarely seen with primary infection in immunocompetent individuals so it is not surprising that virus reactivation can cause disease of the CNS. In AIDS and rarely in cancer patients, CMV can cause ascending sensorimotor neuropathy involving bowel and bladder function. The diagnosis is made by detecting CMV in CSF by culture or DNA amplification. Treatment with antivirals (ganciclovir and/or foscarnet) is generally unsuccessful.

Epstein–Barr virus

CNS lymphoma in AIDS is associated with EBV and the diagnosis is confirmed by specific DNA amplification. In addition, nasopharyngeal carcinoma associated with EBV may invade the CNS.

Adenovirus

Serotypes 7, 12, and 13 cause encephalomyelitis in immunocompromised patients often in association with pneumonia (Flomenberg *et al*. 1994).

Measles virus

Measles in immunosuppressed patients has a very high mortality (Kaplan *et al*. 1992). As many as 40% of patients have no rash, and 20% develop encephalitis. Antibody responses are poor so virus isolation or detection of measles RNA is the key to diagnosis. The encephalitic illness may progress to a chronic form of subacute encephalitis. There is no treatment. Non-immune children with cancer or on chemotherapy exposed to measles must be given hyperimmune globulin.

Mass lesions

Patients will present with focal signs that can develop insidiously. Seizures are more immediate and dramatic. A clear mass lesion on scan must be interpreted in the light of the patient's syndrome. In many individuals this will be a secondary tumour. Radiology may help to distinguish tumour from infection from stroke but lesion biopsy is very important unless it is quite clear clinically from the systemic syndrome and microbiology what is going on. Some causes to be considered are given in Table 10.2.

Pyogenic bacterial abscess

As an abscess develops the radiological signs change over a period of days from focal oedema to the classical well formed abscess (Hagensee *et al*. 1992). Thus early scanning can be misleading and sequential scans are necessary. Eventually a clear ring lesion with ring enhancement and oedema will be shown. An abscess must be aspirated for culture and therapeutic purposes. Appropriate antimicrobials can then be directed to the isolate(s). In healthy individuals, most primary brain abscesses contain mouth flora: a mixture of α-haemolytic streptococci and anaerobes, particularly *Prevotella melaninogenicus*. A few are caused by *Staphylococcus aureus*. In immunosuppressed individuals, however,

Table 10.2 Causes of mass CNS lesions in cancer patients

1. Primary or secondary tumour
2. Infection
   - Bacteria
     —classical pyogenic abscess from oral flora (*Prevotella melaninogenicus* and *Streptococcus milleri*)
     —*Staphylococcus aureus*
     —*Nocardia asteroides*
     —*Mycobacterium tuberculosis*
     —any bacterium
   - Fungi
     —*Candida* spp.
     —*Aspergillus* spp.
     —*Zygomycetes*
     —*Cryptococcus neoformans*
     —*Pneumocystis juroveci*
     —any fungus
   - Parasites
     —*Toxoplasma gondii*

the spectrum of likely micro-organisms is enormously broadened to include any common bacterium seen in bacteraemia. A key part of the management is repeated aspiration of the abscess through the burr hole.

Stroke associated with embolization

It is necessary to exclude endocarditis following bacteraemia associated with long-term intravenous cannulation. Physical examination and trans-oesophageal echocardiogram are essential. Blood cultures should be consistently positive with an indistinguishable organism. However, they are often negative because the patient has already been on broad-spectrum antimicrobials. Then therapy has to be given empirically. Certain valve infections (for example with Gram-negatives or yeasts) cannot be cured by antimicrobials and valve surgery must be planned.

Mycobacterium tuberculosis

Paradoxically, immunosuppression can allow mycobacterial reactivation though granuloma formation can be poor. The tuberculosis, therefore, may not manifest until the recovery phase of periods of immunosuppression. About one half of tuberculosis in the CNS manifests as meningitis and half as granulomatous masses within the neural tissue, whereas relatively few patients have both. The CSF may be quite normal in the latter. The key to the diagnosis of mass lesions, which may be multiple, is to take a biopsy. However, in the context of a patient at high risk of tuberculosis, it may be reasonable to try empirical therapy. However, the differential diagnosis is wide and it is important to diagnose other treatable infections such as nocardiasis and cryptococcosis.

Toxoplasma gondii

T. gondii is a coccidian protozoan parasite of felines. Oocysts are shed in the faeces and contaminate soil. Cysts ingested by animals and humans will invade the gut and enter tissues, including the brain. Except in the newborn, primary infection is asymptomatic or, rarely, a chronic generalized lymphadenitis which may last for months. Organisms replicate intracellularly to form rosettes in host cells of any type. The cells rupture and the parasite enters contiguous cells. After infection is established, the parasite develops into bradyzoites and tissue cysts are formed. The infection is then latent particularly in brain, heart, and skeletal muscle. After primary infection, patients have antibody for life. In severe immunosuppression, the organism may reactivate to cause encephalitis, interstitial pneumonitis, cardiac disease, and chorioretinitis. Disease is seen in about 1% of allogeneic marrow transplant recipients but very rarely in autograft recipients (Martino et al. 2000; Mele et al. 2002). About 90% were seropositive before toxoplasmosis developed and the infection was often delayed until the patient began to show signs of graft versus host disease. The diagnosis of isolated lesions or encephalitis is made by lesion biopsy guided by imaging. Serology is not helpful because IgM antibodies, which are often present and the titre of IgG and neutralizing antibodies, do not necessarily imply active current infection. The mortality of disseminated disease is high. Conventional treatment is with pyrimethamine and sulphadiazine or spiramycin. Clindamycin and azithromycin have been suggested for the prevention of relapse (Nasta and Chiodera 1997; Jacobson et al. 2001). However, they do not cross the blood–brain barrier so are unlikely to be active against cerebral forms of the parasite.

Aspergillus spp. and other moulds

All fungi may disseminate in patients with profound prolonged neutropenia (Figure 10.2). The primary source of most infections is the respiratory tract. The patient may have a classical necrotic lung sequestrum consequent on arteriolar infection. Alternatively, there may be primary sinusitis. Facial pain, headache, and inflammation over the sinus and in the orbit occur, often in patients who have been neutropenic for many weeks. Computerized tomographic scanning of the sinuses is essential to judge the extent of disease and bony destruction. Some patients develop non-pseudomonal ecthyma gangrenosum, which can be easily biopsied, proving that dissemination has occurred. Then perhaps 10–20% of patients will develop mass lesions in the brain with an extremely high mortality. In one series 60% of cerebral mass lesions after allogeneic transplantation were due to *Aspergillus* (Hagensee *et al.* 1994). Lesions are clear on scanning but non-specific. Most patients will have been treated with amphotericin B by the time diagnosis is made, but the results are poor. The drug of choice for aspergillosis is probably voriconazole because it is active and penetrates the blood–brain barrier. Voriconazole is not, however, active against the Mucorales that cause indistinguishable disease. Posaconazole is the latest azole antimicrobial with some activity (Sun *et al.* 2003).

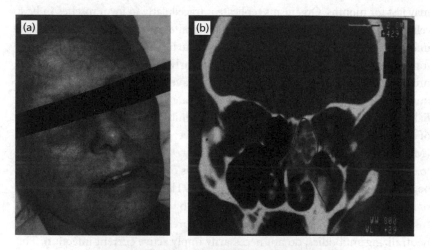

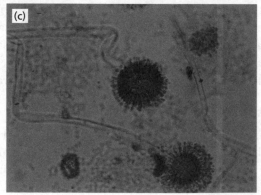

Fig. 10.2 Female 45 AML neutropenic after chemotherapy for 14 days. Sinusitis and brain lesion due to *Aspergillus flavus*. See colour plate section.

Nocardia asteroides

There are many species of the aerobic Gram-positive acid-fast branching rod in the genus *Nocardia* and 13 of 30 have been shown to cause human disease (Lerner 1996). However, discrimination of species is only achievable by RNA hybridization. *Nocardia* spp. are soil- and water-associated organisms probably acquired by inhalation of environmental dust because there are sometimes ward-associated outbreaks. Contamination of hands and fomites may also be important during an outbreak (Houang *et al*, 1980). Direct inoculation especially with *N. braziliensis* can cause local 'mycetoma'. Patients who are immunocompromised may develop disseminated disease (Beaman and Beaman 1994). Whereas most infections are pulmonary (an important differential diagnosis from pulmonary tuberculosis, which it resembles closely), brain abscess is not unusual occurring in just under one half of all cases of nocardiasis. Silent infection in the brain should be sought by imaging in cases with established invasive disease of other organs. Disseminated infections of skin and subcutaneous tissues, retina, joints, kidneys bone, and heart have all been described. The presentation of the brain lesion(s) is dependent on their site. The lesions often develop slowly and mimic tumour so biopsy is essential to establish specific therapy. The preferred agent for therapy is sulphonamide. Trimethoprim is not indicated or necessary. Animal models showed synergy between amikacin and sulphonamide and later imipenem. All strains tested are sensitive to linezolid *in vitro* and there are anecdotal reports of activity (Moylett *et al*. 2003).

Prevention

Cancer patients should be immunized with available conjugate vaccines against pneumococci, meningococci, and *H. influenzae* type b. However, infections with the latter two organisms is very rare. In general, live vaccines are contraindicated as soon as cancer is diagnosed. That precludes administration of measles, live polio, chicken pox, rubella, and BCG vaccines. Serological evaluation early in treatment should include antibody status for herpes viruses, including CMV and varicella zoster, and *Toxoplasma gondii*.

Patients susceptible to infection should be discouraged from visiting countries where they may be exposed to new pathogens. Children non-immune to measles or chicken pox should as far as is reasonable be kept away from those with infection.

The environment for the management of cancer patients should be controlled so that the number of airborne fungal spores is kept to a minimum. Patients should be discouraged from dealing with compost in the garden during inter-chemotherapy periods. Certain foods are also unwise: unpasteurized soft cheeses may be a source of *Listeria*.

Antibiotic prophylaxis would seem sensible. Splenectomized patients should continue to take low doses of penicillin for life except when alternative suitable antibiotics are being given for the treatment of infection. Cotrimoxazole has a broad spectrum of activity and will effectively prevent *Pneumocystis juroveci*, *Nocardia asteroides*, *Listeria monocytogenes*, and many pyogenic bacterial infections. Aciclovir will prevent reactivation herpes simplex and varicella zoster. Ganciclovir is used to prevent CMV infections at periods of greatest susceptibility, especially after bone marrow transplantation. Fluconazole will reduce the risk of *C. albicans* and some other species and itraconazole or posaconazole may reduce the risk of aspergillosis. Problems arise with any form of prophylaxis because of the burden of drugs, potential drug toxicity or hypersensitivity and selection of resistant organisms. Protocols will clearly indicate local preferences and will be related to local antibiotic resistance patterns.

A single dose of an appropriate antibiotic is indicated for neurosurgical procedures. Cefuroxime achieves high tissue concentrations within minutes of administration so is most popular for this purpose. A single large dose (1.5 G) is usually administered after induction of anaesthetic. However, this prophylactic antibiotic must be withheld until after diagnostic biopsy or aspiration for the diagnosis of a CNS mass so as not to confound bacteriological culture. Antimicrobials administered before or after the surgery will paradoxically increase the risk of postoperative infection.

References

Aquino VM, Farah RA, Lee ME, *et al.* (1996). Disseminated Coxsackie A9 infection complicating bone marrow transplantation. *Pediatric Infectious Disease Journal*, **15**, 1053–1054.

Beaman BL and Beaman L. (1994). *Nocardia* species: host-parasite relationships. *Clinical Microbiology Reviews*, **7**, 213–264.

Bennett JE, Dismukes W, Duma RJ, *et al.* (1979). A comparison of amphotericin alone and combined with flucytosine in the treatment of cryptococcal meningitis. *New England Journal of Medicine*, **301**, 126–131.

Biggs DD, Toorkey BC, Carrigan DR, *et al.* (1990). Disseminated echovirus infection complicating bone marrow transplantation. *American Journal of Medicine*, **88**, 421–425.

De Lucca A, Giancola ML, Ammassari A, *et al.* (2000). The effect of potent anti-retroviral therapy and JC virus load in cerebrospinal fluid on clinical outcome of patients with AIDS-associated progressive multifocal leucoencephalopathy. *Journal of Infectious Diseases*, **182**, 1077–1083.

Dockrell DH and Paya CV. (2001). Human herpesvirus-6 and -7 in transplantation. *Reviews in Medical Virology*, **11**, 23–36.

Flomenberg P, Babbit J, and Drobyski WR. (1994). Increasing incidence of adenovirus disease in bone marrow transplant recipients. *Journal of Infectious Diseases*, **169**, 775–781.

Hagensee ME, Bauwens JE, Kjos B, and Bowden RA. (1994). Brain abscess following marrow transplantation: experience at the Fred Hutchinson Cancer Research Center, 1984–1992. *Clinical Infectious Diseases*, **19**, 402–408.

Houang ET, Lovett IS, Thompson FD, *et al.* (1980). *Nocardia asteroids*—a transmissible infection. *Journal of Hospital Infection*, **1**, 31–40.

Jacobson JM, Hafner R, Remington J, *et al.* (2001). ACTG 156 Study Group. Dose escalationphase I/II study of azithromycin and pyrimethamine for the treatment of toxoplasmic encephalitis in AIDS. *AIDS*, **15**, 583–589.

Kaplan LJ, Daum RS, Smarson M, *et al.* (1992). Severe measles in immunocompromised patients. *JAMA*, **267**, 1237–1241.

Leenders AC, Reiss P, Portegies P, *et al.* (1997). Liposomal amphotericin B (Ambisome) compared with amphotericin B followed by oral fluconazole in the treatment of AIDS-associated cryptococcal meningitis. *AIDS*, **11**, 1463–1471.

Lerner PI. (1996). Nocardiosis. *Clinical Infectious Diseases*, **22**, 891–903.

Martino R, Bretagne S, Rovira M, *et al.* (2000). Toxoplasmosis after hematopoietic stem transplantation: report of a 5-y survey from the Infectious Diseases Working Party of the European Group for Blood and Marrow Transplantation. *Bone Marrow Transplantation*, **25**, 1111–1114.

Mele A, Paterson PJ, Prentice HG, *et al.* (2002). Toxoplasmosis in bone marrow transplantation: a report of two cases and systematic review of the literature. *Bone Marrow Transplantation*, **29**, 691–698.

Merle-Melet M, Dossou-Gbete L, Meyer P, *et al.* (1996). Is amoxicillin-cotrimoxazole the most appropriate antibiotic regimen for *Listeria* meningitis? *Journal of Infection*, **33**, 79–85.

Moylett EH, Pacheco SE, Brown-Elliott BA, *et al.* (2003). Clinical experience with linezolid for the treatment of nocardia infection. *Clinical Infectious Diseases*, **36**, 313–318.

Nasta P and Chiodera S. (1997). Azithromycin for relapsing cerebral toxoplasmosis in AIDS. *AIDS*, **11**, 1188.

Rotbart HA. (2002). Treatment of picornavirus infections. *Antiviral Research*, **53**, 83–98.

Safdar A, Papadopoulos EB, and Armstrong D. (2002). Listeriosis in recipients of allogeneic blood and marrow transplantation: thirteen year review of disease characteristics, treatment outcomes, and a new association with cytomegalovirus infection. *Bone Marrow Transplantation*, **29**, 913–916.

Sun QN, Najvar LK, Bocanegra R, *et al.* (2003). In vivo activity of posaconazole against *Mucor.* spp. In an immunosuppressed mouse model. *Antimicrobial Agents and Chemotherapy*, **46**, 2310–2312.

Weber T, Turner RW, Frye S, *et al.* (1994). Specific diagnosis of progressive multifocal leucoencephalopathy by polymerase chain reaction. *Journal of Infectious Diseases*, **169**, 1138–1141.

Whitley RJ and Lakeman F. (1995). Herpes simplex virus of the central nervous system: therapeutic and diagnostic considerations. *Clinical Infectious Diseases*, **20**, 414–420.

Chapter 11

Infections in children

Rachel Dommett, Mike Sharland, and Julia Chisholm

Childhood cancer in perspective

Children and adults with cancer differ in a number of ways. In this section we outline the most important differences, particularly in relation to infectious complications, before discussing in detail areas of interest in the prevention and management of infection in children with cancer.

The spectrum of childhood malignancy

The incidence of cancer in children is fortunately low: in the UK about 1 in 500 children develop a malignancy in the first 15 years of life (Toms 2004). Nevertheless, cancer is a leading cause of childhood death beyond infancy and infection is a significant contributor to cancer deaths. The most important difference between paediatric and adult cancer is in the spectrum of diagnoses seen: in the developed world acute leukaemias (predominantly acute lymphoblastic leukaemia; ALL) form the largest single patient group in children (Figure 11.1). Clinical presentation, response to therapy and outcome also differ in children and adults. Many childhood tumours are highly chemosensitive, so chemotherapy is often the mainstay of treatment with surgery and radiotherapy playing an important role in some patients. During the past 30–40 years there have been marked improvements in outcome with over 70% of children in the USA and Northern and Western Europe remaining disease free beyond 5 years (Gatta *et al.* 2003).

Predisposing factors in childhood cancer

Most children with malignancy have no clearly defined predisposing factors for their disease. Geographical variations in the incidence of different types of paediatric tumours suggest environmental triggers, including infection, for some types of cancers. Incidence varies by population as well as by geography suggesting a genetic influence and there are a number of well documented genetic predisposition syndromes (Stiller 2004).

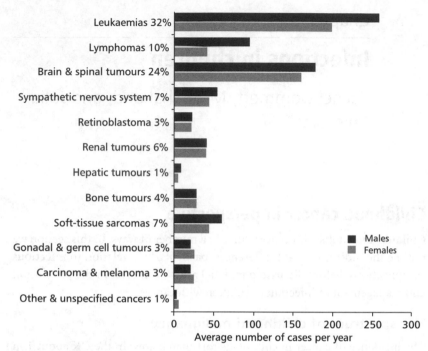

Fig. 11.1 Annual average number of cases of paediatric cancer by diagnostic group and sex, ages 0–14; Great Britain 1989–98. Reproduced from Toms 2004.

It is now clear that viral infections contribute to the aetiology of childhood malignancy (Table 11.1). The association between infection and ALL is of particular interest. There is good evidence that at least some chromosomal translocations associated with ALL arise *in utero* during the expansion of B-cell precursors (Ford *et al*. 1993; Gale *et al*. 1997; Wiemels *et al*. 1999a, b). This event may be sufficient to trigger infant ALL (presentation < 1 year of age with MLL gene rearrangements) but ALL in children aged 2–6 years seems to need at least one further independent, sequential genetic mutation—the 'two-hit' model (Greaves 1999). Infection has been proposed as a potential 'second hit'.

Greaves hypothesized that exposure to common infections in early childhood may protect against ALL by promoting normal maturation of the immune system. Lack of early exposure to infection renders the immune system unmodulated. Subsequent infection with common microbes then occurs in a biologically abnormal time frame for which the immune system is inappropriately programmed, leaving such children at risk of leukaemogenesis (Greaves 1997). A very large UK case–control study looking at day care and social activity during the first year of life as a measure of potential exposure to

Table 11.1 Associations between specific viral infections and paediatric malignancies.

Infection	Tumour types	Comments
Epstein–Barr virus	Burkitt's lymphoma	Endemic in Sub-Saharan Africa
	Hodgkin's disease	Not implicated in all cases
	Nasopharyngeal carcinoma	Common in North Africa and East Asia
	Lymphoproliferative disease	Mainly congenital or acquired immunodeficiency, particularly post-bone marrow or solid organ transplant
Heptatitis B	Hepatocellular carcinoma	Rare in West in children
Hepatitis C	Hepatocellular carcinoma	Rare in West in children
Human immunodeficiency virus	Non-Hodgkin's lymphoma	
Human herpesvirus 8	Kaposi's sarcoma	In association with HIV

infection supports the hypothesis that early exposure to infection reduces the risk of subsequent ALL (Gilham *et al.* 2005).

A second body of evidence from Kinlen and others has shown that transiently increased rates of leukaemia, sometimes occurring in clear geographical clusters, are associated with population movement and mixing (Kinlen 1995). It is postulated that this mixing results in infection in previously unexposed individuals, with an abnormal immune response to such infection (Kinlen and Petridou 1995). Conversely, there is some suggestion that *in utero* exposure to infection might increase the risk of childhood leukaemia (Naumburg *et al.* 2002; Lehtinen *et al.* 2003).

The above lines of evidence suggest that leukaemia can occur as an uncommon response to common pathogens encountered during childhood and perhaps *in utero*. HLA class II polymorphisms, which control response to foreign antigens, may explain part of the association between infection and leukaemia (Taylor *et al.* 2002). An increased susceptibility to infection could contribute to the increased risk of developing leukaemia (particularly ALL) in Down's syndrome (Cuadrado and Barrena 1996). Clearly more work is needed to elucidate the mechanisms of leukaemogenesis and whether preventive strategies are possible.

Infections in children with cancer

Paediatric and adult cancer patients suffer a similar range of infections but children are particularly susceptible to common childhood infections. A very large study of 769 children and 2321 adults with febrile neutropenia showed that significantly fewer children than adults present with a defined site of infection (32% versus 41%; Hann *et al.* 1997). When a specific site was detectable in children it was most commonly upper respiratory tract infection (55%); lower respiratory tract (13%) gastrointestinal tract (GI) (11%), and 'other' (20%) were all much less frequent. By contrast in adults, although upper respiratory tract was also the commonest site (35%), lower respiratory tract (29%) and 'other' (26%) were also very common and GI tract was less common (8%). The relative frequency of some bacterial isolates differed, with children having more streptococcal infections and adults more staphylococcal infections.

The use of central venous catheters (CVCs) is even more widespread in children than in adults (73% versus 60%; Hann *et al.* 1997). The rates of infectious sequelae from different types of devices vary, with external catheters carrying a higher risk of infection than the internalized Port-A-Cath (Mirro *et al.* 1989; Ingram *et al.* 1991; Hengartner *et al.* 2004). Their use has been implicated in a shift in the spectrum of pathogens seen in this patient population towards Gram-positive organisms and has prompted changes in treatment guidelines to incorporate empirical Gram-positive cover.

The commonest Gram-positive bacteraemias in children in the Hann study were streptococci (29%; subgroups not reported), coagulase negative staphylococcus (19%) and *Staphylococcus aureus* (11.5 %; Hann *et al.* 1997). *Viridans streptococci* (VS), α-haemolytic streptococci including *Streptococcus mitis* and *Strep. sanguis*, are now recognized as important pathogens in neutropenic sepsis, causing septic shock and acute respiratory distress syndrome. The most important risk factors for VS bacteraemia in neutropenic children are a diagnosis of acute leukaemia or lymphoma, use of cytarabine-containing chemotherapy, and the presence of pneumonia (Paganini *et al.* 2003). In a large study of 874 children with acute myeloid leukaemia, VS sepsis accounted for 21% of bacteraemias (Gamis *et al.* 2000). The rate of VS infections also increased as intensity of treatment regimens increased. Young children, those with previous VS bacteraemias, those with gut toxicity and those receiving high-dose cytarabine were at particularly high risk of infection.

Gram-negative infections remain the most important cause of septicaemia and septic shock in this patient population, independent of neutrophil count. Sixty three per cent of childhood bacteraemic episodes associated with shock involved one or more Gram-negative isolates and, in the patients requiring ICU transfer, the incidence increased to 83% (Aledo *et al.* 1998). VS was the only group of Gram-positive organisms frequently associated with septic shock.

Antibiotic resistance is a growing problem. Methicillin-resistant *Staphylococcus aureus* (MRSA) is an increasing finding in some centres and the emergence of extended spectrum β-lactamase bacteria (ESBL), sensitive only to carbapenems, is a recent and very worrying trend in many countries.

Fungal infections remain a major problem in children with cancer with the use of increasingly intensive chemotherapy regimens and myeloablative therapy. The fungal species most commonly seen in children are *Candida*, *Aspergillus*, *Mucor*, and Zygomycetes.

Candida may cause skin infection, mucosal infection, severe oesophagitis or systemic disease with fever, jaundice, and pulmonary infiltrates. Hepatosplenic candidiasis is suggested by persistent fever after recovery of neutrophil counts. Patients may complain of abdominal pain associated with hepatosplenomegaly and mild jaundice. Classical radiological findings show 'bull's eye' lesions of hepatosplenic or renal candidiasis and *Candida* may be isolated from blood, urine, or mucosal swabs. Although historically *Candida albicans* has been the most commonly isolated species there is emerging evidence that non-albicans *Candida* (*C. tropicalis*, *C. glabrata*, *C. parapsilosis*, *C. krusei*, *C. lusitaniae*), some of which are insensitive to fluconazole, are more common in paediatric cancer patients (Mullen *et al.* 2003). Explanations for this shift include the increasing use of azole antifungal drugs (fluconazole, itraconazole) for prophylaxis and empirical treatment. This has implications for the antifungal agent of choice in such patients.

Aspergillus infection is most commonly acquired from the external environment and primarily targets the respiratory tract in immunocompromised patients where poorly functioning neutrophils and pulmonary alveolar macrophages are unable to inhibit infection. Children with pulmonary aspergillosis may present with a non-productive cough, pleuritic pain, pleural rub, and haemoptysis but due to neutropenia, fever may be the only sign. It can also target the sinuses and disseminated disease affects the central nervous system, skin, bone, or GI tract.

Computed tomography (CT) is the investigation of choice for suspected chest and sinus disease. CT findings vary depending on the timing of the scan and chest findings can include 'coin lesions', areas of consolidation, interstitial infiltration, or wedge opacities. The CT halo sign, which represents a ring of haemorrhage surrounding nodules, is highly predictive of infection and precedes cavitation by 1–2 weeks. The incidence of cavitation on CT in the paediatric population is reported to be significantly lower than in adults but may relate to the stage of neutrophil recovery in the specific population studied. The absence of cavitation should not prevent diagnosis of this potentially life-threatening condition (Thomas *et al.* 2003).

Diagnosis of *Aspergillus* from a blood culture is rare; bronchoalveolar lavage or biopsy of a suspected lesion are normally required. Newer tests such as aspergillus polymerase chain reaction (Raad *et al.* 2002; Ljungman *et al.* 2005) or galactomannan enzyme immunoassay to detect aspergillus antigen (Mennink-Kersten *et al.* 2004; Maertens *et al.* 2004) may improve diagnostic accuracy for fungal infections in the future.

The burden of viral infections is likely to be underestimated in the paediatric cancer population owing to diagnostic limitations. Children commonly present with upper respiratory tract symptoms, which resolve within a few days. However, some viral infections, which are relatively insignificant in a healthy host, can cause major problems in immunosuppressed patients, particularly after haemopoietic stem cell or bone marrow transplant (BMT). Cytomegalovirus (CMV) can affect ALL patients on continuation chemotherapy who may present with fever, pancytopenia, hepatosplenomegaly, and atypical mononuclear cells in the blood. After BMT, CMV tends to be more aggressive and can cause a severe pneumonitis, hepatitis, retinitis, and infection of the GI tract. Improvements in the diagnosis of CMV (using pp65 antigen detection or real-time polymerase chain reaction methodology; Leruez-Ville *et al.* 2003), the use of CMV-negative blood in susceptible individuals and prophylaxis with aciclovir in at-risk allogeneic transplant recipients have helped to reduce the incidence of infection.

Herpes simplex virus (HSV) can cause significant morbidity but rarely death in cancer patients. Manifestations include skin lesions, which usually remain localized, oral and oesophageal mucositis and encephalitis. Pain is the main problem but mucosal lesions can become secondarily infected with bacteria. More recently recognized, disseminated adenovirus infection in the transplant setting, particularly following T-cell depletion, can cause pneumonitis, fulminant liver failure and rapid death. JC virus and BK virus can cause haemorrhagic cystitis following BMT or stem cell transplant and JC virus may also cause a multifocal leucoencephalopathy in this setting. Chicken pox and measles are extremely important in the paediatric population and are discussed below.

Common respiratory viruses including respiratory syncytial virus, influenza A and B, parainfluenza, adenovirus, and rhinovirus can cause a severe pneumonitis in immunosuppressed patients, particularly following BMT or stem cell transplant. Treatment is largely supportive but ribavirin is available for use in respiratory syncytial virus, adenovirus, and rhinovirus infections and neuraminidase inhibitors can be used to prevent and treat influenza infection during outbreaks in the BMT setting.

The impact of infectious complications on outcome in childhood cancer

Improvements in the prevention and treatment of infections have played a significant part in the improved outcome of treatment for childhood cancer.

This is well illustrated by the results of UK leukaemia trials. A progressive reduction in infection-related deaths was achieved between 1980 and 1997 in UKALL trials VIII, X, and XI and the spectrum of infective agents causing deaths changed (Hargrave *et al.* 2001). Much of the improvement was attributed to the introduction of universal measles immunization, the introduction of cotrimoxazole as prophylaxis against *Pneumocystis carinii* pneumonia (PCP) and recognition of the need for prompt institution of broad-spectrum antibiotics in febrile neutropenia with addition of amphotericin B for persistent fever. Similarly in the Medical Research Council Acute Myeloid Leukaemia Trial 10 trial, treatment-related mortality improved during the trial period (1988–95) as a result of improved supportive care and early treatment of infection (Riley *et al.* 1999).

Improvements in supportive care have enabled oncologists to adopt more aggressive approaches to the treatment of childhood tumours. However, 'dose-intensive' regimens are complicated by more profound immunosuppression and establishing the fine balance between intensifying treatment and tolerable toxicity is an ongoing challenge. Therefore, despite all the advances made, infectious complications remain a major cause of morbidity and mortality in children with cancer.

The child as a patient

The investigation of an infective episode in a very young child is often limited by the child's ability to articulate symptoms. This emphasizes the importance of careful examination, including tympanic membranes, mouth, throat, and central venous access exit site in the clinical assessment of febrile children with cancer along with appropriate laboratory investigations, but even when thorough examination is possible the child will usually lack a detectable clinical focus of infection.

Children are less likely than adults to suffer from coexisting medical conditions that can complicate the management of infectious sequelae of cancer treatment. The obvious exceptions are those with underlying genetic disorders, which may be associated with other congenital anomalies and/or medical conditions. One important example is Down's syndrome, which is associated with an approximately 20-fold increase in the incidence of leukaemia, particularly in children less than 5 years of age (Robison 1992; Hasle *et al.* 2000). Higher mortality from infection during leukaemia treatment has been noted, largely related to increased gut toxicity and mucositis (Wheeler *et al.* 1996; Hargrave *et al.* 2001).

A major difference between adults and children is the maturity of the underlying immune system. Younger patients are naïve immunologically and more susceptible to both common and opportunistic infections. The effect of a diagnosis of cancer and subsequent chemotherapy treatment on a developing immune system is not fully understood. Age at diagnosis, the diagnosis itself (e.g. Hodgkin's disease is associated with immunosuppression), and the details of treatment protocol all influence the degree and nature of immunosuppression during treatment. It also remains to be established exactly how these may affect long-term immune function following cessation of treatment.

Family and social considerations

Paediatricians manage the child in partnership with his or her family. Parents or carers take responsibility for certain aspects of the child's treatment such as oral medication at home and must be aware of the potential complications of therapy. The risk of infection and its presenting symptoms are among the most important issues for a carer to understand. Infection is one of the commonest reasons for an inpatient stay during treatment and can understandably cause major disruptions to normal family life with potential financial repercussions on the household.

Prevention of infection

Treatment for cancer increases the risk of infection in a number of ways. Not only are most patients rendered neutropenic, probably the most significant risk factor for infection, but they also may experience alterations in skin and mucosal barriers, such as mucositis and the presence of an indwelling CVC, and defects in cell-mediated, humoral and innate recognition immunity (Lehrnbecher et al. 1997). A number of strategies are discussed below that may help to reduce the risk of infection but it is not yet possible to eliminate the risk of serious infection in these patients.

Limiting exposure

Parents are commonly concerned that their child may contract an infection from other children, particularly at school or nursery, and ask whether the child should be kept away during periods of neutropenia. In reality most infections contracted in this way are viral upper respiratory tract infections, whereas the most serious potential infections in the immunosuppressed are bacterial, fungal, and opportunistic infections, most of which are likely to arise from the endogenous flora of the neutropenic patient rather than from transmitted infection. The exceptions are chicken pox and measles, highly contagious viral infections, which are potentially fatal in the immunosuppressed patient. A balance is needed so that children continue educational and social activities as normally as possible while avoiding any undue risk. Liaison between the family and the school is important to ensure understanding of the implications of treatment and infection risk. Avoidance of chicken pox contacts in non-immune patients and measles contacts in all patients is important and ideally children should be kept out of school at times of outbreaks. Notification of any contacts among classmates may be helpful in preventing exposure. Avoidance of crowded atmospheres (e.g. crowded trains or buses) is also advocated during periods of neutropenia.

Prophylaxis

Mouth care

Mouth-care protocols have become a routine part of paediatric management to ensure that the mouth remains clean, moist, and free from infection. However, despite existing 'best practice' recommendations there remains a pressing need for evidenced-based oral care guidelines in children receiving chemotherapy (Gibson 2004). Oropharyngeal candidiasis is common, especially in patients with defective T-cell-mediated immunity or those receiving corticosteroids. It may also develop in patients with mucositis or HSV stomatitis particularly if they have received broad-spectrum antibiotics. The routine use of chlorhexidine oral rinse is advised in some patient groups along with prophylactic oral antifungal therapy. Teeth cleaning is of paramount importance in at risk patients as plaque deposits can contain significant bacterial loads and are associated with gingival inflammation (Lucas et al. 1998). The use of soft toothbrushes is recommended with regular replacement as these themselves may become colonized, further exacerbating the problem (Glass and Lare 1986). Dental assessment is important as early treatment of dental disease may reduce the risk of oral infections during cancer treatment (Collard and Hunter 2001).

Pneumocystis carinii

One of the most beneficial prophylactic measures against infection is the use of cotrimoxazole to prevent PCP. Children receiving treatment for certain haematological malignancies, particularly ALL, those undergoing BMT or stem cell transplantation as well as some children with impaired cellular immunity during intensive treatment for solid tumours are particularly susceptible to PCP. The introduction of routine prophylaxis with cotrimoxazole in children with ALL has seen a marked reduction in morbidity and mortality (Hargrave et al. 2001). Cotrimoxazole can lead to poor tolerance of oral maintenance chemotherapy for ALL and alternatives used are nebulized or intravenous pentamidine and dapsone.

Bacterial infections

Many of the pathogens causing infection in patients with cancer form part of their normal flora, acquiring entry via alterations in skin and mucosal barriers. However, routine 'surveillance' cultures are not considered practical or cost-effective in neutropenic patients (Kramer *et al.* 1982).

Routine use of prophylaxis against bacterial infection is uncommon in paediatric oncology practice. Oral quinolones have been used widely as prophylaxis against Gram-negative infections in adults. A meta-analysis of published studies suggests a reduction in the number of Gram-negative infections but not in mortality and it is not clear that oral quinolones decrease the rate of febrile neutropenia (Engels *et al.* 1998). Attempts have been made also to improve Gram-positive prophylaxis by the addition of an agent such as rifampicin to an oral quinolone. Again, while the incidence of Gram-positive infection was reduced, meta-analysis of published studies showed that mortality and some parameters of morbidity were unchanged, with an increase in the incidence of unwanted side-effects of treatment (Cruciani *et al.* 2003).The uncertainty about reduction in morbidity and mortality and the concerns about emergent resistance mean that prophylaxis against bacterial infection is not routinely recommended (Hughes *et al.* 2002).

Quinolones are used with caution in children because of concerns about the risk of arthropathy (Alfaham *et al.* 1987), although the risk is low (about 1%; Grady 2003). Few studies of quinolone prophylaxis in children have been published and the drugs remain unlicensed for general use in children. A recent small study has investigated the limited use of prophylaxis following delayed intensification blocks of the UKALL XI treatment protocol. Patients receiving prophylactic ciprofloxacin had a reduced rate and duration of hospitalization and reduced incidence of Gram-negative bacteraemia (Yousef *et al.* 2004), with the greatest benefit noted during the protracted third, delayed, intensification block. Whether there is a role for oral quinolone prophylaxis in children remains to be established.

Viral infections

Varicella zoster virus (VZV)   Primary varicella can cause serious morbidity or death in patients with impaired cell-mediated immunity. Disseminated infection primarily targets the lungs but other manifestations can include encephalopathy or hepatitis with mortality rates up to 20% in untreated patients. Lesions can be atypical in immunosuppressed patients.

Serum VZV status is routinely tested in newly diagnosed children with cancer. In the event of significant contact with an individual with chicken pox or shingles, patients who remain negative for varicella IgG require prophylactic treatment. Protective quantities of IgG can be acquired from blood transfusions, so patients who are VZV negative at diagnosis should be retested at the time of the varicella contact and undergo passive immunization only if they remain VZV negative. Passive immunization with VZIG or intravenous immunoglobulin (IVIg) as soon as possible after the contact is the treatment of choice but oral aciclovir has also been used in immunocompromised children (Ishida *et al.* 1996; Goldstein *et al.* 2000). Neither treatment completely prevents seroconversion or clinical infection but both can attenuate the disease. Any suggestion of clinical infection requires assessment and intravenous aciclovir. The use of VZIG and early treatment of clinical infection with aciclovir has led to a marked reduction in disseminated infection (Feldman and Lott 1987).

VZV reactivation is one of the most common complications after BMT; up to one half of recipients who survive at least 6 months develop shingles and children appear to develop infection at an earlier stage than adults (Atkinson *et al.* 1980; Kawasaki *et al.* 1996; Sauerbrei *et al.* 1997). Most BMT patients receive prophylactic aciclovir but the duration of treatment is variable and the at-risk period is long. The role of varicella vaccination in post-BMT patients for the provision of long-term prophylaxis is under investigation (Sauerbrei *et al.* 1997).

Measles   Measles can be rapidly progressive in an immunosuppressed child and complications include an interstitial pneumonitis for which there is no effective treatment (Gray *et al.* 1987). Such children may not have an accompanying rash and the diagnosis should therefore be considered in the differential for any 'atypical' pneumonia. The introduction of measles vaccination in the 1980s resulted in virtual eradication of measles but unproven links made between the Measles, Mumps, Rubella (MMR) vaccine and developmental and GI disorders led to reduced vaccine uptake, affecting herd immunity. Currrent UK uptake of MMR is now about 80% (NHS Immunization Statistics, England: 2003–04) instead of the target 95%. Not surprisingly outbreaks have occurred recently in unvaccinated children in areas of low uptake in London (Morgan *et al.* 2003; Atkinson *et al.* 2005). Immunization of siblings and social contacts is paramount if cases are to be avoided in children with cancer. Current guidelines recommend that any patient with a measles contact should have treatment with human normal immunogobulin (HNIG) or IVIg regardless of antibody status, (Gray *et al.* 1987; Royal College of Paediatrics and Child Health 2002) but if measles develops after prophylaxis it is usually fatal.

Herpes simplex virus   HSV infection is seen predominantly in the paediatric BMT population. Patients benefit from aciclovir prophylaxis, which has been demonstrated to reduce the frequency of viral reactivation, prevent viral shedding, and reduce severity of HSV infection (Hann *et al.* 1983; Taylor *et al.* 1990; Epstein *et al.* 1996).

Cytomegalovirus   Anti-CMV strategies used in paediatric BMT recipients include both universal prophylaxis and preemptive therapy. Traditionally, aciclovir is used for prophylaxis in children but newer alternatives include oral valaciclovir, which has recently been found to be more effective than aciclovir in reducing the incidence of CMV infection in a large randomized study (Ljungman *et al.* 2002). The fact that survival was unchanged is probably due to the effectiveness of preemptive therapy. This strategy relies on detection of CMV infection before clinical disease develops, using sensitive and specific virological markers (particularly CMV viral load) and initiation of treatment in patients with evidence of CMV reactivation.

Fungal infections

Antifungal prophylaxis is used in specific diagnostic groups dependent on treatment regimen. Fluconazole is the commonest drug used and is well absorbed orally but administration is restricted in order to prevent the emergence of resistant *Candida* species (Wingard 1994). Itraconazole prophylaxis reduces invasive fungal infection in adult patients with haematological malignancy (Glasmacher *et al.* 2003) and is commonly used in BMT patients where prevention of *Aspergillus* infection is the primary aim. More recently voriconazole has been used in the same way. Liposomal amphotericin prophylaxis in BMT patients reduces the risk of fungal colonization but not of invasive fungal infection (Tollemar *et al.* 1993; Kelsey *et al.* 1999) and is best reserved for the patients at highest risk (e.g. previous invasive fungal infection).

Immunizations

Immunizations in children with cancer can be given provided the vaccine can be delivered safely (Royal College of Paediatrics and Child Health 2002), although response during immunosuppressive therapy may be impaired. Live vaccines carry the risk of vaccine-induced infection and are normally avoided during, and up to, 6 months after the completion of conventional chemotherapy or until there is evidence of immune reconstitution following stem cell or BMT. It is recommended that administration of non-live vaccines should continue during chemotherapy treatment in young children with cancer according to the universal childhood immunization schedule (using inactivated polio vaccine and avoiding MMR), provided that the child's general condition is stable.

Most of the vaccines in the universal childhood vaccination programme do not contribute significantly to protection against infections commonly problematic in the immunosuppressed patient in the Western world. Exceptions are *Haemophilus influenza* B and pneumococcal immunization; both infections show increased prevalence in children with ALL. In some parts of the world hepatitis B is also problematic. Varicella zoster vaccine is not administered routinely in the UK but is part of the universal vaccination programme in healthy children in the USA, Canada, Germany, and Sweden. Universal immunization of healthy children would dramatically reduce the incidence of VZV seronegativity in children at the time of the diagnosis of cancer. A small recent study has demonstrated that a two-dose regimen of live attenuated vaccine is effective in non-immune children during continuation treatment for ALL or > 3 months following the completion of intensive chemotherapy for solid tumours. One of the 17 subjects developed widespread varicella skin lesions that responded to aciclovir, possibly related to the administration of steroids 4 weeks prior to vaccination (Leung *et al.* 2004). Ongoing studies are required to evaluate its safety during chemotherapy but use of the vaccine in seronegative family members (especially siblings) may be important in providing indirect protection for susceptible children.

Influenza can cause morbidity, delays in chemotherapy, and occasional mortality in children with cancer and is particularly serious when outbreaks occur in the BMT setting. Trivalent split virion influenza vaccine is safe and reasonably effective in children receiving treatment for both haematological malignancy and solid tumours (Chisholm *et al.* 2001, 2003; Porter *et al* 2004) and is recommended annually prior to the influenza season during chemotherapy, within 6 months of completing chemotherapy and following BMT or stem cell transplant (Royal College of Paediatrics and Child Health 2002).

Immunosuppressive therapy can impair pre-existing vaccine-induced immunity (Reinhardt *et al.* 2003) and for this reason it is recommended that additional boosters of all the components of the primary immunization schedule are administered 6 months after the end of chemotherapy treatment. Children who have undergone BMT or stem cell transplant should have a complete set of primary immunizations once the immune system has recovered (Royal College of Paediatrics and Child Health 2002).

Colony stimulating factors

Granulocyte colony-stimulating factor (G-CSF) and granulocyte macrophage-CSF (GM-CSF) are both CSFs that increase circulating neutrophils, GM-CSF also increasing eosinophils, macrophages, and sometimes lymphocytes. Use of G-CSF as primary prophylaxis in children has been found to reduce the duration of neutropenia, lower rates of neutropenic fever, decrease use of antibiotics, and diminish the need for hospitalization in most, but not all, studies (Riikonen *et al.* 1994; Lehrnbecher and Welte 2002; Sung *et al.* 2004b). These are potential advantages to the child and family but to date no study has shown a reduction in mortality, the most significant outcome measure. In addition, CSFs are very costly and in a randomized, cross-over study of G-CSF primary prophylaxis following intensification treatment in children with ALL and T-NHL treated on the UKALL XI protocol, the observed reduction in hospital admission from 91 to 74% was not associated with a demonstrable cost–benefit (Little *et al.* 2002).

Current guidelines do not recommend routine G-CSF primary prophylaxis following chemotherapy (Lehrnbecher and Welte 2002). Primary prophylaxis may be considered where the expected incidence of febrile neutropenia is above 40%, for example high-risk or relapsed ALL and dose-intensive solid tumour protocols such as high-risk neuroblastoma. There may come a point where benefits outweigh the costs as chemotherapy regimens continue to intensify and wider routine prophylactic usage becomes indicated. Ongoing studies are needed in this area.

Secondary prophylaxis may benefit children who have experienced at least one previous episode of prolonged (> 7 days) or severe neutropenia with proven bacterial or fungal infection, which led to modification of their chemotherapy regimen or two previous episodes of prolonged and severe neutropenia with or without infection (Schaison *et al.* 1998). By contrast with prophylaxis, most clinicians would have no hesitation in using CSFs in neutropenic children with established severe infection (e.g. pneumonia, soft tissue infection, fungal infection, overwhelming sepsis), although benefit in these circumstances has not been demonstrated directly (Lehrnbecher and Welte 2002).

Management of infection

A number of factors must be considered when assessing and managing a child with a suspected infection. From the time of diagnosis to the end of treatment and beyond, patients are susceptible to both common paediatric pathogens and more unusual opportunistic infective agents. A patient may not always have a high fever and importantly the 'ill' neutropenic child should be treated as if septic whether febrile or not. Common clinical manifestations of infection such as pus or soft tissue swelling may not be apparent during neutropenia. The outcome of infection in children has improved dramatically with the introduction of standardized empirical antibiotic regimens for febrile neu-tropenia (Chanock and Pizzo 1996) but guidelines for the management of infections in the febrile non-neutropenic child are less standardized (Salzer et al. 2003).

The initial assessment of any patient with suspected infection requires a careful history and detailed clinical examination (including the ears, throat, and CVC exit site). Blood cultures from all lumens of the CVC should be taken. The importance of this practice was emphasized by a study which found that 43% of positive isolates from double lumen catheters came from only one of the lumens (Adamkiewicz et al. 1999). The same study demon-strated limited usefulness of peripheral cultures in patients with a CVC and this is not considered routine practice in children. Urine microscopy and cul-ture is mandatory as classic symptoms of urinary tract infection may not be evident from the history. Viral serology, swabs from sites of apparent clinical infection and stool samples are taken as appropriate. Routine chest radio-graphy is no longer undertaken unless the patient has symptoms or signs of chest infection (Feusner et al. 1988; Collins et al. 2001). Other diagnostic tests such as C-reactive protein and cytokines may be used but are rarely specific (Riikonen et al 1992; Heney et al. 1992; Santolaya et al. 1994; Kallio et al. 2000).

Progressive, planned approach to the management of infection in the neutropenic child

The largest published series of outcome of febrile neutropenia suggests mor-tality from infection of about 1% in children compared with 4% in adults (Hann et al. 1997). Any febrile, neutropenic child may have significant and potentially life-threatening sepsis, so investigation and treatment of the febrile, neutropenic child is always urgent. Neutropenia is defined as neu-trophils $< 1.0 \times 10^9/l$ but the greatest risk of sepsis is when neutrophils are below $0.5 \times 10^9/l$ (severe neutropenia) and some centres differentiate these groups in their management protocols. Current European guidelines define significant fever as $> 38\,°C$ on two occasions over a 12-hour period or a single spike above $38.5\,°C$ (Cometta et al. 1996).

The key initial consideration in febrile neutropenia is to prevent severe mor-bidity or mortality from Gram-negative infection. The early recommendations for febrile neutropenia in the 1970s included routine use of combination antibiotic regimens to provide 'double' Gram-negative cover and this approach remains common in paediatrics. Combinations of aminoglycoside with a β-lactam remain a popular choice. The β-lactam also gives broad-spectrum Gram-positive cover and aminoglycosides have activity against most Staph. aureus. The reduction in Gram-negative bacteraemic episodes has prompted some groups to question the continued use of aminoglycosides with their attendant toxicities in the paediatric age group.

The high incidence of Gram-positive infections seen in paediatric cancer patients during the 1980–90s, most of which are resistant to β-lactam antibiotics, has resulted in the increased use of vancomycin and teicoplanin. The inclusion of a glycopeptide in the first-line antibiotic combination has been debated. The relatively low virulence of most Gram-positive bacteria means that many centres feel such antibiotics can be withheld until microbiological confirmation is available. A recent survey of practice in the USA has found that the increase in vancomycin-resistant enterococcus infections seen in centres that have used vancomycin as a first-line antibiotic has resulted in a change of practice in response to this worrying yet predictable finding (Kline and Baorto 2004).

Any safe modification to reduce treatment burden is welcomed when treating children. Monotherapy has been widely evaluated in both adult and paediatric populations with third-generation cephalosporins and carbapenems offering potential promise. The main concern is the emergence of resistance to individual agents, especially by *Pseudomonas* species (Hughes *et al.* 2002) and failure of empirical therapy, with potentially serious or fatal consequences. Available evidence suggests that monotherapy is at least as effective and safe as combination therapy (Furno *et al.* 2002) but in practice it may be more appropriate to reserve monotherapy for patients at lower risk of serious complications such as those with a short anticipated duration of neutropenia or who are clinically stable at presentation (Klastersky 2004).

The crucial factor in choosing safe, effective empirical antibiotic regimens is close monitoring of bacterial isolates and resistance patterns in the local paediatric cancer population in collaboration with the microbiology team. By continued surveillance, changing patterns of isolates and resistance can be determined and antibiotic strategies modified as needed. Even with defined local guidelines the empirical antibiotic regimen may be modified according to clinical circumstances, such as the addition of vancomycin for an obvious CVC tunnel infection or metronidazole when significant gut pathology (not just diarrhoea) is suspected.

The median time from the start of empirical antibiotic therapy to defervescence of fever in childhood febrile neutropenia is 3 days (Hann *et al.* 1997) but in practice a wide range is noted. Once empirical antibiotic therapy has commenced the child should be reassessed at 48 hours with blood culture results and treatment modified according to positive cultures and sensitivities. Any child remaining febrile should have repeat blood cultures regularly until the cessation of fever. Previous practice had been to await neutrophil recovery

($> 0.5 \times 10^9/l$) before discontinuing intravenous antibiotics after resolution of fever but studies in the 1990s showed that in the well child with negative blood cultures, in whom local infection is controlled and there is some evidence of marrow recovery, intravenous antibiotics can be safely discontinued regardless of neutrophil count 24–48 hours after resolution of fever (Mullen and Buchanan 1990; Cohen *et al.* 1995; Aquino *et al.* 1997).

More recently the focus of interest has moved to the area of risk stratification in which patients at low risk of serious infection may have their antimicrobial treatment appropriately reduced, with management at least in part in the ambulatory setting. This approach potentially reduces the risk of nosocomial infection and the development of bacterial resistance and has obvious cost-benefits, enabling children to spend more time at home with their families.

The early work on risk stratification by Talcott focused on adult cancer patients. He reviewed 261 medical records of patients with febrile neutropenia and identified four subgroups of patients, three of which were considered to be at higher risk of infection (patients already hospitalized when fever developed, outpatients with comorbidity and outpatients with cancer 'not in remission') and one group of 'low-risk' patients (Talcott *et al.* 1988). The risk prediction model utilized clinical information available on the first day of febrile neutropenia and was validated in a prospective trial involving 444 patients with febrile neutropenia. Thirty four per cent of patients in one of the high-risk groups were found to suffer from serious medical complications compared with only 5% in the low-risk group (Talcott *et al.* 1992). However the criteria, although effective at predicting adverse outcome, were not sufficient to discriminate between bacterial infections and other causes of fever. More recently, the Multinational Association for Supportive Care in Cancer (MASCC) developed a new clinical risk index, which identifies adult patients at low risk of medical complications during resolution of fever (Klastersky *et al.* 2000). The criteria used cannot be directly translated into paediatric practice, but several studies have been conducted in paediatric populations addressing the same issues (Aquino *et al.* 1997; Klaassen *et al.* 2000; Santolaya *et al.* 2004). To date there is no universally agreed, validated, set of parameters for identifying low-risk paediatric patients. Current models include stratification on the basis of clinical variables that include predicted degree and duration of neutropenia, type and status of underlying disease, associated systemic symptoms such as hypotension that indicate risk of severe infection, proven bacteraemia, and fever and neutrophil count at the time of presentation. As our understanding of aspects of innate immunity (such as mannose-binding lectin) and infection risk improves, genetic factors may be found to contribute to risk stratification and management strategies in febrile neutropenia (Neth *et al.* 2001).

A recent report assessing parental preferences to inpatient versus outpatient management of low-risk paediatric febrile neutropenia found that only 53% of parents would choose outpatient oral antibiotic management if it was offered (Sung *et al.* 2004a). This highlights the need to consider perceived parental confidence as well as medical factors and compliance when making management decisions.

The risk of fungal infection increases significantly as the duration of fever with profound neutropenia increases. Underlying diagnosis (especially acute myeloid leukaemia), treatment schedule (especially allogeneic BMT), immunosuppression with steroids and severe graft versus host disease also contribute to risk. However, the detection of invasive fungal infection is notoriously difficult. For this reason it is now standard to introduce antifungal treatment after several days of persistent fever where no other cause has been identified and early investigation with abdominal ultrasound scan, chest X-ray and sometimes CT is indicated. Historically conventional amphotericin B has been the treatment of choice for persistent fever of unknown origin owing to its broad spectrum of activity but its use is limited by side-effects including nephrotoxicity. It has been the preferred treatment for documented infection with non-albicans *Candida*, hepatosplenic candidiasis, aspergillosis, and other fungal infections, while fluconazole is active in other *C. albicans* infections. The development of lipid formulations of amphotericin B, which have reduced toxicity and can be given at higher doses, has improved management and outcome in these infections (Hann and Prentice 2001). Newer agents such as caspofungin, a member of the echinocandin family, and voriconazole, a new azole, are now available but are not licensed in children.

Both caspofungin (Walsh *et al.* 2004) and voriconazole (Walsh *et al.* 2002) have equal efficacy and a better toxicity profile than amphotericin B in the management of persistent febrile neutropenia in adults and teenagers. Voriconazole was shown in one randomized study to give better response rates and a better toxicity profile than conventional amphotericin B against invasive aspergillosis (Herbrecht *et al.* 2002) and caspofungin is as effective as conventional amphotericin in invasive candidiasis and candidaemia (Mora-Duarte *et al.* 2002). These agents have been used in combination with amphotericin preparations with promising results (Elanjikal *et al.* 2003; Cesaro *et al.* 2004; Castagnola *et al.* 2004; Lassaletta *et al.* 2004). Further investigation is required to define how best to use these agents to treat invasive fungal infection in this population.

Conclusions

While outcome of treatment for paediatric malignancy continues to improve and deaths from infection have fallen, children who are immunosuppressed by chemotherapy still remain at significant risk of serious infection. In the future it is hoped that a combination of improved preventive strategies, new antimicrobial agents to counteract emerging bacterial resistance and to treat difficult fungal and viral pathogens, coupled with a better understanding of how to use such agents will result in a continued decline in deaths from infection in this patient population. Conversely, better identification of those at low risk of serious infection may allow reduction in the intensity of treatment for fever in carefully selected low-risk patients.

References

Adamkiewicz TV, Lorenzana A, Doyle J, and Richardson S. (1999). Peripheral vs. central blood cultures in patients admitted to a pediatric oncology ward. *Pediatric Infectious Disease Journal*, 18, 556–558.

Aledo A, Heller G, Ren L, *et al.* (1998). Septicemia and septic shock in pediatric patients: 140 consecutive cases on a pediatric hematology-oncology service. *Journal of Pediatric Hematology and Oncology*, 20, 215–221.

Alfaham M, Holt ME, and Goodchild MC. (1987). Arthropathy in a patient with cystic fibrosis taking ciprofloxacin. *British Medical Journal*, 295, 699.

Aquino VM, Buchanan GR, Tkaczewski I, and Mustafa MM. (1997). Safety of early hospital discharge of selected febrile children and adolescents with cancer with prolonged neutropenia. *Medical and Pediatric Oncology*, 28, 191–195.

Atkinson K, Meyers JD, Storb R, Prentice RL, and Thomas ED. (1980). Varicella-zoster virus infection after marrow transplantation for aplastic anemia or leukemia. *Transplantation*, 29, 47–50.

Atkinson P, Cullinan C, Jones J, Fraser G, and Maguire H. (2005). Large outbreak of measles in London: reversal of health inequalities. *Archives of Diseases in Childhood*, 90, 424–425.

Castagnola E, Machetti M, Cappelli B, *et al.* (2004). Caspofungin associated with liposomal amphotericin B or voriconazole for treatment of refractory fungal pneumonia in children with acute leukaemia or undergoing allogeneic bone marrow transplant. *Clinical Microbiology & Infection*, 10, 255–257.

Cesaro S, Toffolutti T, Messina C, *et al.* (2004). Safety and efficacy of caspofungin and liposomal amphotericin B, followed by voriconazole in young patients affected by refractory invasive mycosis. *European Journal of Haematology*, 73, 50–55.

Chanock SJ and Pizzo PA. (1996). Fever in the neutropenic host. *Infectious Disease Clinics of North America*, 10, 777–796.

Chisholm JC, Devine T, Charlett A, Pinkerton CR, and Zambon M. (2001). Response to influenza immunisation during treatment for cancer. *Archives of Diseases in Childhood*, 84, 496–500.

Chisholm J, Howe K, Taj M, and Zambon M. (2003). Influenza immunisation in children with solid tumours. *Medical and Pediatric Oncology*, 41, 256.

Cohen KJ, Leamer K, Odom L, Greffe B, and Stork L. (1995). Cessation of antibiotics regardless of ANC is safe in children with febrile neutropenia. A preliminary prospective trial. *Journal of Pediatric Hematology and Oncology*, 17, 325–330.

Collard MM and Hunter ML. (2001). Oral and dental care in acute lymphoblastic leukaemia: a survey of United Kingdom children's cancer study group centres. *International Journal of Paediatric Dentistry*, 11, 347–351.

Collins C, Fenton M, and Phillips B. (2001). Are routine chest x-rays helpful in the management of febrile neutropenia? *Archives of Diseases in Childhood*, 85, 253.

Cometta A, Calandra T, Gaya H, *et al.* (1996). Monotherapy with meropenem versus combination therapy with ceftazidime plus amikacin as empiric therapy for fever in granulocytopenic patients with cancer. The International Antimicrobial Therapy Cooperative Group of the European Organization for Research and Treatment of Cancer and the Gruppo Italiano Malattie Ematologiche Maligne dell'Adulto Infection Program. *Antimicrobial Agents and Chemotherapy*, 40, 1108–1115.

Cruciani M, Malena M, Bosco O, Nardi S, Serpelloni G, and Mengoli C. (2003). Reappraisal with meta-analysis of the addition of Gram-positive prophylaxis to fluoro-quinolone in neutropenic patients. *Journal of Clinical Oncology*, 21, 4127–4137.

Cuadrado E and Barrena MJ. (1996). Immune dysfunction in Down's syndrome: primary immune deficiency or early senescence of the immune system? *Clinical Immunology & Immunopathology*, 78, 209–214.

Elanjikal Z, Sorensen J, Schmidt H, *et al.* (2003). Combination therapy with caspofungin and liposomal amphotericin B for invasive aspergillosis. *Pediatric Infectious Disease Journal*, 22, 653–656.

Engels EA, Lau J, and Barza M. (1998). Efficacy of quinolone prophylaxis in neutropenic cancer patients: a meta-analysis. *Journal of Clinical Oncology*, 16, 1179–1187.

Epstein JB, Ransier A, Sherlock CH, Spinelli JJ, and Reece D. (1996). Acyclovir prophylaxis of oral herpes virus during bone marrow transplantation. *European Journal of Cancer Part B Oral Oncology*, 32B, 158–162.

Feldman S and Lott L. (1987). Varicella in children with cancer: impact of antiviral therapy and prophylaxis. *Pediatrics*, 80, 465–472.

Feusner J, Cohen R, O'Leary M, and Beach B. (1988). Use of routine chest radiography in the evaluation of fever in neutropenic pediatric oncology patients. *Journal of Clinical Oncology*, 6, 1699–1702.

Ford AM, Ridge SA, Cabrera ME, *et al.* (1993). In utero rearrangements in the trithorax-related oncogene in infant leukaemias. *Nature*, 363, 358–360.

Furno P, Bucaneve G, and Del Favero A. (2002). Monotherapy or aminoglycoside-containing combinations for empirical antibiotic treatment of febrile neutropenic patients: a meta-analysis. *Lancet Infectious Diseases*, 2, 231–242.

Gale KB, Ford AM, Repp R, *et al.* (1997). Backtracking leukemia to birth: identification of clonotypic gene fusion sequences in neonatal blood spots. *Proceedings of the National Academy of Science USA*, 94, 13950–13954.

Gamis AS, Howells WB, DeSwarte-Wallace J, Feusner JH, Buckley JD, and Woods WG. (2000). Alpha hemolytic streptococcal infection during intensive treatment for acute myeloid leukemia: a report from the Children's cancer group study CCG-2891. *Journal of Clinical Oncology*, 18, 1845–1855.

Gatta G, Corazziari I, Magnani C, Peris-Bonet R, Roazzi P, and Stiller C. (2003). Childhood cancer survival in Europe. *Annals of Oncology*, 14 (Suppl. 5), v119–v127.

Gibson F. (2004). Best practice in oral care for children and young people being treated for cancer: can we achieve consensus? *European Journal of Cancer*, 40, 1109–1110.

Gilham C, Peto J, Simpson J, *et al.* (2005). Day care in infancy and risk of childhood acute lymphoblastic leukaemia: findings from UK case-control study. *British Medical Journal*, 330, 1279–1280.

Glasmacher A, Prentice A, Gorschluter M, *et al.* (2003). Itraconazole prevents invasive fungal infections in neutropenic patients treated for hematologic malignancies: evidence from a meta-analysis of 3,597 patients. *Journal of Clinical Oncology*, 21, 4615–4626.

Glass RT and Lare MM. (1986). Toothbrush contamination: a potential health risk? *Quintessence International*, 17, 39–42.

Goldstein SL, Somers MJ, Lande MB, Brewer ED, and Jabs KL. (2000). Acyclovir prophylaxis of varicella in children with renal disease receiving steroids. *Pediatric Nephrology*, 14, 305–308.

Grady R. (2003). Safety profile of quinolone antibiotics in the pediatric population. *Pediatric Infectious Disease Journal*, 22, 1128–1132.

Gray MM, Hann IM, Glass S, Eden OB, Jones PM, and Stevens RF. (1987). Mortality and morbidity caused by measles in children with malignant disease attending four major treatment centres: a retrospective review. *British Medical Journal*, 295, 19–22.

Greaves MF. (1997). Aetiology of acute leukaemia. *Lancet*, 349, 344–349.

Greaves M. (1999). Molecular genetics, natural history and the demise of childhood leukaemia. *European Journal of Cancer*, 35, 1941–1953.

Hann IM and Prentice HG. (2001). Lipid-based amphotericin B: a review of the last 10 years of use. *International Journal of Antimicrobial Agents*, 17, 161–169.

Hann IM, Prentice HG, Blacklock HA, *et al.* (1983). Acyclovir prophylaxis against herpes virus infections in severely immunocompromised patients: randomised double blind trial. *British Medical Journal*, 287, 384–388.

Hann I, Viscoli C, Paesmans M, Gaya H, and Glauser M. (1997). A comparison of outcome from febrile neutropenic episodes in children compared with adults: results from four EORTC studies. International Antimicrobial Therapy Cooperative Group (IATCG) of the European Organization for Research and Treatment of Cancer (EORTC). *British Journal of Haematology*, 99, 580–588.

Hargrave DR, Hann II, Richards SM, *et al.* (2001). Progressive reduction in treatment-related deaths in Medical Research Council childhood lymphoblastic leukaemia trials from 1980 to 1997 (UKALL VIII, X and XI). *British Journal of Haematology*, 112, 293–299.

Hasle H, Clemmensen IH, and Mikkelsen M. (2000). Risks of leukaemia and solid tumours in individuals with Down's syndrome. *Lancet*, 355, 165–169.

Heney D, Lewis IJ, Evans SW, Banks R, Bailey CC, and Whicher JT. (1992). Interleukin-6 and its relationship to C-reactive protein and fever in children with febrile neutropenia. *Journal of Infectious Diseases*, 165, 886–890.

Hengartner H, Berger C, Nadal D, Niggli FK, and Grotzer MA. (2004). Port-A-Cath infections in children with cancer. *European Journal of Cancer*, 40, 2452–2458.

Herbrecht R, Denning DW, Patterson TF, *et al.* (2002). Voriconazole versus amphotericin B for primary therapy of invasive aspergillosis. *New England Journal of Medicine*, 347, 408–415.

Hughes WT, Armstrong D, Bodey GP, *et al.* (2002). 2002 guidelines for the use of antimicrobial agents in neutropenic patients with cancer. *Clinical Infectious Diseases*, 34, 730–751.

Ingram J, Weitzman S, Greenberg ML, Parkin P, and Filler R. (1991). Complications of indwelling venous access lines in the pediatric hematology patient: a prospective comparison of external venous catheters and subcutaneous ports. *American Journal of Pediatric Hematology and Oncology*, 13, 130–136.

Ishida Y, Tauchi H, Higaki A, Yokota-Outou Y, and Kida K. (1996). Postexposure prophylaxis of varicella in children with leukemia by oral acyclovir. *Pediatrics*, 97, 150–151.

Kallio R, Surcel HM, Bloigu A, and Syrjala H. (2000). C-reactive protein, procalcitonin and interleukin-8 in the primary diagnosis of infections in cancer patients. *European Journal of Cancer*, 36, 889–894.

Kawasaki H, Takayama J, and Ohira M. (1996). Herpes zoster infection after bone marrow transplantation in children. *Journal of Pediatrics*, 128, 353–356.

Kelsey SM, Goldman JM, McCann S, *et al.* (1999). Liposomal amphotericin (AmBisome) in the prophylaxis of fungal infections in neutropenic patients: a randomised, double-blind, placebo-controlled study. *Bone Marrow Transplantation*, 23, 163–168.

Kinlen LJ. (1995). Epidemiological evidence for an infective basis in childhood leukaemia. *British Journal of Cancer*, 71, 1–5.

Kinlen LJ and Petridou E. (1995). Childhood leukemia and rural population movements: Greece, Italy, and other countries. *Cancer Causes Control*, 6, 445–450.

Klaassen RJ, Goodman TR, Pham B, and Doyle JJ. (2000). 'Low-risk' prediction rule for pediatric oncology patients presenting with fever and neutropenia. *Journal of Clinical Oncology*, 18, 1012–1019.

Klastersky J. (2004). Management of fever in neutropenic patients with different risks of complications. *Clinical Infectious Diseases*, 39 (Suppl. 1), S32–S37.

Klastersky J, Paesmans M, Rubenstein EB, *et al.* (2000). The Multinational Association for Supportive Care in Cancer risk index: a multinational scoring system for identifying low-risk febrile neutropenic cancer patients. *Journal of Clinical Oncology*, 18, 3038–3051.

Kline RM and Baorto EP. (2004). Treatment of pediatric febrile neutropenia in the era of vancomycin-resistant microbes. *Pediatric Blood and Cancer*, 44, 205–206.

Kramer BS, Pizzo PA, Robichaud KJ, Witesbsky F, and Wesley R. (1982). Role of serial microbiologic surveillance and clinical evaluation in the management of cancer patients with fever and granulocytopenia. *American Journal of Medicine*, 72, 561–568.

Lassaletta A, Perez A, Diaz MA, Sevilla J, Gonzalez-Vicent M, and Madero L. (2004). Successful treatment of invasive aspergillosis with oral voriconazole following intravenous liposomal amphotericin in a child with acute lymphoblastic leukemia. *Journal of Pediatric Hematology and Oncology*, 26, 117–119.

Lehrnbecher T and Welte K. (2002). Haematopoietic growth factors in children with neutropenia. *British Journal of Haematology*, 116, 28–56.

Lehrnbecher T, Foster C, Vazquez N, Mackall CL, and Chanock SJ. (1997). Therapy-induced alterations in host defense in children receiving therapy for cancer. *Journal of Pediatric Hematology and Oncology*, 19, 399–417.

Lehtinen M, Koskela P, Ogmundsdottir HM, *et al.* (2003). Maternal herpesvirus infections and risk of acute lymphoblastic leukemia in the offspring. *American Journal of Epidemiology*, 158, 207–213.

Leruez-Ville M, Ouachee M, Delarue R, *et al.* (2003). Monitoring cytomegalovirus infection in adult and pediatric bone marrow transplant recipients by a real-time PCR assay performed with blood plasma. *Journal of Clinical Microbiology*, 41, 2040–2046.

Leung TF, Li CK, Hung EC, *et al.* (2004). Immunogenicity of a two-dose regime of varicella vaccine in children with cancers. *European Journal of Haematology*, 72, 353–357.

Little MA, Morland B, Chisholm J, *et al.* (2002). A randomised study of prophylactic G-CSF following MRC UKALL XI intensification regimen in childhood ALL and T-NHL. *Medical and Pediatric Oncology*, 38, 98–103.

Ljungman P, de La CR, Milpied N, *et al.* (2002). Randomized study of valacyclovir as prophylaxis against cytomegalovirus reactivation in recipients of allogeneic bone marrow transplants. *Blood*, 99, 3050–3056.

Ljungman P, von Dobeln L, Ringholm L, Lewensohn-Fuchs I, Klingspor L, and Sparrelid E. (2005). The value of CMV and fungal PCR for monitoring for acute leukaemia and autologous stem cell transplant patients. *Scandinavian Journal of Infectious Diseases*, 37, 121–127.

Lucas VS, Roberts GJ, and Beighton D. (1998). Oral health of children undergoing allogeneic bone marrow transplantation. *Bone Marrow Transplantation*, 22, 801–808.

Maertens J, Theunissen K, Verbeken E, *et al.* (2004). Prospective clinical evaluation of lower cut-offs for galactomannan detection in adult neutropenic cancer patients and haematological stem cell transplant recipients. *British Journal of Haematology*, 126, 852–860.

Mennink-Kersten MA, Donnelly JP, and Verweij PE. (2004). Detection of circulating galactomannan for the diagnosis and management of invasive aspergillosis. *Lancet Infectious Diseases*, 4, 349–357.

Mirro J Jr, Rao BN, Stokes DC, *et al.* (1989). A prospective study of Hickman/Broviac catheters and implantable ports in pediatric oncology patients. *Journal of Clinical Oncology*, 7, 214–222.

Mora-Duarte J, Betts R, Rotstein C, *et al.* (2002). Comparison of caspofungin and amphotericin B for invasive candidiasis. *New England Journal of Medicine*, 347, 2020–2029.

Morgan OW, Meltzer M, Muir D, *et al.* (2003). Specialist vaccination advice and pockets of resistance to MMR vaccination: lessons from an outbreak of measles. *Communicable Diseases and Public Health*, 6, 330–333.

Mullen CA and Buchanan GR. (1990). Early hospital discharge of children with cancer treated for fever and neutropenia: identification and management of the low-risk patient. *Journal of Clinical Oncology*, 8, 1998–2004.

Mullen CA, Abd El-Baki H, Samir H, Tarrand JJ, and Rolston KV. (2003). Non-albicans Candida is the most common cause of candidemia in pediatric cancer patients. *Supportive Care in Cancer*, 11, 321–325.

Naumburg E, Bellocco R, Cnattingius S, Jonzon A, and Ekbom A. (2002). Perinatal exposure to infection and risk of childhood leukemia. *Medical and Pediatric Oncology*, 38, 391–397.

Neth O, Hann I, Turner MW, and Klein NJ. (2001). Deficiency of mannose-binding lectin and burden of infection in children with malignancy: a prospective study. *Lancet*, 358, 614–618.

NHS Immunisations Statistics, England: 2003–04. Available at *www.publications.doh.gov.uk*

Paganini H, Staffolani V, Zubizarreta P, Casimir L, Lopardo H, and Luppino V. (2003). Viridans streptococci bacteraemia in children with fever and neutropenia: a case-control study of predisposing factors. *European Journal of Cancer*, 39, 1284–1289.

Porter CC, Edwards KM, Zhu Y, and Frangoul H. (2004). Immune responses to influenza immunization in children receiving maintenance chemotherapy for acute lymphoblastic leukemia. *Pediatric Blood and Cancer*, 42, 36–40.

Raad I, Hanna H, Sumoza D, and Albitar M. (2002). Polymerase chain reaction on blood for the diagnosis of invasive pulmonary aspergillosis in cancer patients. *Cancer*, 94, 1032–1036.

Reinhardt D, Houliara K, Pekrun A, Lakomek M, and Krone B. (2003). Impact of conventional chemotherapy on levels of antibodies against vaccine-preventable diseases in children treated for cancer. *Scandinavian Journal of Infectious Diseases*, 35, 851–857.

Riikonen P, Saarinen UM, Teppo AM, Metsarinne K, Fyhrquist F, and Jalanko H. (1992). Cytokine and acute-phase reactant levels in serum of children with cancer admitted for fever and neutropenia. *Journal of Infectious Diseases*, 166, 432–436.

Riikonen P, Saarinen UM, Makipernaa A, *et al*. (1994). Recombinant human granulocyte-macrophage colony-stimulating factor in the treatment of febrile neutropenia: a double blind placebo-controlled study in children. *Pediatric Infectious Disease Journal*, 13, 197–202.

Riley LC, Hann IM, Wheatley K, and Stevens RF. (1999). Treatment-related deaths during induction and first remission of acute myeloid leukaemia in children treated on the Tenth Medical Research Council acute myeloid leukaemia trial (MRC AML10). The MCR Childhood Leukaemia Working Party. *British Journal of Haematology*, 106, 436–444.

Robison LL. (1992). Down syndrome and leukemia. *Leukemia*, 6 (Suppl. 1), 5–7.

Royal College of Paediatrics and Child Health. (2002). Immunisation of the Immunocompromised Child. Best Practice Statement. Available at www.rcpch.ac.uk.

Salzer W, Steinberg SM, Liewehr DJ, Freifeld A, Balis FM, and Widemann BC. (2003). Evaluation and treatment of fever in the non-neutropenic child with cancer. *Journal of Pediatric Hematology and Oncology*, 25, 606–612.

Santolaya ME, Cofre J, and Beresi V. (1994). C-reactive protein: a valuable aid for the management of febrile children with cancer and neutropenia. *Clinical Infectious Diseases*, 18, 589–595.

Santolaya ME, Alvarez AM, Aviles CL, *et al*. (2004). Early hospital discharge followed by outpatient management versus continued hospitalization of children with cancer, fever, and neutropenia at low risk for invasive bacterial infection. *Journal of Clinical Oncology*, 22, 3784–3789.

Sauerbrei A, Prager J, Hengst U, Zintl F, and Wutzler P. (1997). Varicella vaccination in children after bone marrow transplantation. *Bone Marrow Transplantation*, 20, 381–383.

Schaison G, Eden OB, Henze G, *et al*. (1998). Recommendations on the use of colony-stimulating factors in children: conclusions of a European panel. *European Journal of Pediatrics*, 157, 955–966.

Stiller CA. (2004). Epidemiology and genetics of childhood cancer. *Oncogene* 23, 6429–6444.

Sung L, Feldman BM, Schwamborn G, *et al*. (2004a). Inpatient versus outpatient management of low-risk pediatric febrile neutropenia: measuring parents' and healthcare professionals' preferences. *Journal of Clinical Oncology*, 22, 3922–3929.

Sung L, Nathan PC, Lange B, Beyene J, and Buchanan GR. (2004b). Prophylactic granulo-cyte colony-stimulating factor and granulocyte-macrophage colony-stimulating factor decrease febrile neutropenia after chemotherapy in children with cancer: a meta-analysis of randomized controlled trials. *Journal of Clinical Oncology*, 22, 3350–3356.

Talcott JA, Finberg R, Mayer RJ, and Goldman L. (1988). The medical course of cancer patients with fever and neutropenia. Clinical identification of a low-risk subgroup at presentation. *Archives of Internal Medicine*, 148, 2561–2568.

Talcott JA, Siegel RD, Finberg R, and Goldman L. (1992). Risk assessment in cancer patients with fever and neutropenia: a prospective, two-center validation of a prediction rule. *Journal of Clinical Oncology*, 10, 316–322.

Taylor CE, Sviland L, Pearson AD, et al. (1990). Virus infections in bone marrow transplant recipients: a three year prospective study. *Journal of Clinical Pathology*, 43, 633–637.

Taylor GM, Dearden S, Ravetto P, et al. (2002). Genetic susceptibility to childhood common acute lymphoblastic leukaemia is associated with polymorphic peptide-binding pocket profiles in HLA-DPB1*0201. *Human Molecular Genetics*, 11, 1585–1597.

Thomas KE, Owens CM, Veys PA, Novelli V, and Costoli V. (2003). The radiological spectrum of invasive aspergillosis in children: a 10-year review. *Pediatric Radiology*, 33, 453–460.

Tollemar J, Ringden O, Andersson S, Sundberg B, Ljungman P, and Tyden G. (1993). Randomized double-blind study of liposomal amphotericin B (Ambisome) prophylaxis of invasive fungal infections in bone marrow transplant recipients. *Bone Marrow Transplantation*, 12, 577–582.

Toms JR (ed.). (2004). *Cancer Stats Monograph*. London: Cancer Research UK.

Walsh TJ, Pappas P, Winston DJ, et al. (2002). Voriconazole compared with liposomal amphotericin B for empirical antifungal therapy in patients with neutropenia and persistent fever. *New England Journal of Medicine*, 346, 225–234.

Walsh TJ, Teppler H, Donowitz GR, et al. (2004). Caspofungin versus liposomal amphotericin B for empirical antifungal therapy in patients with persistent fever and neutropenia. *New England Journal of Medicine*, 351, 1391–1402.

Wheeler K, Chessells JM, Bailey CC, and Richards SM. (1996). Treatment related deaths during induction and in first remission in acute lymphoblastic leukaemia: MRC UKALL X. *Archives of Diseases in Childhood*, 74, 101–107.

Wiemels JL, Cazzaniga G, Daniotti M, et al. (1999a). Prenatal origin of acute lymphoblastic leukaemia in children. *Lancet*, 354, 1499–1503.

Wiemels JL, Ford AM, Van Wering ER, Postma A, and Greaves M. (1999b). Protracted and variable latency of acute lymphoblastic leukemia after TEL-AML1 gene fusion in utero. *Blood*, 94, 1057–1062.

Wingard JR. (1994). Infections due to resistant Candida species in patients with cancer who are receiving chemotherapy. *Clinical Infectious Diseases*, 19 (Suppl. 1), S49–S53.

Yousef AA, Fryer CJ, Chedid FD, Abbas AA, Felimban SK, and Khattab TM. (2004). A pilot study of prophylactic ciprofloxacin during delayed intensification in children with acute lymphoblastic leukemia. *Pediatric Blood and Cancer*, 43, 637–643.

Chapter 12

Eye infections

Hari Jayaram and Elizabeth Graham

Cancer and its treatments increase the risk of developing infection and also create a risk from opportunistic pathogens that would not cause disease in normal individuals. The aim of this chapter is to highlight those conditions that may be encountered in the eye in the immunocompromised cancer patient, and facilitate early recognition, referral and initiation of treatment.

Adnexal infections

Herpes zoster ophthalmicus (HZO)

HZO occurs due to infection of the ophthalmic branch of the trigeminal nerve by the varicella zoster virus (VZV), which often lies latent in the trigeminal ganglion. HZO is rarely seen under the age of 50 years in the normal population, but may present in younger patients in this cohort.

Erythema, swelling, and pain of the periocular tissues occur in a distinctive dermatomal distribution, and are followed by crops of vesicles that erupt and crust over in a characteristic manner. Lesions on the lateral aspect of the nose (Hutchinson's sign) in the distribution of the external nasal nerve signify potential intraocular involvement due to the nasociliary nerve, and should prompt referral to an ophthalmologist.

There may be an associated red eye due to:

- Conjunctivitis; often follicular in nature or due to secondary bacterial infection.
- Corneal involvement (keratitis) in two-thirds of cases (Liesegang 1985), characterized by thick ropey elevated dendrites, which stain minimally with fluorescein and are usually self-limiting.
- Uveitis, often associated with high intraocular pressure, occurs more commonly in the presence of external nasal nerve involvement and causes symptoms of brow-ache and photophobia.

Immunosuppressed patients are at increased risk of developing recurrent keratitis and uveitis with a protracted course, which is unusual in the normal population (Ragozzino *et al.* 1982), and the consequent inflammatory damage is related to the level of immune compromise.

Systemic antiviral therapy should ideally be commenced within 72 hours of onset. Oral famciclovir is preferable to aciclovir due to an increased oral bioavailability and prolonged half-life of its active metabolite. The value of topical antiviral treatment is unclear, although antibiotic therapy is often used to prevent a secondary bacterial infection. There is no evidence that early high-dose systemic steroids are beneficial in the prevention of trigeminal neuralgia (Esmann *et al.* 1987).

The treatment of uveitis includes topical corticosteroids and mydriatics.

Cutaneous herpes simplex infection

Herpes simplex virus (HSV) affects the eyelids of children in the normal population, but occurs throughout life and with increased severity in those patients with a compromised immune system. Crops of small vesicles are seen on the eyelid associated with inflammation of the lid margin. The vesicles rupture, crust, and heal over a few days. There may be an associated ipsilateral conjunctivitis. Treatment is with topical aciclovir ointment.

Molluscum contagiosum

Molluscum contagiosum is caused by a large DNA pox virus. Multiple pale, shiny umbilicated nodules 2–3 mm in diameter are seen on the eyelid margin. Shedding of viral particles may produce an ipsilateral conjunctivitis. Aggressive local spread may occur in immuno-compromised individuals with lesions being progressive and recurrent. Lubricants can alleviate symptoms and if natural regression does not occur promptly, treatment by shave excision, cautery, or cryotherapy can be effective.

Conjunctiva and cornea

Bacterial conjunctivitis

This condition classically presents with redness, irritation, and a mucopurulent discharge that causes crusting of the eyelids on waking. The commonest responsible pathogens are *Staphylococcus aureus, Streptococcus pneumoniae*, and *Haemophilus influenzae* (Mannis 1990). It is important to examine the eyelids to exclude a secondary cause, such as blepharitis ('dandruff' of the eyelids).

Primary empirical treatment with a broad-spectrum topical antibiotic such as chloramphenicol is recommended initially. Cultures for organism identification and sensitivities are wise in the immuno-compromised patient, as the incidence of bacterial conjunctivitis is higher and may often be due to atypical and recalcitrant pathogens.

Blepharitis is treated with regular lid hygiene. This involves cleaning the eyelid margin with a weak solution of baby shampoo or sodium bicarbonate.

Infectious keratitis

Compromise of the normal host defence mechanisms to external pathogens may occur in association with contact lens wear and disruption of the ocular surface, for example due to dry eye or corneal exposure.

Local or systemic immune compromise in the oncology patient, either due to the malignancy, immunosuppressive therapies, or poor nutrition may compound this risk, and also contribute to a more aggressive course. Causative organisms may be bacterial, viral, fungal, or parasitic.

Presentation is with reduced vision, ocular pain, photophobia, and lacrimation. The eye will be red with white infiltrates visible on the corneal surface. Fluorescein staining may highlight the associated epithelial defect, or in the case of HSV, reveal a characteristic dendritic ulcer (Figure 12.1).

Bacterial keratitis can be due to Gram positive and negative organisms. *Pseudomonas* spp. is frequently seen with contact lens related keratitis in the immunocompetent patient and is known to be an important cause of infection in cancer patients with a compromised immune system (Rolston and

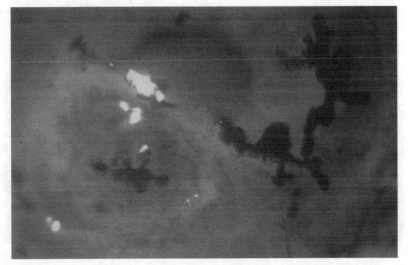

Fig. 12.1 Dendritic ulcers due to HSV, stained with Rose Bengal. See colour plate section.

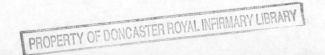

Bodey 1992). HSV and VZV keratitis in this group exhibit a fulminant course and can lead to corneal scarring, neovascularization, and blindness.

Prompt referral to an ophthalmologist for assessment and treatment is recommended due to the potential blinding complications of this condition. These patients may require daily supervision by the ophthalmologist in the acute stage.

Endophthalmitis

Endophthalmitis is a devastating condition involving infection of the intraocular contents that inevitably has a poor visual outcome. In the context of the cancer patient, organisms enter the eye via haematogenous spread and the endophthalmitis is endogenous in nature. Frequent culprits are intravenous lines, wound infections and urinary tract infections.

In the immunocompromised individual the causative organisms may understandably vary, although bacteria and fungi are most frequently implicated. Oncology patients *per se* are known to be predisposed to this condition (Tanaka *et al.* 2001; Jackson *et al.* 2003).

Patients usually present with reduced vision, floaters, and variable ocular pain, all of which may be bilateral in a quarter of cases. The affected eye may not initially be very injected, which can lead to a delay in diagnosis in the critically ill patient. Conjunctival hyperaemia and hypopyon (Figure 12.2) are seen more frequently in bacterial endophthalmitis. Visualization of the fundus is often very difficult due to the infective material throughout the eye. In the early stages, retinal examination may reveal Roth spots (Figure 12.3), which have a white centre surrounded by haemorrhage, and point to a bacterial aetiology.

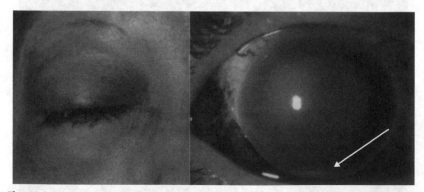

Fig. 12.2 Hypopyon (arrow) due to endophthalmitis in an elderly lady with metastatic disease. The cornea is hazy and the contents of the eye look yellow due to severe inflammation caused by the infection. See colour plate section.

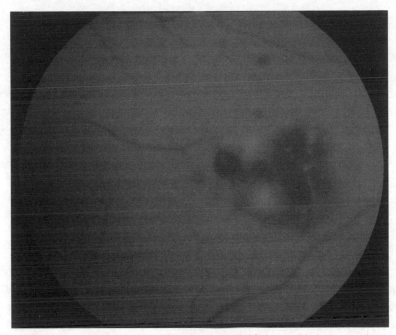

Fig. 12.3 Roth Spots seen in a case of endophthalmitis in an elderly man with cerebral glioma. See colour plate section.

Fungal endophthalmitis may exhibit white fluffy balls within the vitreous overlying retinal and choroidal infiltrates (Figure 12.4). Sources of fungaemia are usually intravenous lines (Schelenz and Gransden 2003) with *Candida albicans* being the most prevalent pathogen, but in the severely ill *Aspergillus, Fusarium* (Figure 12.5), *Nocardia,* or *Cryptococcus* may be seen. However, *Cryptococcus* more commonly presents to an ophthalmologist in patients with meningitis who have blurred vision and diplopia with papilloedema because of raised intracranial pressure.

The visual prognosis of all cases of endophthalmitis is poor, but can be improved by prompt ophthalmological attention. Investigation involves Gram stain, microscopy, and culture of samples of aqueous humour and vitreous. In patients with underlying cancer, particularly haematological, fresh samples should be sent for histological analysis in order to exclude recurrence within the eye rather than infection.

Mandatory investigations include 24-hour temperature monitoring, blood cultures, mid-stream urine analysis, echocardiography, and magnetic resonance imaging of the brain as there is a small mortality from metastatic abscesses.

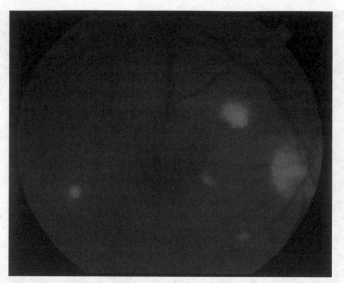

Fig. 12.4 Candida lesions of the retina in a 56 year old woman recovering from major bowel surgery for malignancy. See colour plate section.

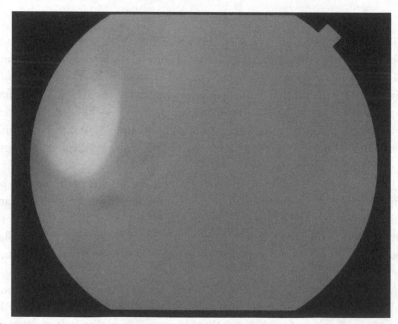

Fig. 12.5 Fusarium retinitis in a teenager with leukaemia. See colour plate section.

Broad-spectrum intravenous antibiotic therapy should be initiated. Intravitreal antibiotics, usually vancomycin and ceftazidime or amikacin, are given at the time of vitreous biopsy. Intravitreal amphotericin B may be administered if there is a strong clinical suspicion of fungal infection.

Posterior segment infections

Cytomegalovirus retinitis

Cytomegalovirus (CMV) is a common opportunistic infection seen in the immunocompromised host. CMV retinitis is a progressive and destructive infection, which if left untreated will lead to blindness. It may occur *de novo* or as a reactivation of latent infection, and commonly occurs with a CD4 lymphocyte count of less than 50 cells/mm^3. CMV viraemia or uraemia is often detected in such patients.

Presentation is insidious and patients are often asymptomatic in the absence of macula or optic nerve involvement.

Slit-lamp examination reveals moderate anterior uveitis and cells in the vitreous. Fulminant CMV retinitis is characterized by full thickness retinal necrosis (whitening) associated with haemorrhage (Figure 12.6), retinal

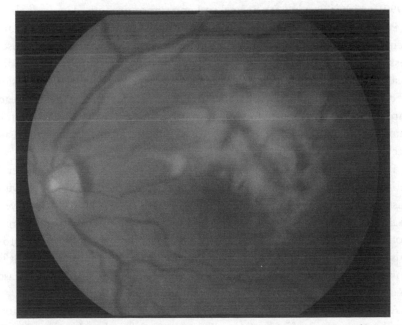

Fig. 12.6 CMV Retinitis in a 60 year old man on systemic immunosuppression. See colour plate section.

arteriolar sheathing, and fluffy sheathing of the retinal veins. A granular variant is more difficult to identify and is often confused with treated disease. Prompt recognition and treatment are required in order to prevent visual loss due to optic nerve or macula involvement, and to minimize the area of affected retina in order to reduce the risk of retinal detachment, which may be seen in up to half of cases (Freeman *et al.* 1993).

Treatment may be systemic or local administration of antiviral therapy, usually ganciclovir or foscarnet. In patients who cannot tolerate systemic therapy or in whom there is no evidence of systemic disease, intravitreal injection or sustained release drug implants (Musch *et al.* 1997) may be considered. Reduction of immunosuppression, if possible, is also important to increase host defences.

There is no evidence to support routine screening of patients at risk, but referral to an ophthalmologist is recommended in the presence of extraocular CMV disease or positive blood or urine cultures, especially in the presence of unexplained visual symptoms.

Acute retinal necrosis (herpes simplex virus or varicella zoster virus retinitis)

VZV and HSV cause a fulminant retinitis (Culbertson *et al.* 1986; Duker *et al.* 1990), which is seen in both normal and immunocompromised individuals.

Patients with acute retinal necrosis typically present with blurred vision, ocular pain, photophobia and floaters. A diminished immune response causes less intraocular inflammation, and hence less redness and pain. Fundal examination in acute retinal necrosis shows extensive yellow white areas of necrosis involving the peripheral retina. Untreated, some of these spread rapidly in a circumferential manner, sparing the posterior pole within the major vascular arcades. There is evidence of intraocular inflammation and an occlusive retinal vasculitis.

There is a spectrum of disease ranging from involvement of the peripheral retina only with preserved vision, to fulminant rapidly progressive disease with ensuing blindness. Progressive outer retinal necrosis (PORN) is the name given to a particularly severe form characterized by minimal intraocular inflammation and no retinal vascular disease, which occurs in severely immunocompromised patients (Figure 12.7), e.g. following bone marrow transplantation. It is unknown which host and viral factors are important in the severity of disease in either immunocompetent or immunocompromised patients.

All patients should undergo vitreous biopsy for polymerase chain reaction confirmation of the offending virus. Treatment involves the administration of intravenous aciclovir (Blumenkranz *et al.* 1986) followed by oral agents for

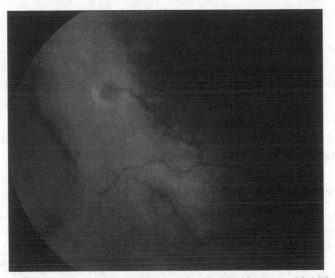

Fig. 12.7 PORN complicated by a retinal tear in a leukamic patient with leukopenia. See colour plate section.

3 months to reduce the risk of involvement of the fellow eye, as untreated disease becomes bilateral in up to 80% of cases. However, the incidence of blindness in the affected eye remains at 40% due primarily to retinal detachment.

The visual prognosis of PORN is universally poor and optimum therapy is unclear. Cidofovir and foscarnet are often used as most affected patients have been on long term aciclovir treatment.

Toxoplasma chorioretinitis

Ocular toxoplasmosis is caused by the intracellular protozoan *Toxoplasma gondii*. The condition is predominantly congenital in origin in the immuno-competent individual, but clearly compromised patients are at risk of acquired infection.

The protozoan has a neurotrophic predilection and attacks the retina as well as other central nervous system tissues. Active disease in the retina tends to be focal and unilateral, although immunocompromised patients may show bilateral and multifocal disease, and are at risk from disseminated central nervous system involvement.

Patients present with increased floaters and blurring of vision. Fundal examination typically shows white fluffy lesions adjacent to an isolated pigmented chorioretinal scar. There is localized inflammation of the vitreous and when severe gives rise to the 'headlight in the fog' appearance. In patients with a compromised immune system ocular toxoplasmosis may be focal, multifocal, or diffuse and present in one or both eyes.

In the normal subject the condition is self-limiting and treatment is only initiated if central vision, major retinal vessels or the optic nerve are threatened.

In the context of the immunocompromised cancer patient, treatment should be started for any active lesion due to the risk of systemic dissemination. A typical treatment regimen involves oral clindamycin and pyrimethamine with folinic acid, although the latter should be used with caution as it may worsen bone marrow suppression.

References

Blumenkranz MS, Culbertson WW, Clarkson JG, and Dix R. (1986). Treatment of the acute retinal necrosis syndrome with intravenous acyclovir. *Ophthalmology*, **93**, 296–300.

Culbertson WW, Blumenkranz MS, Pepose JS, Stewart JA, and Curtin VT. (1986). Varicella zoster virus is a cause of the acute retinal necrosis syndrome. *Ophthalmology*, **93**, 559–569.

Duker JS, Nielsen JC, Eagle RC, Jr., Bosley TM, Granadier R, and Benson WE. (1990). Rapidly progressive acute retinal necrosis secondary to herpes simplex virus, type 1. *Ophthalmology*, **97**, 1638–1643.

Esmann V, Geil JP, Kroon S, *et al.* (1987). Prednisolone does not prevent post-herpetic neuralgia. *Lancet*, **ii**, 126–129.

Freeman WR, Friedberg DN, Berry C, *et al.* (1993). Risk factors for development of rhegmatogenous retinal detachment in patients with cytomegalovirus retinitis. *American Journal of Ophthalmology*, **116**, 713–720.

Jackson TL, Eykyn SJ, Graham EM, and Stanford MR. (2003). Endogenous bacterial endophthalmitis: a 17-year prospective series and review of 267 reported cases. *Survey of Ophthalmology*, **48**, 403–423.

Liesegang TJ. (1985). Corneal complications from herpes zoster ophthalmicus. *Ophthalmology*, **92**, 316–324.

Mannis MJ. (1990). Bacterial conjunctivitis. In: *Duane's Clinical Ophthalmology* (eds W Tasman and EA Jaeger), pp. 5:3–5:7. Philadelphia, PA: JB Lippincott.

Musch DC, Martin DF, Gordon JF, Davis MD, and Kuppermann BD. (1997). Treatment of cytomegalovirus retinitis with a sustained-release ganciclovir implant. The Ganciclovir Implant Study Group. *New England Journal of Medicine*, **337**, 83–90.

Ragozzino MW, Melton LJ, 3rd, Kurland LT, Chu CP, and Perry HO. (1982). Population-based study of herpes zoster and its sequelae. *Medicine (Baltimore)*, **61**, 310–316.

Rolston KV and Bodey GP. (1992). Pseudomonas aeruginosa infection in cancer patients. *Cancer Invest*, **10**, 43–59.

Schelenz S and Gransden WR. (2003). Candidaemia in a London teaching hospital: analysis of 128 cases over a 7-year period. *Mycoses*, **46**, 390–396.

Tanaka M, Kobayashi Y, Takebayashi H, Kiyokawa M, and Qiu H. (2001). Analysis of predisposing clinical and laboratory findings for the development of endogenous fungal endophthalmitis. A retrospective 12-year study of 79 eyes of 46 patients. *Retina*, **21**, 203–209.

Chapter 13

Infections in patients with cancer at the end of life

Caroline McLoughlin and Max Watson

We shall have to learn to refrain from doing things merely because we know how to do them.
Theodore Fox 1899–89: speech to Royal College of Physicians (18 October 1965)

Introduction

The treatment of patients in the last stages of life has been spotlighted in recent years with debates surrounding euthanasia, physician-assisted suicide, advance directives, and issues relating to 'do not resuscitate' orders. The use of antimicrobials in patients with advanced malignancy has become part of this contentious discussion, in which there is a tendency for their true efficacy to be over, or under emphasized in the heat of debate.

Thus, managing infection in patients with advanced malignancy requires both clinical skill, as well as wisdom and flexibility to help patients and their families negotiate this very important part of life which, '. . . has a significance out of all proportion to its duration' (Dame Cicely Saunders 1918–2005).

This chapter, focusing on patients with cancer at the end of life, attempts to describe the frequency of infection; the associated risk factors; the most common sites; the range of common infectious organisms encountered; the resulting symptoms; the efficacy of antimicrobials and other interventions; and the management of common infections. It concludes with some algorithms for antimicrobial use.

Successfully managing infection at the end of life requires a patient-centred rather than a disease-centred approach.

Definitions

WHO definition of palliative care

Palliative care is an approach that improves the quality of life of patients and their families facing the problem associated with life-threatening illness, through the prevention and relief of suffering by means of early identification and impeccable assessment and treatment of pain and other problems, physical, psychosocial, and spiritual. Palliative care affirms life and regards dying as a normal process. It intends to neither hasten or postpone death and aims to enhance quality of life—this may also influence the course of the illness. It is also applicable early in the course of illness, in conjunction with other therapies that are intended to prolong life such as chemotherapy or radiotherapy and includes those investigations needed to better understand and manage distressing clinical complications (WHO 2002).

Treatment goals

The goals of patient management change as the patient progresses along their disease journey. Three phases in palliative care illustrate this changing of management goals.

- *palliative care phase*: goal to preserve quantity and quality of life for as long as possible;
- *hospice care phase*: goal to preserve quality of life; and
- *terminal care phase*: goal to maximize comfort, dignity, and support of patients and relatives, and minimize the medicalization of dying.

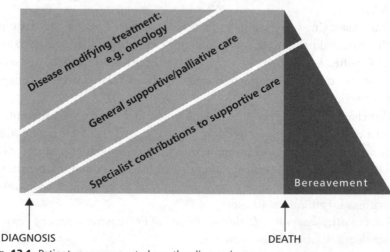

Fig. 13.1 Patient management along the disease journey.

Introduction

The diagnosis and management of infection in patients with cancer at the end of life is complicated by the need to ensure that treatment is appropriate both the particular infection but also for the patient's stage of illness and changing treatment goals.

Diagnosis

Pyrexia may be induced by a variety of non-infectious stimuli including underlying malignancy (particularly lymphoma), certain medications (such as tamoxifen), accelerated tumour growth or necrosis, or hepatic or central nervous system spread (Nagy-Argen and Haley 2002). Raised or lowered white cell counts can both result from advanced disease or iatrogenic causes such as chemotherapy, radiotherapy, or corticosteroids. Corticosteroids, commonly prescribed in cancer patients at the end of life, can inhibit pyrexia and produce a leucocytosis in the absence of local or systemic infection. Additionally, as oncology treatment protocols are changing, patients are often treated later in their diseases requiring increased vigilance and awareness of potential side-effects even in those who have only a few days to live. Also, as a result of cognitive impairment, secondary to disease, medications, or other co-morbid factors, symptoms of infection may not be reported by patients with advanced disease (Pereira *et al.* 1997).

Treatment

Once diagnosed, the treatment of infection is often far from straightforward. The underlying diagnosis, the stage of the illness, the level of multisystem deterioration, uncontrolled pain, or other symptoms, and the patient's and family's own wishes will all influence the application of more or less aggressive interventions (Pereira *et al.* 1998).

Ethical responsibilities

For the physician in the acute hospital setting unused to diagnosing dying, and trained to treat acute illness, not actively treating infection can seem like a dereliction of duty (Nagy-Agren and Haley 2002) particularly as the use of an antimicrobial is commonly seen as a simple intervention, which is thus difficult to justify withholding.

In the light of this it is not surprising that the use of antimicrobials, after the point where they can be realistically expected to have any positive impact, as a 'last resort' in dying patients has been described (Ahronheim *et al.* 1996; Bauduer *et al.* 2000). Among this group of patients, empiric antimicrobials were prescribed more frequently than pathogen-directed therapy and antimicrobial administration was commonly initiated in the absence of documented infection.

Deciding not to give antimicrobials does not mean 'not treating' and symptom control may actually be the most appropriate treatment of choice for many such patients.

Conversely, as patients at the end of life may have multiple distressing symptoms and co-morbidities, the treatment of any potentially reversible factor, such as infection, could significantly reduce their symptom burden.

Particular care needs to be taken to ensure that the staff, patient, and family are made aware of the goal of using antimicrobials in the palliative care context.

Without adequate explanation patients who no longer want any 'active treatment' may refuse antimicrobials aimed at reducing their symptom burden, or alternatively patients or families may lose confidence in healthcare professionals when antimicrobials don't produce the 'cure' for which they are unrealistically hoping.

It is also necessary to be aware of the potential burden of prescribing antimicrobials to patients, particularly those with advanced disease. Repeated venesections for laboratory monitoring of antimicrobial levels, 'commitment' to other diagnostic tests, antimicrobial side-effects, drug interactions, and intravenous access can all be sources of distress for the patient approaching the end of life (Ahronheim *et al.* 1996).

Ethics of isolation policies at the end of life

Vancomycin-resistant enterococci (VRE), bacteria that produce extended-spectrum β-lactamases (ESBL) and methicillin-resistant *Staphylococcus aureus* (MRSA) have had a major impact in the hospital and hospice setting on patients with advanced malignancy (Ali *et al.* 2005). The ethical difficulties are most pronounced when patients who are in advanced stages of their illness are involved. For such dying patients these infections pose limited direct impact apart from the measures implemented to prevent cross-infection to other patients and staff.

Infection control policies, including use of side rooms, restricting patient activity in the ward, and gloving and gowning of all staff and visitors can increase the sense of isolation in the vulnerable patient. These infections can also delay admission to the hospital or hospice if side rooms are required and the time taken to clean the room after discharge will also reduce the number of available beds.

Frequency of infection

The rate of infection in patients with advanced malignancy is high. A Medline review from January 1976 through to January 2001 identified eight reports describing infections in 957 patients with advanced cancer (Nagy-Agren and Haley 2002). (Articles focusing on the management of neutropenic sepsis and other infections associated with active oncology treatment were excluded.) The overall infection rate was 41.6%—with rates varying from 29 to 83%. With the exception of Homsi (Homsi *et al.* 2000), who required a positive culture as evidence of infection and subsequently produced the lowest frequency, the studies diagnosed infection on clinical grounds with bacteriological confirmation in some patients.

Such infection rates are significantly higher than those reported in acute medical, surgical, and rehabilitation units and reflect the increased susceptibility to infection in patients with cancer at the end of life. A number of disease-related and treatment-induced factors have been implicated for this increased susceptibility.

Disease factors

Impaired immunity, with alterations in white cells and cytokine levels, poor healing, general debility, weight loss, and asthenia mediated again by cytokines either directly from the tumour or by cytokines that have been altered by the tumour's presence, are illustrative of the many pathological processes in advanced disease that promote infection.

Patient factors

Decreased level of consciousness, immobility, depression, incontinence, inability to clear chest secretions or keep clean, poor appetite and dehydration etc.(Pereira *et al.* 1998)

Treatment factors

Foreign bodies

Urinary catheters, Hickman catheters, syringe driver butterflies, and intravenous cannulae can all increase the risk of developing infection.

Medication

Corticosteroids, antibiotics, anticholinergics, and benzodiazepines are just a few of the groups of medications commonly used in palliative care that can adversely effect a patient's resistance to infection.

Chemotherapy and radiotherapy

All healthcare professionals in contact with cancer patients who have recently had oncological treatment need to be aware of the risks of a lowered immune response. Typically this happens in the second week after chemotherapy, the 'nadir' period, although this can occur earlier or later. Manifestation of sepsis in a patient who is undergoing oncological treatment can be minimal, and there should be a high index of suspicion. The routine signs of a raised temperature, a fast pulse, or sweating may be absent. Without such vigilance, patients may suddenly deteriorate and become septicaemic which, for a significant proportion, will be fatal.

Sites of infection

In studies of bacterial infection sites in patients in the palliative care setting, the two most common are the urinary and respiratory tracts—and have accounted respectively for up to 42.5% and 36.5% of all infections in cancer patients at the end of life. Skin and subcutaneous site infections occur in 12.5–22%. Other sites of infection, each accounting for less than 5%, include blood/septicaemia; colostomy/gastrostomy stomata; and the parotid gland (Pereira *et al.* 1998).

Causative organisms

In reviews of organisms implicated in infections in patients in the palliative care setting the most common bacteriological organisms encountered are *Escherichia coli, Staphylococcus aureus*, and *Enterococcus*.

In urinary tract infections *E. coli, Klebsiella pneumoniae*, and *Enterococcus* are most commonly responsible while respiratory tract infections are usually due to *Staph. aureus, Haemophilus influenzae*, and *Pseudomonas aeruginosa. Staph. aureus* was also most commonly responsible for the majority of skin and sub-cutaneous infections (Pereira *et al.* 1998; Nagy-Agren and Haley 2002).

There is limited information on the frequency of VRE and ESBL in patients with cancer at the end of life. Prentice studied admissions to 118 beds in three hospices in south London and noted that between 4% and 8% of patients were MRSA positive (Prentice *et al.* 1998); 16% of these patients subsequently suffered clinically significant MRSA infections. Another study by Ali and Sykes found that 5.8% of 120 patients admitted to St Christopher's Hospice when swabbed were positive for MRSA, but over the course of their admission none developed associated symptomatic infection. The authors conclude that the burden placed on this vulnerable group by conventional eradication may be disproportionate to any benefit derived (Ali *et al.* 2005).

In the mouth, where infection is a very common cause of morbidity in those with advanced disease, *Candida*, which is found in the normal oral flora of 50% of the population, is present in up to 80% of patients (Back 2001).

Common symptoms

A range of symptoms are produced by infections at the end of life. These include headache, delirium, pain, oral problems, breathlessness, dysuria, frequency and incontinence, diarrhoea, malodour, pyrexia, fatigue, and ultimately deterioration and death. Such a range of symptoms will cause different patients different degrees of morbidity; a dry mouth may be insignificant to one patient and a total preoccupation for another. The clinician involved with caring for patients with advanced malignancy must thus temper interventions to individual patient's symptom burden.

Efficacy of antimicrobials

Although there are limited data, a review of the current literature reveals an overall 'positive' response to antimicrobials in approximately 40–50% of patients with advanced cancer and infection (Vitetta *et al.* 2000; Clayton *et al.* 2003).

In these studies a response was deemed positive if the patient's overall condition improved; there was a return to previous functional status; the symptoms or signs of infection improved or the patient's symptoms improved even if their overall condition deteriorated.

It was also noted that a positive response was more common in terminal and stable phase patients than in deteriorating or acute phase patients (Clayton *et al.* 2003). Also, when bacteriological sensitivities were available, the outcome of antimicrobial use was more commonly associated with a positive response than when microbiology results were unavailable.

More specifically, White discussed antimicrobial options with 309 consecutive patients with advanced cancer and predicted prognosis of less than 6 months, and subsequently documented the use and effects of antimicrobials in this patient population (White *et al.* 2003). While the response rate varied with the antimicrobial used, there was a positive symptom response in up to 92% of patients with urinary tract infections and up to 50% in patients with respiratory tract infections. Lower response rates were noted in skin and subcutaneous infections and in bacteraemia.

Patient's overall survival and infection-related deaths were not significantly affected by the use of antimicrobials.

In case studies, considerable improvement in pain control following aggress-ive infection management and antimicrobial treatment has been noted (Bruera and MacDonald 1986; Mackey *et al.* 1995).

Such positive responses must be balanced against treatment burdens to the patient.

Prescribing

Before prescribing antimicrobials to patients with advanced malignancy it is important to clarify the goal of treatment, how the antimicrobial can be monitored, and the risk of side-effects and drug interactions.

Once these questions have been answered, the multidisciplinary team need to ensure that the treatment decision encompasses the patient's and family's wishes. It may also be appropriate at the outset to negotiate with the patient and family a trial period after which, if there is no improvement, treatment would be discontinued.

Goals of end of life care

The ultimate goal of end of life care is to relieve the patient and family's physical, emotional, and spiritual suffering. To achieve this goal it is essential to consider the evidence base for effective care; the point reached on the disease journey; the patient and family's wishes, and ethical and legal concerns.

While the evidence base for the effective treatment of infection has been discussed earlier in the chapter, this section focuses on the latter points.

Point reached on the disease journey

Three distinct phases have been recognized at the end of life:

- the *palliative care phase* the goal is to preserve the quality and quantity of life for as long as possible.
- In the *hospice care phase* the goal is to preserve the quality of life.
- In the *terminal care phase* the goal is to maximize comfort, dignity and support of patients and relatives and minimize the medical interventions of dying.

On this basis, the rationale for treating infection in patients in the palli-ative care phase of their illness may differ to that for patients in the termi-nal phase.

The patient and family's wishes

Exploring attitudes to and concerns regarding death and dying is inherent to end of life care. This can be extremely challenging—particularly in a society that is increasingly death denying.

Public expectations regarding the treatment of disease can lead to the perception that all disease should be curable and all life prolonged, and if such is not the case then, 'somebody must be to blame'.

Withholding antimicrobials may be perceived by the patient and/or the family as hastening death. However, with good communication, and an honest, open, and trusting relationship between patient/family and professional these issues can be discussed sensitively, confusion unravelled, and fears exposed.

Legal concerns

Requests for euthanasia or the application of formal advanced directives, which can include instructions on the use of antimicrobials, must be discussed sensitively. In practice, such requests may be just the visible tip of an iceberg of unresolved issues. Exploration of these issues in association with effective symptom control often diminishes the desire for a deliberate ending of life.

Ethical concerns

In direct contrast infection can also be perceived by some as a common and appropriate cause of death in cancer patients—'an old man's best friend'. This perception may make patients and families reluctant to accept antimicrobial treatment even when it is the most suitable means of obtaining improved symptom control.

An ethical framework upon which to base such challenging management decisions is invaluable. The most widely used ethical framework in health issues in the West is summarized below.

◆ *autonomy*: to inform and involve the patient in decision making
◆ *beneficence*: to do good
◆ *non-maleficence*: to do no harm
◆ *justice*: to balance the needs of individuals with those of society.

Focusing on patient autonomy, White discussed antimicrobial options with patients who had confirmed advanced disease. Patients were asked to select one of three options (White *et al.* 2003).

Table 13.1 Patient choices and antimicrobial use

Patient choices and antimicrobial use	%
Full use (A)	20.8
Symptomatic use only (B)	48.2
No antimicrobials (C)	31.0

- *option A*: full antimicrobial use for suspected or established infections as would be done in acute medical or surgical care;
- *option B*: antimicrobial use for symptomatic treatment only;
- *option C*: no antimicrobial use.

The choices were made after a full disclosure and discussion of the potential advantages and disadvantages of treatment. The majority of patients chose either not to use antimicrobials or limit their use to symptomatic infections (Table 13.1).

The choice of the restricted use of antimicrobials was more common among patients who were older and had a lower performance status.

This choice was independent of the type of malignancy, gender, caregiver or spousal status, previous treatment, healthcare payer, or medications for pain, depression or anxiety.

In cancer patients at the end of life it is not always possible to guarantee that antimicrobial therapy will result in improved symptom control. Therefore, when attempting to do good and to do no harm, (beneficence and non-maleficence), it may be reasonable to initiate a therapeutic trial of antimicrobial therapy. If deterioration then occurs, despite treatment, it would be reasonable to discontinue therapy.

Management of common infections

The antimicrobials selected by the treating physician should be in line with local hospital policies. Local surveillance of pathogenic patterns and susceptibility to antimicrobials is essential when determining infectious trends. *E. coli, Staph. aureus,* and *Enterococcus* are the most commonly noted infectious organisms in hospices—suggesting that patients with advanced cancer may have common patterns of infection at the end of life. Good practice dictates that urine, sputum, faeces, blood, and other relevant samples should be collected for culture prior to antimicrobial treatment. Although desirable, this is not always practical in advanced cancer as many hospices lack on site laboratory support and repeated blood cultures may be both distressing and inappropriate for patients in the hospice and terminal care phase.

Selection of an appropriate antibiotic at this stage must take account not only of the likely sensitivies of the organisms involved but the potential burden to the patient of the particular antimicrobial and its means of administration.

Patient journey

The following account tracks one patient through the closing stages of his disease journey and illustrates how different management strategies are required for the different stages of advanced illness. In practice it is often difficult to determine the point the patient has reached and the opinions of the multidisciplinary team and the patient and family should be sought.

Mr X is a 65-year-old gentleman with a Dukes' C colorectal carcinoma and liver metastases—Stage IV. He was not suitable for metastectomy (multiple metastases in both lobes) and received a course of palliative chemotherapy 3 months ago. He has no significant co-morbidities. He has a good performance status, Karnofsky 70–80%, and smokes 20 cigarettes per day. He was admitted to his local district general hospital with pyrexia, dehydration, vomiting, tachycardia, and a productive cough. A lower respiratory tract infection (LRTI) is diagnosed on clinical grounds.

Palliative care phase

The goal in this phase is to preserve the quality and quantity of life for as long as possible.

In view of the patient's previously good performance status and lack of significant co-morbidities it would be appropriate, after exploring the patient's and family's wishes, and performing routine haematological, bacteriological, and radiological investigations, to commence intravenous fluids and antibiotics. If Mr X improves he can be converted to oral fluids and antibiotics. If his condition deteriorates specialist microbiological advice should be sought and treatment changed appropriately. If he deteriorates further an open, honest, sensitive discussion with the patient, (if possible), the family and the multidisciplinary team will be necessary to reach a decision regarding possible antibiotic withdrawal.

Mr X improves with intravenous fluids and antibiotics and is successfully discharged. Several months later his condition globally deteriorates and a repeat computed tomography scan confirms marked disease progression with lung metastases. His performance status falls to 40–50%. He develops a further LRTI and is readmitted to the local district general hospital where the palliative care team are asked to review him.

Hospice care phase

The goal of this phase is to preserve quality of life.

At this stage it is appropriate to identify and treat any potentially reversible factors contributing to Mr X's deterioration. After the necessary investigations, a trial of antibiotics is again appropriate to control pyrexia and cough and to reduce sputum production. If the patient improves then the antibiotic course should be completed. If further deterioration occurs it is important to consider if this is the beginning of the terminal phase. However, depending on the consensus of the patient, family, and multidisciplinary further microbiological advice may be appropriate.

A chest X ray reveals widespread patchy consolidation throughout both of Mr X's lung fields. Mr X is very distressed by his shortness of breath and is unable to tolerate oral medications. A course of intravenous co-amoxyclav is commenced, and within 48 hours Mr X becomes less breathless and anxious and is able to eat again, much to his family's relief.

He slowly recovers and is transferred to the hospice for rehabilitation for a few days prior to being discharged back to the care of his own GP and the community palliative care team.

Terminal care phase

The goal of this phase is to maximize comfort, dignity, and support of the patient and family, and minimize the medical intervention of dying.

Unfortunately after 3 weeks at home he develops another chest infection, which confines him to bed. His GP discusses readmitting him to hospital but Mr X and his family requests that he be admitted to the hospice instead.

On arrival at the hospice staff note a marked deterioration since his discharge. Mr X fails to improve despite further antibiotics and remains bed bound. He is unable to tolerate oral medications and can only manage sips of water. He occasionally spikes temperatures and is increasingly sleeping. The hospice team diagnose that Mr X is dying (Ellershaw and Murphy 2005) and having explained this to the family placing him on the Integrated Care Pathway for the Dying (Ellershaw and Murphy 2005).

At this stage further antibiotic treatment is unlikely to have a positive impact on Mr X's life. A course of antibiotics has recently been completed, the temperatures may well be secondary to widespread malignant disease and the shortness of breath may be due to lung metastases. Also as he is unable to manage oral medications, antibiotic treatment would require intravenous cannulation and administration—potentially a further treatment burden, especially in a patient who is so weak. Therefore, if the pyrexia and shortness of breath are distressing they can be controlled with regular paracetamol, rectally if necessary, and low doses of parenteral opioids while hyoscine hydrobromide or glycopyronium can be used for respiratory secretions.

These decisions are discussed openly, honestly and sensitively with the patient and family and their opinion sought.

Mr X continued to deteriorate and died peacefully with his family in attendance.

The steps necessary to reach these decisions are summarized in the algorithms in Figures 13.2–13.5.

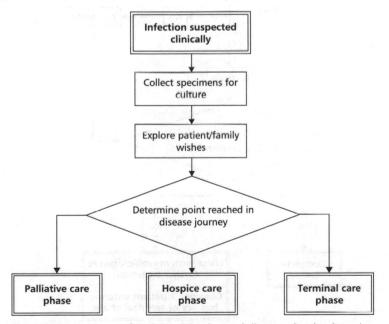

Fig. 13.2 Initial assessment of patient with advanced disease who develops signs and symptoms of infection.

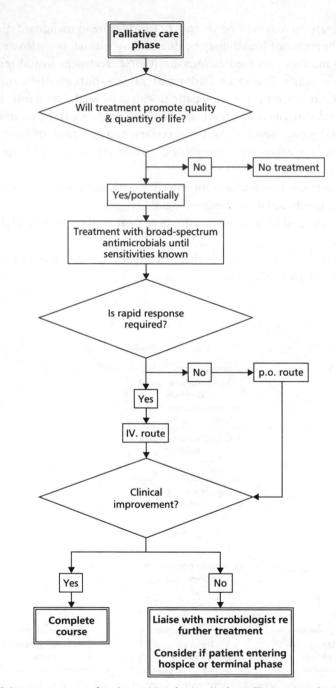

Fig. 13.3 Management of patient with infection in the palliative care phase.

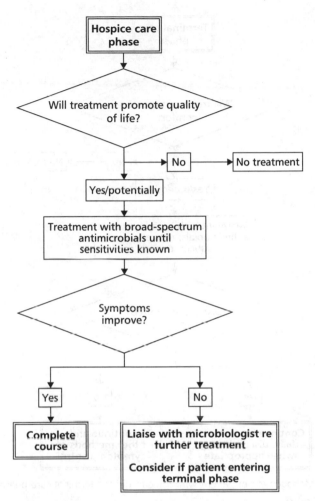

Fig. 13.4 Management of patient with infection in the hospice care phase.

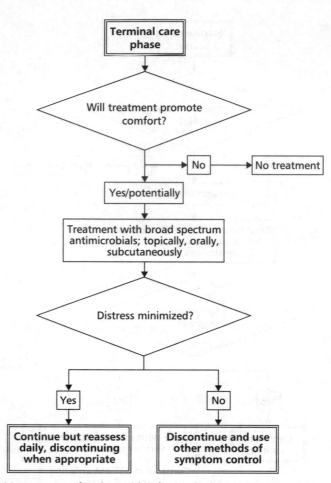

Fig. 13.5 Management of patient with infection in the terminal care phase.

References

Ahronheim JC. (1996). Nutrition and hydration in the terminal patient. *Clinics in Geriatric Medicine*, 12, 379–391.

Ahronheim JC, Morrison RS, Baskin SA, Morris J, and Meier DE. (1996). Treatment of the dying in the acute care hospital; advanced dementia and metastatic cancer. *Archives of Internal Medicine*, **156**, 2094–2100.

Ali S, Sykes N, Flock P, Hall E, and Buchan J. (2005). An investigation of MRSA infection in a hospice. *Palliative Medicine*, **19**, 188–196.

Back IN. (2001). Palliative Medicine Handbook. Cardiff: BPM.

Bauduer F, Capdupuy C, and Renoux M. (2000). Characteristics of deaths in a department of oncohaematology within a general hospital; a study of 81 cases. *Support Care Cancer*, **8**, 302–306.

Bruera E, and MacDonald N. (1986). Intractable pain in patients with advanced head and neck tumors: a possible role of local infection. *Cancer Treatment Reports*, **70**, 691–692.

Clayton J, Fardell B, Hutton-Potts J, Webb D, and Chye R. (2003). Parenteral antibiotics in a palliative care unit: prospective analysis of current practice. *Palliative Medicine*, **17**, 44–48.

Ellershaw JE, and Murphy D. (2005). The Liverpool Care Pathway (LCP) influencing the UK national agenda on care of the dying. *International Journal of Palliative Nursing*, **11**, 132–134.

Homsi J, Walsh D, Panta R, Lagman R, Nelson KA, and Longworth DL. (2000). Infectious complications of advanced cancer. *Support Care Cancer*, **8**, 487–492.

Mackey JR, Birchall I, and MacDonald N. (1995). Occult infection as a cause of hip pain in a patient with metastatic breast cancer. *Journal of Pain and Symptom Management*, **10**, 569–572.

Nagy-Agren S, and Haley H. (2002). Management of infections in palliative care patients with advanced cancer. *Journal of Pain and Symptom Management*, **24**, 64–70.

Pereira J, Hanson J, and Bruera E. (1997). The frequency and clinical course of cognitive impairment in patients with terminal cancer. *Cancer*, **79**, 835–842.

Pereira J, Watanabe S, and Wolch G. (1998). Methicillin-resistant Staphylococcus aureus infection in palliative care. *Journal of Pain and Symptom Management*, **16**, 374–381.

Prentice W, Dunlop R, Armes PJ, Cunningham DE, Lucas C, and Todd J. (1998). Methicillin-resistant Staphylococcus aureus infection in palliative care. *Palliative Medicine*, **12**, 443–449.

Vitetta L, Kenner D, and Sali A. (2000). Bacterial infections in terminally ill hospice patients. *Journal of Pain and Symptom Management*, **20**, 326–334.

Watson M, Lucas C, Hoy A, and Back I. (2005). Oxford Handbook of Palliative Care. Oxford: Oxford University Press.

White PH, Kuhlenschmidt HL, Vancura BG, and Navari RM. (2003). Antimicrobial use in patients with advanced cancer receiving hospice care. *Journal of Pain and Symptom Management*, **25**, 438–443.

WHO (2002). World Health Organization National Cancer Control Programmes, Policies and Managerial Guidelines. Geneva: World Health Organization.

Index